OB/GYN SECRETS

Second Edition

HELEN L. FREDERICKSON, MD
Gynecologic Oncologist
Saint Joseph Hospital
Denver, Colorado

LOUISE WILKINS-HAUG, MD, PhD
Assistant Professor
Department of Obstetrics,
  Gynecology and
  Reproductive Biology
Brigham and Women's Hospital
Harvard Medical School
Boston, Massachusetts

HANLEY & BELFUS, INC./ Philadelphia

Publisher: **HANLEY & BELFUS, INC.**
Medical Publishers
210 South 13th Street
Philadelphia, PA 19107
(215) 546-7293; 800-962-1892
FAX (215) 790-9330

OB/GYN SECRETS, 2nd edition   ISBN 1-56053-205-X

Library of Congress catalog card number 96-79704

Last digit is the print number: 9 8 7 6 5 4 3 2

CONTENTS

II. REPRODUCTIVE ENDOCRINOLOGY AND INFERTILITY

III. GYNECOLOGIC ONCOLOGY

IV. GENERAL OBSTETRICS

V. MATERNAL COMPLICATIONS

CONTRIBUTORS

Jean T. Abbott, M.D., F.A.C.E.P.
Associate Professor, Division of Emergency Medicine, Department of Surgery, University of Colorado Health Sciences Center, Denver, Colorado

Sam E. Alexander, M.D.
Private practice, Denver, Colorado

Richard Allen, M.D.
Residency Director, Department of Obstetrics and Gynecology, Saint Joseph Hospital, Denver; Clinical Associate Professor, Department of Obstetrics and Gynecology, University of Colorado Health Sciences Center, Denver, Colorado

Susan Arnold-Aldea, M.D.
Instructor, Department of Obstetrics and Gynecology, Harvard Medical School, Boston, Massachusetts

Elizabeth L. Aronsen, M.D.
Clinical Assistant Professor of Medicine, University of Colorado Health Sciences Center, Denver, Colorado

Kevin Bachus, M.D.
Private practice, Rocky Mountain Center for Reproductive Medicine, Fort Collins, Colorado

Vanessa A. Barss, M.D.
Associate Professor of Obstetrics and Gynecology, Department of Obstetrics, Gynecology and Reproductive Biology, Harvard Medical School, Boston, Massachusetts

Lynn A. Barta, M.D.
Department of Obstetrics and Gynecology, Kaiser Permanente of Colorado, Denver, Colorado

Scott M. Barton, M.D.
Staff Physician, Department of Obstetrics and Gynecology, Colorado Permanente Medical Group, Denver; Boulder Community Hospital, Boulder; Saint Joseph Hospital, Denver, Colorado

Sally E. Berga, Ph.D., M.D.
Department of Obstetrics and Gynecology, Saint Joseph Hospital, Denver, Colorado

Jonathan C. Berman, M.D.
Assistant Clinical Professor, Department of Anesthesiology, University of Colorado Health Sciences Center, Denver, Colorado

Susan Berman, M.D., M.B.A.
Instructor, Department of Obstetrics and Gynecology, Harvard Medical School, Boston, Massachusetts

Dell Bernstein, M.D.
Assistant Professor of Obstetrics and Gynecology, University of Colorado Health Sciences Center, Denver, Colorado

George Betz, M.D., Ph.D.
Clinical Professor, University of Colorado Health Sciences Center, Denver; Head, Reproductive Endocrinology, Kaiser Permanente Medical Group, Denver, Colorado

Nina M. Boe, M.D.
Assistant Professor, Department of Obstetrics and Gynecology, University of California at Davis, Sacramento, California

Mary Langer Bowman, M.D.
Resident Physician, Department of Obstetrics and Gynecology, Saint Joseph Hospital, Denver, Colorado

D. Ware Branch, M.D.
Associate Professor, Department of Obstetrics and Gynecology, University of Utah, Salt Lake City, Utah

Joanna Bures, M.D.
Instructor in Psychiatry, Harvard Medical School, Boston; Director, Perinatal Psychopharmacology, Brigham and Women's Hospital, Boston, Massachusetts

Nadine A. Burrington, M.D.
Chairman, Department of Obstetrics and Gynecology, Affiliated Health Services, Mount Vernon, Washington

Grace Chang, M.D.
Department of Medicine, Brigham and Women's Hospital, Boston, Massachusetts

Deborah Cohen, R.N.
Brigham and Women's Hospital, Boston, Massachusetts

Matthew B. Cort, M.D.
Assistant Clinical Professor, Department of Obstetrics and Gynecology, University of Colorado Health Sciences Center, Denver, Colorado

Kim Cox, M.D.
Private practice, Pocatello, Idaho

Susan A. Davidson, M.D.
Assistant Professor, Director of Gynecologic Oncology, Department of Obstetrics and Gynecology, University of Colorado Health Sciences Center, Denver, Colorado

Kevin Paul Davis, M.D.
Assistant Clinical Professor, Department of Gynecologic Oncology, Division of Obstetrics and Gynecology, University of Colorado Health Sciences Center, Denver, Colorado

L. Dorine Day, M.D.
Perinatologist, Saint Joseph Hospital, Denver; Assistant Clinical Professor, University of Colorado Health Sciences Center, Denver, Colorado

Corinne Dix, M.D.
Private practice, Denver, Colorado

Kathleen Ann Doyle, M.D., M.P.H.
Clinical Faculty, Department of Obstetrics and Gynecology, Saint Joseph Hospital, Denver, Colorado

Bruce C. Drummond, M.D.
Department of Obstetrics and Gynecology, Saint Joseph Hospital, Denver, Colorado

Jean E. Dwinnell, M.D.
Clinical Instructor, Department of Obstetrics and Gynecology, University of Colorado Health Sciences Center, Denver, Colorado

Danny J. Eicher, M.D.
Assistant Clinical Professor, Department of Obstetrics and Gynecology, University of Colorado Health Sciences Center, Denver, Colorado

Patrick English, M.D.
Kaiser Permanente Medical Center, Santa Rosa, California

Miriam Erick, M.S., R.D., C.D.E.
Lecturer on Obstetrics, Gynecology, Reproductive Biology, Harvard Medical School, Boston; Department of Nutrition, Brigham and Women's Hospital, Boston, Massachusetts

Ty Bolton Erickson, M.D.
Private practice, Idaho Falls, Idaho

Kenneth A. Faber, M.D.
Assistant Clinical Professor, Department of Obstetrics and Gynecology, University of Colorado Health Sciences Center, Denver, Colorado

Scott Farhart, M.D.
Private practice, San Antonio, Texas

Edward D. Frederickson, M.D.
Clinical Assistant Professor of Medicine, Division of Nephrology, Emory University School of Medicine, Atlanta, Georgia

Helen L. Frederickson, M.D.
Gynecologic Oncologist, Saint Joseph Hospital, Denver, Colorado

Gretchen Frey, M.D.
Private practice, Denver, Colorado

Randy S. Glassman, M.D.
Director, Women's Psychiatric Services, Division of Psychiatry, Brigham and Women's Hospital, Boston; Instructor in Psychiatry, Harvard Medical School, Boston, Massachusetts

Robert C. Goodlin
Retired

Marshall Ray Gottesfeld, M.D.
Clinical Instructor, Department of Obstetrics and Gynecology, University of Colorado Health Sciences Center, Denver, Colorado

Michael F. Greene, M.D.
Associate Professor of Obstetrics, Gynecology and Reproductive Biology, Department of Obstetrics and Gynecology, Harvard Medical School, Boston; Director, Maternal Fetal Medicine, Massachusetts General Hospital, Boston, Massachusetts

Debra Gussman, M.D.
Assistant Clinical Professor, Department of Obstetrics and Gynecology, University of Colorado Health Sciences Center, Denver, Colorado

John Alan Harrington, D.O.
Clinical Assistant Professor, Department of Reproductive Endocrinology, University of Colorado Health Sciences Center, Denver; Kaiser Permanente Medical Group, Denver, Colorado

Craig Haug, M.D.
Assistant Professor, Department of Surgery, Tufts University School of Medicine, Boston, Massachusetts

Albert D. Haverkamp
Perinatologist, Department of Obstetrics and Gynecology, Kaiser Permanente Medical Group, Denver, Colorado

Kent D. Heyborne, M.D.
Director, Perinatal Services, Columbia/Swedish Medical Center, Englewood, Colorado

Mark D. Iafrati, M.D.
Instructor, Department of Surgery, Tufts University School of Medicine, Boston, Massachusetts

Jolene K. Johnson, M.D.
Assistant Clinical Professor of Medicine, Department of Internal Medicine, Louisiana State University, Baton Rouge, Louisiana

Terry Johnson, M.D.
Department of Obstetrics and Gynecology, Saint Joseph Hospital, Denver, Colorado

Debra Klaisle, M.D.
Private practice, Modesto, California

Thomas B. Landry, M.D.
Department of Obstetrics and Gynecology, Kaiser Permanente Medical Group, Denver, Colorado

Sharon Langendoerfer, M.D.
Associate Professor, Department of Pediatrics, University of Colorado School of Medicine, Denver, Colorado

Mervyn L. Lifschitz, M.D.
Private practice, Denver, Colorado

Judith McCarthy, M.D.
Department of Obstetrics and Gynecology, Kaiser Permanente Medical Group, San Rafael, California

Don McClure, M.D.
Pathologist, Saint Joseph Hospital, Denver, Colorado

Robert S. McDuffie, Jr., M.D.
Chief of Perinatology, Department of Obstetrics and Gynecology, Kaiser Permanente Medical Group, Denver, Colorado

John G. McFee, M.D.
Associate Professor of Obstetrics and Gynecology, University of Colorado Health Sciences Center, Denver; Associate Director of Obstetrics and Gynecology, Denver Health Medical Center, Denver, Colorado

James A. McGregor, M.D., C.M.
Professor and Vice Chair, Department of Obstetrics and Gynecology, University of Colorado Health Sciences Center, Denver, Colorado

Stacy Mellum, M.D.
Private practice, Reno, Nevada

Thomas W. Montag, M.D.
Department of Obstetrics and Gynecology, Division of Gynecologic Oncology, Mountain Area Health Education Center, Asheville, North Carolina

Sue Anne Murahata, M.D.
Assistant Professor, Department of Obstetrics and Gynecology, University of Colorado Health Sciences Center, Denver, Colorado

Mary E. Norton, M.D.
Instructor of Obstetrics and Gynecology, Department of Obstetrics, Gynecology and Reproductive Science, Harvard Medical School, Boston, Massachusetts

Errol R. Norwitz, M.D., Ph.D.
Clinical Instructor, Department of Obstetrics and Gynecology, Harvard Medical School, Boston, Massachusetts

Martin E. Nowick, M.D.
Clinical Assistant Professor, Department of Obstetrics and Gynecology, University of Colorado Health Sciences Center, Denver, Colorado

Donna Okuda, M.D.
Clinical Instructor, Department of Obstetrics and Gynecology, Saint Joseph Hospital, Denver, Colorado

Susan K. Palmer, M.D.
Associate Professor of Anesthesiology, University of Colorado Health Sciences Center, Denver, Colorado

Polly E. Parsons, M.D.
Associate Professor, Department of Medicine, University of Colorado Health Sciences Center, Denver, Colorado

Jeffrey Pickard, M.D.
Clinical Associate Professor, Department of Medicine, University of Colorado Health Sciences Center, Denver, Colorado

Jean C. Ryan, M.D.
Clinical Instructor of Obstetrics and Gynecology, Harvard Medical School, Boston, Massachusetts

Mark O. Saunders, M.D.
Aurora Presbyterian Hospital, Aurora Regional Medical Center, Aurora, Colorado

William B. Schoolcraft, M.D.
Director, The Center for Reproductive Medicine, Englewood, Colorado

Thomas D. Shipp, M.D.
Instructor of Obstetrics, Gynecology, and Reproductive Biology, Harvard Medical School, Boston, Massachusetts

Robert M. Silver, M.D.
Assistant Professor, Department of Obstetrics and Gynecology, University of Utah, Salt Lake City, Utah

Shailini Singh, M.D.
Clinical Associate Professor of Obstetrics and Gynecology, and Director of Maternal-Fetal Medicine, Georgetown University Medical Center, Washington, D.C.

Timothy L. Sorrells, M.D.
Saint Joseph Hospital, Denver, Colorado

Lyman B. Spaulding, M.D., Ph.S.
Private practice, Fort Morgan, Colorado

Craig F. Stark, M.D.
Department of Obstetrics and Gynecology, Kaiser Permanente Medical Group, Denver, Colorado

Catherine Stevens-Simon, M.D.
Associate Professor of Pediatrics and Adolescent Medicine, University of Colorado Health Sciences Center, Denver, Colorado

Stephen L. Stoll, M.D.
Aurora Regional Medical Center, Aurora, Colorado

E. Stewart Taylor, M.D.
Emeritus Professor and Chairman, Department of Obstetrics and Gynecology, University of Colorado Health Sciences Center, Denver, Colorado

David M. Terry, M.D.
Department of Obstetrics and Gynecology, Saint Joseph Hospital, Denver, Colorado

Heidi Tessler, M.D.
Department of Medicine, Rose Medical Center, Denver, Colorado

Michael W. Trierweiler, M.D.
Private practice, North Platte, Nebraska

Robert E. Wall, M.D.
Chairman, Department of Obstetrics and Gynecology, Columbia Rose Medical Center, Denver; Associate Clinical Professor, Department of Obstetrics and Gynecology, University of Colorado Health Sciences Center, Denver, Colorado

Robert J. Wester, M.D.
Clinical Instructor, Department of Obstetrics and Gynecology, Saint Joseph Hospital, Denver, Colorado

Marsha Wheeler, M.D.
Assistant Professor, Department of Obstetrics and Gynecology, Denver Health Medical System, Denver, Colorado

Louise Wilkins-Haug, M.D., Ph.D.
Assistant Professor, Department of Obstetrics, Gynecology, and Reproductive Biology, Harvard Medical School, Boston, Massachusetts

William B. Wilson, Jr., M.D.
Retired. Formerly, Assistant Professor, Department of Obstetrics and Gynecology, Denver Health Medical System, Denver, Colorado

Carolyn M. Zelop, M.D.
Assistant Professor of Obstetrics and Gynecology, University of Chicago, Chicago, Illinois

PREFACE TO THE FIRST EDITION

This book continues the tradition of The Secrets Series® by presenting an overview of obstetrics and gynecology in question and answer format. Comprehensive coverage is more properly the domain of the major textbooks in the field. *Ob/Gyn Secrets* is intended to be a handy reference that emphasizes the common problems encountered in gynecologic and obstetric practice and that simplifies a vast amount of information without being overly simplistic.

A wide range of topics in obstetrics and gynecology is addressed, with sections on general gynecology, reproductive endocrinology and infertility, gynecologic oncology, general obstetrics, maternal complications, the fetus, the placenta, and labor and delivery.

Some questions have more than one right answer. Some questions have no right answer. Some answers are controversial. The authors have attempted to ask key questions and provide their best answers based on the current information available.

It is hoped that the reader will find this text enjoyable and practically useful and that the patient will be its ultimate benefactor.

PREFACE TO THE SECOND EDITION

In this second edition, we have tried to incorporate changes in practice management, address new technologies, and provide up to date information and references.

We want to thank the contributing authors for their time and effort. Linda Belfus, our publisher, deserves special thanks for her patience and perseverance, for without her this second edition would never have been finished.

We hope our readers will enjoy this format and that their patients will benefit from our efforts.

Helen L. Frederickson, M.D.
Louise Wilkins-Haug, M.D., Ph.D.

DEDICATION

The second edition of OB/GYN Secrets is dedicated to Charles Abernathy, the creator of The Secrets Series®, who passed away in 1994. He will always be remembered by all of us who "crossed his path" in medicine for his superb clinical skills (scientific and humanistic), his stimulating teaching and his enthusiasm for life.

I. General Gynecology

1. VULVOVAGINITIS

Mark O. Saunders, M.D.

1. What are the characteristics of a normal physiologic vaginal discharge?

A physiologic vaginal discharge consists of cervical and vaginal secretions, epithelial cells, and bacterial flora. The normal vaginal pH is 3.8–4.2. A physiologic vaginal discharge is usually white and odorless and does not cause itching, burning, or other discomfort. The amount of discharge varies with the day of the menstrual cycle.

2. What comprises normal vaginal flora?

Lactobacillus sp. (Doderlein's bacilli), an aerobic gram-positive rod, is the most common bacteria. Other bacterial flora include streptococci, staphylococci, diphtheroids, *Gardnerella vaginalis*, *Escherichia coli*, and several anaerobic organisms. *Candida* and *Mycoplasma* spp. are also commonly found.

3. What is vulvovaginitis? What are its symptoms?

Vulvovaginitis is inflammation and irritation of the vagina and vulva, most commonly caused by microbiologic agents. Usually the infection originates in the vagina. The most common symptoms are vulvovaginal itching and/or burning, abnormal odor, and increased discharge. Not all inflammatory conditions of the vagina (vaginitis) necessarily cause vulvar irritation. Patients with chlamydial infections of the cervix also may present with increased vaginal discharge as a chief complaint. Atrophic vaginitis is a noninfectious cause of vaginal irritation in postmenopausal women that occurs secondary to estrogen deficiency.

4. Name three common causes of vaginitis.

(1) *Candida* sp. (yeast, Monilia), (2) *Trichomonas vaginalis*, and (3) synergistic bacterial infection (bacterial vaginosis).

5. How is a definitive diagnosis made?

The definitive diagnosis is made by culturing the vaginal discharge, although the value of vaginal cultures is limited by the large variety of normal bacterial flora. Vaginal pH is useful in that a normal value is < 4.5 and no patient with a normal pH has bacterial vaginosis. Specific etiologic agents may be suspected from the presenting signs and symptoms. All discharges should be examined microscopically after being suspended in separate solutions of normal saline and 10–15% potassium hydroxide (KOH). The latter facilitates identification of yeast pseudohyphae by lysing cellular components of the discharge.

6. What are the characteristic features of yeast vaginitis?

The most common symptom is vaginal and vulvar pruritus. There may also be some dysuria. The discharge is usually white and commonly has a cottage-cheese appearance. Microscopic examination of the KOH smear reveals characteristic pseudohyphae, the absence of which does not rule out yeast vaginitis. Culturing the discharge in Sabouraud's or Nickerson's medium detects a significant percentage that otherwise would be missed.

7. How is yeast vaginitis treated?

Numerous topical antifungal agents are available: clotrimazole (Mycelex), miconazole (Monistat), butoconazole (Femstat), and terconazole (Terazol). Some of these agents are now sold over-the-counter without a prescription. They are administered in a cream or suppository form nightly for 3–7 days and sometimes longer. New oral preparations are available with one-dose therapy (fluconazole). When the problem is recurrent, work-up should include a screening for diabetes mellitus and HIV. Alternate treatment regimens include topical gentian violet or boric acid suppositories.

8. What are the characteristic features of trichomonal vaginitis?

The main symptom is a profuse, usually malodorous vaginal discharge that is greenish-gray in color and has a frothy appearance. Microscopic examination of the saline smear reveals many white blood cells and the pathognomonic unicellular flagellated organism.

9. How is trichomonal vaginitis treated?

Because trichomonal vaginitis is a sexually transmitted disease, treatment of both the patient and her sexual partner is necessary. Metronidazole is the drug of choice, 500 mg orally twice daily for 7 days for both the patient and her partner or a one-time dose of metronidazole, 2 gm orally for each. Metronidazole prohibits metabolism of ethanol; thus these two agents should not be mixed. An alternative to metronidazole is topical clotrimazole for 7–14 days, but it is much less effective.

10. What are the characteristic features of bacterial vaginosis?

The main symptom is a slightly increased discharge with an odor. The discharge is usually gray in color. Microscopic examination of the saline smear shows characteristic clue cells, which are vaginal epithelial cells studded with coccobacilli, obscuring the cell borders. Application of 10–15% KOH to a smear of this discharge results in a fishy odor (positive whiff test). The responsible organism is *Gardnerella vaginalis*.

11. How is bacterial vaginosis treated?

There are several effective treatment regimens for bacterial vaginosis. These include metronidazole, 500 mg orally twice daily for 7 days, and clindamycin, 300 mg orally twice daily for 7 days. In addition, there are intravaginal regimens of 0.75% metronidazole gel applied twice daily for 5 days and 2% clindamycin cream applied once daily for 7 days. While there is debate about whether the sexual partner should also be treated, most authorities definitely recommend treatment of the partner in cases of recurrent infections.

Bacterial vaginosis has been associated with pregnancy complications, including preterm labor and preterm premature rupture of membranes; therefore, it should be treated aggressively during pregnancy. Use of metronidazole is contraindicated during the first trimester.

12. What are the characteristic features of a chlamydial infection?

Chlamydia trachomatis causes mucopurulent cervicitis, and the patient's chief complaint may be vaginal discharge. Although *C. trachomatis* does not cause vaginitis per se, one should be aware of it when evaluating a patient with a vaginal discharge. Speculum examination usually reveals mucopurulent discharge from a sometimes friable cervix. *C. trachomatis* is an intracellular organism, and chlamydial infection is diagnosed by tissue culture or other tests for detection of chlamydial antigen. Chlamydial infections should be suspected when microscopic examination of the saline smear reveals numerous white blood cells but no clue cells, yeast, or trichomonads.

13. How is chlamydial infection treated?

Chlamydial infections may be treated with one of several regimens: doxycycline, 100 mg orally twice daily for 7 days; azithromycin, 1 mg orally as a single dose; erythromycin, 500 mg orally 4 times daily for 7 days; or ofloxacin, 300 mg orally twice daily for 7 days. Because these infections are sexually transmitted, the partner should also be treated.

14. What are the characteristic features of atrophic vaginitis?

The estrogen deficiency that typically occurs after menopause may cause atrophy and subsequent inflammation of the vaginal mucosa. Common symptoms are vaginal dryness and itching, dyspareunia, and occasionally vaginal bleeding. Inspection of the vagina usually reveals a dry, thin vaginal mucosa with little or no rugations.

15. How is atrophic vaginitis treated?

Atrophic vaginitis is treated with estrogen replacement in oral form or with an estrogen vaginal cream. In women who cannot use hormonal therapy, nonhormonal lubricants are available (Replens).

BIBLIOGRAPHY

1. American College of Obstetricians and Gynecologists Technical Bulletin #226: Vaginitis. July 1996.
2. Eschenbach DA: Vaginitis including bacterial vaginosis. Curr Opin Obstet Gynecol 6:389, 1994.
3. Foster DC: Vulvitis and vaginitis. Curr Opin Obstet Gynecol 5:726, 1993.
4. Hay PE, Lamont RF, Taylor-Robinson D, et al: Abnormal bacterial colonization of the genital tract and subsequent preterm delivery and late miscarriage. BMJ 308:295, 1994.
5. Lenison ME, Trestmen I, Quach R, et al: Quantitative bacteriology of the vaginal flora in vaginitis. Am Obstet Gynecol 133:139, 1979.
6. Maccato ML, Kaufman RH: Fungal vulvovaginitis. Curr Opin Obstet Gynecol 3:849, 1991.
7. McKay M: Vulvodynia. Arch Dermatol 125:256, 1989.
8. Schydlower M, Shafer M-A: *Chlamydia trachomatis* infections in adolescents. Adolesc Med State Art Rev 1:615–628, 1990.
9. Sobel JD, Brooker D, Stein E, et al: Single oral dose fluconazole compared with conventional clotrimazole topical therapy of *Candida* vaginitis. Am J Obstet Gynecol 172:1263, 1995.
10. Spinillo A, Pizzoli G, et al: Epidemiologic characteristics of women with idiopathic recurrent vulvovaginal candidiasis. Obstet Gynecol 51:721, 1993.

2. HERPES GENITALIS

James A. McGregor, M.D., C.M.

1. What are herpes viruses?

Herpes viruses are a large family of double-stranded DNA viruses that are widely distributed in nature. Herpes simplex infection was well described by Ptolomy. Herpes means "creep" in Latin; each of these viruses may be spread by close bodily contact.

2. Name six common herpes viruses that may infect humans.

Herpes simplex virus 1 (HSV-1), herpes simplex virus 2 (HSV-2), cytomegalovirus (CMV), varicella zoster virus (VZV), Epstein-Barr virus (EBV), and human herpes virus type 6 (HHV-6).

3. What is viral tropism?

Different kinds of herpes viruses have a strong predilection for infecting certain types of cells. Both HSV-1 and HSV-2 may primarily infect genital or orofacial skin or epithelia. Roughly 90% of genital infections are HSV-2 and 10% are HSV-1; the reverse is true for orofacial herpes.

4. What is the difference between primary, initial, and recurrent genital herpes?

Initial infection occurs the first time an individual is infected with that specific virus, i.e., HSV-1 or HSV-2. Initial infections may be highly variable. Many initial infections are asymptomatic. The classic "primary" clinical episode of genital herpes occurs in approximately one-third of individuals with no antibodies to HSV-1 or 2. Many patients may have severe, painful, "primary" but noninitial episodes of genital herpes. HSV-1 or 2 rapidly infects and mediates prolonged (for the life of the individual?) latent infection of the innervating root ganglia cells, e.g., S-3-4 in the genital area. "Primary" genital herpes is often widely spread, prolonged (12–21 days to heal) and associated with systemic signs and symptoms (malaise, fever, headache, and findings of aseptic meningitis), whereas recurrent herpes is circumscribed and lasts 2–4 days.

5. What are fever blisters?

Fever blisters are recurrent episodes of orolabial herpes. Causes include generalized illness with a fever, immunosuppression, or ill-understood stimuli to the infected nerve root ganglia cell, e.g., sun exposure, surgical manipulation of the nerve, and various other stresses. Recurrent genital HSV is similar to "fever blisters," including menses-associated changes and sometimes trauma to the skin during coitus.

6. What is a herpetic prodrome?

Activation of HSV infection in the infected cells of the cord, trigeminal nerve, or autonomic ganglia can cause altered sensation or neurologic function in an affected area that is most often perceived as hypesthesia, burning, itching, tingling, or lancinating pain. The presence of a herpetic prodrome is sometimes associated with viral shedding from the affected epidermal area, i.e., vulva, vagina, cervix, or penis.

7. What is the difference between HSV-1 and HSV-2?

While these viruses are quite different (> 50% difference in genome), HSV-1 and HSV-2 may infect similar body sites, cause similar clinical manifestations, and elicit cross-reacting antibody responses (using less specific serologic tests). Newer serologic tests for glycoprotein G-1 for HSV-1 and glycoprotein G-2 for HSV-2 do not cross-react and can give specific antibody responses. Clinically, HSV-2 tends to cause more severe and recurrent genital tract infection, whereas HSV-1 infections are milder and recurrences rapidly diminish in frequency.

8. Can people have genital herpes and not know it?

Yes. Use of HSV-2 specific G2 antibody tests show that about one-third of sexually active adults have serologic evidence of HSV-2 infection. Less than 5% have a past history of genital HSV.

9. Describe herpetic skin lesions.

Classically, they appear as clusters of "dew drops on a rose petal," i.e., clusters of clear or yellow fluid-filled vesicles with erythematous bases. Such lesions are less common in the genital area; painful ulcerations, papules, or even folliculitis-like lesions are more common. Herpetic cervicitis commonly causes a white-gray area of necrosis, and may be mistaken for cervical cancer. All of these lesions are infectious to susceptible contacts.

10. How infectious is genital herpes?

Transmission of infection depends upon factors such as inoculum, immunity to HSV-1 or 2 (which may be partially protective against the alternate viruses), and the extent of epithelial trauma (HSV does not appear to infect intact epithelium). Infection occurs in approximately 50% or more of close sexual contacts. Rates may be higher during activities such as competitive wrestling (traumatic herpes or herpes gladiatorum).

11. Can genital herpes be spread without contact with clinically apparent herpetic lesions?

Yes. Recent studies suggest that 25% or more of new infections are mediated by contact with an asymptomatic individual who is shedding HSV from genital tract skin. As many as 1% of individuals may have HSV-2 recovered from genital tract sites at any one time.

12. Which two viruses can be commonly identified in reproductive tract squamous cell carcinomas involving the cervix, vagina, vulva, or penis?

HSV-2 and various human papillomaviruses (HPVs).

13. How might couples in which one partner has genital HSV infection reduce the risk of spread to the other?

Avoidance of direct sexual contact when the infected individual has a lesion or is experiencing a prodrome can greatly reduce transmission. Routine use of female or male condoms is theoretically effective. Anti-HSV vaccination trials of seronegative partners are under way.

14. How does acyclovir work against HSV-1 or 2 infection?

Acyclovir is one of three orally absorbed agents that are effective against HSV infection. Within infected cells, acyclovir is activated by HSV-determined thymidine kinase. Mammalian cell thymidine kinase activates acyclovir little, if at all. Activated acyclovir acts to interfere with production of new viruses within the host cell nucleus. Valcyclovir is the valine ester of acyclovir. This agent, along with famcyclovir, possesses superior pharmacokinetics, which allows twice daily dosing.

15. Is treatment with acyclovir always indicated for patients with genital HSV recurrence?

No. Most individuals suffer recurrent HSV-2 lesions that last only several days. These patients require supportive care: keeping the area clear and dry and applying comforting soaks or compresses (used teabag compresses are a common folk remedy) may relieve pain. Local (5% xylocaine jelly or ointment) or mild analgesics may be of benefit.

16. Can autoinoculation with HSV-1 or 2 occur?

Definitely. Even though individuals may possess antibodies from prior genital or orofacial herpes, the virus may infect other sites, e.g., acute herpetic eye infection if contact lenses are inserted after contact with infectious secretions from contaminated fingers or saliva.

17. Should primary episodes of genital HSV be treated?

Generally, acyclovir effectively terminates HSV replication, but it may take 1 or 2 days for symptoms to improve. If lesions and symptoms appear to be clearing, supportive care is appropriate. Otherwise, oral acyclovir (200 mg capsules 5 times a day orally, omitting a dose in the middle of the night) should be started and continued for 10 days. Given the availability of oral therapy, topical acyclovir does not appear to be useful for primary or recurrent herpes.

18. What are the indications for hospitalization and treatment with intravenous acyclovir?

Patients with severe systemic symptoms and nausea and vomiting may be unable to take oral acyclovir. Patients with findings of aseptic meningitis (severe headache, nuchal rigidity, photophobia) or encephalopathy should be seen in consultation with a neurologist or infectious disease specialist and given parenteral acyclovir. Patients with presumed HSV hepatitis should also receive parenteral acyclovir, i.e., 5 mg/kg acyclovir intravenously every 8 hours along with adequate hydration. Serum creatinine should be determined daily to detect any renal impairment that may be associated with high, prolonged doses of acyclovir.

19. When is intermittent oral treatment with acyclovir appropriate?

When recurrence develops infrequently ($\leq$ 2 each year), various doses (400 mg twice daily or 200 mg 5 times daily) given promptly at the onset of the prodrome or lesion for 5–10 days reduces pain, time to healing, and viral shedding. Prophylaxis with similar doses of acyclovir may be used on an individualized basis, i.e., prior to trigeminal nerve manipulation, immunosuppression, or some other predictable antecedent of recurrent disease.

20. When is suppression of HSV infection with acyclovir indicated?

Patients with frequent recurrences ($\geq$ 6 per year) may be helped dramatically by use of a daily suppressive dose (800 mg of acyclovir orally once or 400 mg twice daily).

21. How long may acyclovir suppression be continued?

Although the FDA-approved indication remains 6 months of continued suppression, an increasingly large number of patients have been followed for 1 or more years without toxicity.

While acyclovir is not implicated as a teratogen, prudence suggests provision of effective contraception while the patient receives acyclovir.

22. Does resistance to acyclovir occur?
Yes. Since the initiation of use of acyclovir, several HSV strains appear to be resistant to acyclovir. Development of resistance may be prevented by always using acyclovir in full doses.

23. Can prevention or treatment of genital HSV (and other genital ulcer-producing infections) reduce risks of HIV transmission?
Presumably. Studies show that transmission of the AIDS-associated virus HIV-1 is increased many fold by the presence of genital ulcer-associated infections, such as genital herpes, chancroid, and syphilis. Prevention or treatment of these disorders may greatly reduce risk of HIV transmission during intercourse.

BIBLIOGRAPHY

1. Baker DA: Herpes simplex virus infections. Curr Opin Obstet Gynecol 4:676, 1992.
2. Brown ZA, Benedetti JK, Watts DH, et al: A comparison of detailed and simple histories in the diagnosis of genital herpes complicating pregnancy. Am J Obstet Gynecol 172:1295–1309, 1955.
3. Corey L: The current trend in genital herpes. Progress in prevention. Sex Transm Dis 21(Suppl 2):S38, 1994.
4. Haddad J, Larger B, Astruc D, et al: Oral acyclovir and recurrent genital herpes during late pregnancy. Obstet Gynecol 82:102–104, 1993.
5. Kinghorn GR: Genital herpes: Natural history and treatment of acute episodes. J Med Virol (Suppl 1):33, 1993.
6. Kinghorn GR: Epidemiology of genital herpes. J Int Med Res 22(Suppl 1):14A, 1994.
7. Lavoie SR, Kaplowitz LG: Management of genital herpes infection. Semin Dermatol 13(4):248, 1994.
8. Maccato M: Herpes in pregnancy. Clin Obstet Gynecol 36:896, 1993.
9. Praber GG, Coney L, Brown ZA, et al: The management of pregnancies complicated by genital infections with herpes simplex virus. Clin Infect Dis 15:1031–1038, 1992.
10. Scott LL, Sanchez J, Jackson GC, et al: Acyclovir suppression to prevent cesarean section delivery after first episode genital herpes. Obstet Gynecol 87:69–73, 1996.

3. PELVIC INFLAMMATORY DISEASE

Thomas B. Landry, M.D.

1. What is pelvic inflammatory disease?
Pelvic inflammatory disease (PID) is an infection of the upper genital tract in women. The infection usually starts in the lower genital tract and ascends to involve the upper genital tract. It usually involves sexually transmitted organisms but may be caused by organisms endogenous to the lower genital tract.

2. What structures are involved in PID?
The infection originates in the vagina and cervix. It ascends to involve the endometrium, fallopian tubes, ovaries, and peritoneum. Parametrial tissues are also involved. In serious infections, microorganisms migrate along the peritoneum to the upper abdomen. Perihepatic adhesions are a sequelae of upper abdominal involvement. These adhesions extend from the liver capsule to the diaphragm. This condition is referred to as Fitz-Hugh–Curtis syndrome. Adhesions are described as "violin strings."

3. What is silent PID?
Occasionally, an infection of the upper genital tract is asymptomatic. Silent PID is believed to be common with chlamydial infections and helps to explain damage to the fallopian tubes without a previous history of PID.

4. What is the difference between PID and acute salpingitis?

The terms are used interchangeably to describe ascending infections of the upper genital tract.

5. How common is PID?

The exact number of cases of PID per year is unknown. It is thought that 3% of women have PID during their lifetime. However, if laparoscopy is performed when PID is suspected, the diagnosis is confirmed in only about 60% of patients.

6. What is the effect of PID on office visits, hospital admissions, and operative procedures in the United States?

PID generates approximately 2.5 million visits to physicians annually. There are approximately 250,000–300,000 inpatient hospital admissions and 150,000 operative procedures in the United States annually for conditions directly related to PID.

7. What causes PID?

PID is usually caused by an ascending infection from the vagina and cervix. The primary organisms involved are *Neisseria gonorrhoeae* and *Chlamydia trachomatis*. Various aerobic and anaerobic organisms are usually also present and may be endogenous to the lower tract. The resultant damage to the cervix may permit organisms to move upward.

8. Is PID always considered a sexually transmitted disorder?

No. Instrumentation of the uterus can introduce organisms into the upper genital tract causing PID. Examples include endometrial biopsies, dilation and curettage, insertion of an intrauterine device, intrauterine insemination, hysteroscopy and uterine sounding. Five thousand cases of PID occur per year from pregnancy termination. Prophylactic antibiotics are advocated in high-risk patients.

9. How are menstrual periods related to PID?

It is rare for women not having menstrual periods to acquire PID. This includes pregnant, premenopausal, and postmenopausal women. Also, acquiring PID is more likely during menstruation, probably because of the absence of a barrier and because blood is a good culture medium.

10. Is PID possible during pregnancy?

PID is possible during pregnancy. Once the gestational sac is large enough to form an effective barrier to ascending infection (at 6 weeks' gestation), new onset PID is unlikely. PID is also possible in pregnancy with possible hematogenous spread as well as acute exacerbation of chronic salpingitis. The preoperative diagnosis in a pregnant patient with PID is usually appendicitis.

11. Can douching cause PID?

Some studies have indicated an increased rate of PID in patients who douche, especially around their menses. Pressure at the cervical os may facilitate the transport of infectious organisms into the uterine cavity.

12. What are the risk factors for PID?

Women at risk for acquiring any sexually transmitted disease are at high risk for developing PID. Risks include multiple sexual partners, intrauterine device, previous episode of PID, or a partner with a sexually transmitted disease.

13. What is the relationship between chlamydial infection, gonorrhea, and PID?

It is estimated that two-thirds of patients with PID have one or both of these organisms. Patients with gonococcal PID tend to have an abrupt onset of symptoms with distinct signs of local infection and systemic illness. PID caused by chlamydial infection, however, has a gradual onset and may go undetected and cause ongoing damage.

14. Besides *C. trachomatis* and *N. gonorrhoeae*, what other organisms are commonly isolated in patients with PID?

Aerobic:	*Gardnerella vaginalis*	Anaerobic:	*Bacteroides* sp.
	Escherichia coli		*Peptococcus* sp.
	Streptococcus sp.		*Peptostreptococcus* sp.
	Haemophilus influenzae		
	Proteus mirabilis		
	Klebsiella sp.		
	Other *Enterobacteriaceae*		

15. What is the recurrence rate of PID?
The recurrence rate of PID is about 25%.

16. What is the most common complaint with acute PID?
Lower abdominal pain.

17. Is cervical motion tenderness diagnostic of PID?
Cervical motion tenderness may be elicited in any patient with an acute peritoneal inflammatory process. Thus it may be present in patients with ectopic pregnancy, intraperitoneal bleeding, appendicitis, and adnexal torsion, among other disorders. The "chandelier sign" is the term commonly applied to describe the pain experienced when peritoneal motion is elicited.

18. What laboratory tests should be done for a patient suspected of having PID?
All patients should have a pregnancy test, complete blood count with differential, urinalysis, erythrocyte sedimentation rate, and cervical cultures for *C. trachomatis* and *N. gonorrhoeae*. White count elevation suggests infectious process, whereas anemia suggests intraperitoneal bleeding. Urinalysis rules out urinary tract infection. An elevated erythrocyte sedimentation rate is suggestive of an acute inflammatory process. Patients also may benefit from a Gram stain of purulent discharge to identify gram-negative intracellular diplococci, indicating the presence of *N. gonorrhoeae*.

19. How is the diagnosis of PID made?
The triad of lower abdominal pain and tenderness, cervical motion tenderness and adnexal tenderness along with one of the following:
Febrile illness (> 38° Celsius)
Leukocytosis (> 10,500 white blood cells/cubic mm)
Adnexal mass on pelvic exam or ultrasound
Purulent material on culdocentesis
Gram stain of discharge suggestive of gonorrhea (intracellular gram-negative diplococci)

20. Is the erythrocyte sedimentation particularly useful in establishing the diagnosis?
Erythrocyte sedimentation rate ≥ 15 mm/hr is helpful in establishing the diagnosis. Studies have also indicated that ESR in combination with C-reactive protein may help to discern the severity of PID (ESR ≥ 40 mm/hr and C-reactive protein ≥ 60 mg/l). Results may help to choose a treatment regimen (i.e., inpatient vs. outpatient).

21. What additional test may be useful?
Ultrasound is useful if pain is severe enough to prevent an adequate pelvic exam or if a pelvic mass is suspected.

22. Does laparoscopy play a role in the diagnosis of PID?
Laparoscopy should be used as a diagnostic tool in patients with severe lower pain of uncertain etiology. Laparoscopy may be useful in differentiating between PID and appendicitis as well as identifying other causes for pelvic pain. It may help to direct treatment in certain patients, thus saving time and money. Laparoscopy is useful in patients who do not improve after 48–72 hours of intravenous antibiotics. Pelvic abscesses can be identified and drained.

23. What is the differential diagnosis of PID?

Acute appendicitis

Endometriosis

Adnexal torsion

Ruptured ovarian cyst

Renal disorders (nephrolithiasis, pylonephritis)

Urinary tract infections

Gastrointestinal disorders

Pelvic adhesions

Lower lobe pneumonias

24. What information is useful in differentiating acute appendicitis from PID?

Clinical indicators favoring appendicitis include the presence of anorexia and onset of pain later than day 14 of the menstrual cycle. Indicators favoring PID include a history of vaginal discharge, urinary symptoms, prior episode of PID, tenderness outside the right lower quadrant, cervical motion tenderness, vaginal discharge on pelvic exam, and positive urinalysis. Despite these clinical indicators, differentiating acute appendicitis from PID remains a dilemma.

25. What are the sequelae of PID?

The sequelae of PID include ectopic pregnancy, infertility, chronic pelvic pain, hydrosalpinx, tuboovarian abscess, and chronic dyspareunia.

26. How does PID affect ectopic pregnancy?

The risk of ectopic pregnancy after at least one episode of PID is 6–10 times greater than among controls.

27. How does PID affect fertility?

After one episode of PID, approximately 30% of women become infertile compared with 3% of women without a previous episode of PID. Women who delay seeking treatment are at an even higher risk of damage leading to infertility and ectopic pregnancy.

28. Can PID be lethal?

Yes. Delay of diagnosis and treatment can lead to life-threatening sepsis. Ruptured tuboovarian abscess can lead to sepsis. Also, ectopic pregnancies are responsible for up to 20% of maternal deaths. One-half of women with ectopic pregnancies have a history of PID.

29. Are there ways to prevent PID?

Barrier methods of birth control (condoms, diaphragms, and spermicidal preparations) are effective both as mechanical obstructive devices and as chemical barriers. Bacteria are known to attach to spermatozoa and may be carried past the cervical mucous barrier. Any practice that prevents sperm from ascending therefore helps to prevent PID.

30. Do oral contraceptives have a role in preventing PID?

The use of oral contraceptives does not reduce the risk of infections of the lower genital tract and in fact may encourage behavior that enhances spread of lower genital tract infections. However, oral contraceptives may exert a protective effect against PID by altering the cervical mucus and endometrium and thus retarding the ascending infection.

31. How does tubal ligation affect PID?

PID is rare in patients with previous tubal ligation. PID may occur in patients with a tubal ligation, but generally such patients are clinically more symptomatic and may be septic. More severe infections are necessary to cause peritonitis because the tubes are blocked.

32. How do intrauterine devices (IUDs) affect PID?

The incidence of PID is increased in women using IUDs for birth control. This increase is limited to the first 4 months after insertion. Unilateral tuboovarian abscesses are more common with IUD use.

33. Should IUDs be removed in a patient with PID?

The IUD should be removed after adequate levels of antibiotics are achieved (approximately 48 hr).

34. How does human immunodeficiency virus (HIV) affect PID?

HIV-positive women more often have a temperature > 38°C, a genital ulcer, and tuboovarian abscess. Such patients also are more likely to require surgery and hospitalization. There is no difference in the incidence of chlamydial infection or gonorrhea in HIV-positive women compared with controls. HIV is associated with more severe clinical manifestations of PID but does not affect the microbial cause or response to therapy.

35. How is PID treated?

Outpatient

Cefoxitin, 2.0 gm intramuscularly, with probenecid, 1.0 gm
   or
Ceftriaxone, 250 mg intramuscularly
   or
Equivalent cephalosporin
   plus
Doxycycline, 100 mg orally 2 times daily for 10–14 days

Patients not responding within 48–72 hours should be hospitalized for parenteral therapy. It is necessary to see patients within 48–72 hours to evaluate their condition.

Inpatient

Regimen A	Regimen B
Doxycycline, 100 mg every 12 hours orally or intravenously	Clindamycin, 900 mg intravenously every 8 hours
plus	plus
Cefoxitin, 2.0 gm every 6 hours intravenously or Cefotetan, 2.0 gm every 12 hours intravenously	Gentamicin, 2.0 mg/kg intravenous loading dose followed by maintenance dose of 1.5 mg/kg every 8 hours

Regimen A or B should be continued for 48 hours after the patient improves clinically. The patient should then be continued on doxycycline, 100 mg orally twice daily, plus metronidazole, 500 mg orally twice daily for 10–14 days.

36. When is hospitalization required?

Hospitalization is required in all nulliparous patients having their first episode of PID. Aggressive therapy may reduce the degree of injury to the fallopian tubes and thus prevent infertility and future ectopic pregnancies. This benefit is lost with subsequent episodes of PID. Other indications for hospitalization:

Intolerance of oral medications	Uncertain diagnosis
Presence of a pelvic mass	Failure to respond to oral antibiotics
Presence of an IUD	Noncompliance
Upper abdominal pain	Pregnancy

37. Does the treatment of PID differ for pregnant patients?

Erythromycin is used to treat pregnant women in whom tetracycline is contraindicated. All pregnant patients should be treated as inpatients.

38. How does the treatment differ for patients with tuboovarian abscesses?

If PID is accompanied by tuboovarian abscesses, metronidazole or clindamycin should be used because of their ability to penetrate abscesses. If no improvement is noticed in 72 hours, surgical intervention is indicated. If the abscess fills the posterior cul-de-sac and is seen as a point in the posterior vaginal fornix, colpotomy may be performed for drainage.

39. Summarize the principles of managing PID.

1. Rule out pregnancy.
2. Use standard clinical criteria to guide, not dictate, diagnosis.
3. Err on the side of overdiagnosis of PID to prevent sequelae.
4. Treat early with broad-spectrum antibiotics.
5. Reassess the patient in 48–72 hrs after initiating treatment.
6. Identify and treat or refer sexual partners.
7. Screen and treat lower genital infections in both men and women.
8. Encourage the use of barrier contraceptive with spermicide.

Shafer MA, Sweet RL: Pelvic inflammatory disease in adolescent females. Adolesc Med State Art Rev 1:545–546, 1990.

BIBLIOGRAPHY

1. Ault Ka, Faro S: Pelvic inflammatory disease. Current diagnostic criteria and treatment guidelines. Postgrad Med 93(2):85–86, 89–91, 1993.
2. Burkman RT Jr: Noncontraceptive effects of hormonal contraceptives: Bone mass, sexually transmitted disease and pelvic inflammatory disease, cardiovascular disease, menstrual function and future fertility. Am J Obstet Gynecol 170(5 Pt 2):1569–1575, 1994.
3. Centers for Disease Control: 1989 Sexually transmitted disease treatment guidelines. MMWR 38(5–8): 31–33, 1989.
4. Herbst AI, Mishell DR, Stenchever MA, Droegemueller W: Comprehensive Gynecology, 2nd ed. Mosby, 1992, pp 691–720.
5. Hillis SD, Joesoef R, Marchbanks PA, et al: Delayed care of pelvic inflammatory disease as a risk factor for impaired infertility. Am J Obstet Gynecol 168:1503–1509, 1993.
6. Kamenga MC, De Cock KM, St. Louis ME, et al: The impact of human immunodeficiency virus infection on pelvic inflammatory disease: A case-control study in Abdijan, Ivory Coast. Am J Obstet Gynecol 172:919–925, 1995.
7. Miettinen AK, Heinonen PK, Laippala P, Paavonen J: Test performance of erythrocyte sedimentation rate and C-reactive protein in assisting the severity of acute pelvic inflammatory disease. Am J Obstet Gynecol 169:1143–1149, 1993.
8. Scholes D, Daling JR, Stergachis A, et al: Vaginal douching as a risk factor for acute pelvic inflammatory disease. Obstet Gynecol 81:601–606, 1993.
9. Shafer MA, Sweet RL: Pelvic inflammatory disease in adolescent females. Adolesc Med State Art Rev 1:545–546, 1990.
10. Washington AE, Katz P: Cost of and payment source for pelvic inflammatory disease, trends and projections, 1993 through 2000. JAMA 266:2565–2569, 1991.
11. Webster DP, Schneider CN, Cheche S, et al: Differentiating acute appendicitis from pelvic inflammatory disease in women of childbearing age. Am J Emerg Med 11:569–572, 1993.

4. DYSMENORRHEA

Stephen L. Stoll, M.D.

1. A female patient arrives in the office seeking relief for recurrent cramping that occurs with her menstrual flow. What is the cause of her discomfort?

This patient is probably suffering from one of the most common problems treated by physicians—dysmenorrhea. Dysmenorrhea, from Greek, means painful monthly flow.

2. Are all types of period cramping the same?

No! Dysmenorrhea is usually classified as either primary or secondary. However, it may be confused with chronic pelvic pain. A complete evaluation will assist the physician in making the diagnosis and planning the proper course of treatment.

3. What is the difference between primary and secondary dysmenorrhea?

Primary dysmenorrhea is pelvic pain that occurs in the absence of pelvic disease. Secondary dysmenorrhea, on the other hand, always has an underlying cause.

4. Are there other types of dysmenorrhea?

You may see the word dysmenorrhea used with other descriptive terms that refer to the cause of painful periods. However, these can be separated into the two main groups of primary and secondary dysmenorrhea. Listed below are several different types of dysmenorrhea that may be encountered when reading about dysmenorrhea.

Primary Dysmenorrhea	Secondary Dysmenorrhea		
Essential	Acquired	Mechanical	Membranous
Psychogenic	Congestive	Tubal	Obstructive
Spasmodic	Inflammatory	Uterine	Ovarian

5. What is the incidence of dysmenorrhea?

It is the most common gynecologic problem. Between 30 and 75% of women suffer from dysmenorrhea. The figure generally quoted is slightly more than 50%. Different studies show a wide range of incidence, depending on how the study was done and which ages were studied.

6. Although it is a common problem, is it a serious one?

About 10% of women with dysmenorrhea are forced to miss from 1–3 days of school or work each month.

7. How does the physician decide if the dysmenorrhea is primary or secondary?

The following may be useful in making a diagnosis: (1) history, (2) physical exam, (3) ultrasound, (4) hysterosalpingogram, (5) laparoscopy, (6) hysteroscopy, and (7) dilatation and curettage.

8. How do these studies help?

They allow the physician to confirm the presence or absence of pelvic disease. Treatment plans can then be tailored to alleviate the condition causing pain.

9. How do these studies help in making the diagnosis of primary dysmenorrhea?

In primary dysmenorrhea, all of the above studies will be negative. However, one may obtain some clues from the history.

10. What is the typical history in primary dysmenorrhea?

Pelvic cramping usually occurs after ovulation has begun, usually 6–12 months after menarche. The pain generally starts several hours before or with menstrual flow, lasts from hours to days, and abates within 48–72 hours.

11. How is the pain described?

The pain is usually spasmodic, is located in the lower abdomen, and might be described as resembling labor pains.

12. Are there any other areas that might be affected?

The pain frequently radiates to either the back or upper thighs. Radiation to other areas is unusual in primary dysmenorrhea.

13. What other symptoms might be seen?

Nausea and vomiting, 90%   Lower backache, 60%
Fatigue, 85%   Headache, 45%
Diarrhea, 60%
Fainting, dizziness, and nervousness have also been described in severe cases.

14. What would the physician expect to find on the physical exam of a patient with primary dysmenorrhea?

The physical exam should be completely normal. The abdomen should show no masses, and pelvic and rectovaginal exams likewise will be normal. If the exam is being carried out during the time of pelvic cramping, the uterus and cervix may be mildly tender to pressure and movement. However, the physician would expect all other aspects of the pelvic exam to be normal.

Precaution: When evaluating a first episode of pain, the patient must be evaluated for pelvic infection and pregnancy.

15. If no pelvic disease is found in primary dysmenorrhea, what is the cause of the pain?

A variety of factors have been implicated, including behavioral and psychological factors, uterine ischemia, and prostaglandins. The latter two are thought to be the major causes, with the patient's individual response to the pain playing a minor role. Behavioral and psychological factors will influence the patient's reaction to the discomfort that she is experiencing. Cultural factors, prior experience with pain, and the individual situation all play a role in the patient's reaction.

16. How do prostaglandins cause pain?

There is good correlation between the amount of prostaglandin production and cramps. It is now thought that as prostaglandin production increases, there is increased uterine cramping that results in uterine ischemia and pain. Studies have shown that prostaglandin production increases during the first 48–72 hours of menstrual flow. Decreasing prostaglandin production with medications can decrease the pain.

17. Other than uterine cramping with ischemia, are there any other ways that prostaglandins cause discomfort?

Prostaglandins may also cause hypersensitization of pain terminals to both physical and chemical stimuli.

18. How is the patient with dysmenorrhea managed?

The first step in any evaluation is the history and physical evaluation. If the physical exam is normal and the history is consistent with primary dysmenorrhea, either birth control pills (oral contraceptives) or antiprostaglandins may be considered.

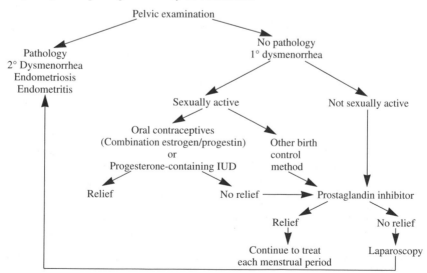

Evaluation and treatment of dysmenorrhea. (From Litt IF: Menstrual problems during adolescence. Pediatr Rev 4:203, 1983, with permission.)

19. How does one decide which course of therapy to try?

If the patient has no contraindications to the use of birth control pills, this is usually the first step tried. For the patient requiring birth control, it is a very good choice. However, if the patient is very young, there may be objections from the parents. For this group of patients, it is often helpful to have a joint meeting with the parents, patient, and physician when choosing a course of therapy.

20. How do birth control pills reduce cramping?

Birth control pills decrease the thickness of the endometrium and change the hormone status to the same levels as those found in the early proliferative stage. This stage has the lowest level of prostaglandin production. By lowering prostaglandin levels, cramping, uterine ischemia, and pain are decreased.

21. How is the patient followed?

After two or three menstrual cycles, the patient is evaluated again and adjustments in medication are made, if necessary. Approximately 90% of patients can be helped by the use of birth control pills alone, but some patients will require the addition of prostaglandin synthetase inhibitors. For patients who do not want to take or cannot take birth control pills, prostaglandin synthetase inhibitors are the first choice of treatment.

22. How do prostaglandin synthetase inhibitors work?

Five chemical groups of inhibitors work by two different mechanisms. Both groups reduce the amount of prostaglandin that can act on the myometrium. By reducing the amount of prostaglandin, normal uterine activity returns.

23. How are these medications administered?

The medication is started on the first day of cramping. Patients are told to initiate the medication with the first signs of discomfort and to continue it over the next 2–3 days. The dosage interval will vary according to the type of medication used. The medication should be continued over the next several months and then reevaluated for effectiveness.

24. How effective is this type of treatment?

Studies have shown that prostaglandin synthetase inhibitors are more than 70% effective in relieving primary dysmenorrhea.

25. Can anything be done to improve relief from dysmenorrhea if this method is not completely effective?

At times, it may be necessary to change to another type of inhibitor. Some patients respond better to one medication than to another. Another approach is to start the medication about 24 hours prior to the expected onset of cramping. This works best for patients who have regular cycles where the cramping can be anticipated. This treatment is then continued for 2–3 days after the flow has started.

26. How do you treat the very young patient who does not want to take birth control pills?

This patient can be started on a prostaglandin synthetase inhibitor. She should be encouraged to continue her normal activities if possible. Gentle abdominal massage, local heat, pelvic tilts and stretching exercises may also be helpful. Regular exercise seems to help to decrease the amount of cramping. Obese women appear to have an increased incidence of dysmenorrhea.

27. Are there any activities that seem to make the cramping worse?

A lack of sleep, stress, and caffeine are all thought to increase the intensity of cramping.

28. What can be done for the young patient who has only minimal relief from antiprostaglandins?

If the patient does not obtain adequate relief from the use of several different antiprostaglandins, she is encouraged to try a course of birth control pills along with the antiprostaglandin medication. If she continues to have problems in spite of conservative therapy, evaluation for other causes of dysmenorrhea is warranted.

29. Are there any patients who should not take antiprostaglandins?

Patients who have hypersensitivity to aspirin or similar compounds should not use this class of drugs. Patients with ulcers or gastrointestinal upset are not good candidates for the use of antiprostaglandins. Taking the medication with food or milk may be helpful.

30. How do you evaluate the patient who continues to have problems?

Continued problems may indicate a need to evaluate the patient for other types of pelvic disease. Ultrasound and laparoscopy may be helpful during this stage of evaluation. Psychological evaluation may also be indicated.

31. If all studies are normal, how should the patient be managed?

Psychological testing, if not already done, may be helpful. Although the pain may not be completely eliminated, the patient may be able to manage the discomfort better. The use of codeine may be helpful for a few days each month. However, because of the potential dangers associated with the use of narcotics, this should only be used for a short period of time. The total amount of medication needs to be followed closely. If other physicians are involved in the care of the patient, it is helpful to speak to them directly so that only one person is managing this aspect of the patient's care. The patient should be told that refills of medications can be done only during office hours so that the chart can be reviewed.

32. Are there any other treatment options?

Acupuncture has been described as being helpful for some patients, although there are only a few studies in this area. Calcium antagonists are also being studied and appear to hold some promise. The use of transcutaneous electrical nerve stimulation (TENS) has also been described.

34. What facts in the history might lead to a search for secondary causes?

Histories that show recurrent infections of the pelvis, IUD usage, recent pelvic operations, heavy periods, or irregular cycles should always initiate a search for other causes. A recent change in sexual partners or multiple partners should prompt careful evaluation.

33. The patient with suspected primary dysmenorrhea who does not respond to conservative therapy needs evaluation for secondary dysmenorrhea. Which other patients need this type of evaluation?

The history usually offers some clues. Patients with secondary dysmenorrhea are often older patients, with the onset of symptoms occurring several years after the first period. However, this is not always true. Some very young patients can have endometriosis, pelvic inflammatory disease, pregnancy, or other causes for their discomfort. It should not be assumed that all young patients have primary dysmenorrhea or that all older patients have secondary dysmenorrhea.

35. How important is the physical exam in secondary dysmenorrhea?

A careful physical examination is a mandatory part of the evaluation. An abnormal pelvic exam often leads to the cause for secondary dysmenorrhea. Pelvic inflammatory disease, leiomyomata, ovarian cysts, and endometriosis can often be diagnosed from the physical exam.

36. What other diseases should be considered when evaluating secondary dysmenorrhea?

Endometriosis/endometritis (see table)	Ruptured ectopic pregnancy
Ruptured ovarian cyst	Appendicitis
Chronic pelvic pain	Pelvic inflammatory disease
Miscarriage (both threatened and actual abortion)	Intestinal colic
Hemorrhage from or into ovarian cyst	Renal or biliary colic
Torsion of ovary	Adenomyosis

Causes of Secondary Dysmenorrhea

	ENDOMETRIOSIS	ENDOMETRITIS
Pain		
Location	Pelvic	Pelvic
Pattern	Recurrent, with menses	Acute episode begins with menses, continues thereafter
		Pain may extend to involve entire abdomen, particularly right upper quadrant (perihepatitis)
Associated Findings	None	Fever
		Elevated WBC
		Elevated ESR
		Purulent discharge at onset
Pelvic Examination	Mild tenderness on palpation of involved area	Exquisite tenderness on palpation of uterus and on motion of cervix if fallopian tubes have become involved
	May have thickening, beading of rectovaginal septum and/or suspensory ligaments	
	May find ovarian cyst ("chocolate")	Purulent cervical discharge
	No vaginal discharge	

From Litt IF: Evaluation of the Adolescent Patient. Philadelphia, Hanley & Belfus, 1990, p 99, with permission.

37. How are patients with secondary dysmenorrhea evaluated?

A complete blood count and erythrocyte sedimentation rate are helpful. If infection is suspected, the cervix is cultured for sexually transmitted diseases.

38. What is the next step in the evaluation?

A pelvic ultrasound and/or hysterosalpingography (HSG) is then done. Hysterosalpingography is helpful when intrauterine scarring or leiomyomata are suspected. It is not used for every patient and is not done as a routine part of the evaluation. However, it is one way to evaluate the interior structure of the uterus and tubes.

39. What other methods of evaluation are available for secondary dysmenorrhea?

In evaluating secondary dysmenorrhea, the use of laparoscopy, hysteroscopy, or dilatation and curettage usually provides a diagnosis. The specific procedure selected depends on the history and physical examination. With the newer equipment available for both hysteroscopy and laparoscopy, corrective surgery can often be performed at the time of the diagnostic procedure. Modern pelviscopy equipment, coupled with laser and video cameras, has greatly extended the range of conditions that can be treated at the time of the diagnostic procedure.

40. How is secondary dysmenorrhea treated?

The treatment of secondary dysmenorrhea depends on the condition causing the pain. Once a diagnosis is made, the appropriate treatment can be planned. The key to the treatment of both primary and secondary dysmenorrhea is making the correct diagnosis. This may take several months, but most patients can be helped.

BIBLIOGRAPHY

1. American College of Obstetricians and Gynecologists: Dysmenorrhea. ACOG Tech Bull 68, 1988.
2. Avant RF: Dysmenorrhea. Prim Care 15:549, 1988.
3. Caufriez A: Menstrual disorders in adolescence: Pathophysiology and treatment. Horm Res 36:156, 1991.
4. Akerlund M: Vascularization of human endometrium. Uterine blood flow in healthy conditions and in primary dysmenorrhea. Ann NY Acad Sci 734:47, 1994.
5. Smith RP: Cyclic pelvic pain and dysmenorrhea. Obstet Gynecol Clin North Am 20:753, 1993.

6. Dawood MY: Nonsteroidal anti-inflammatory drugs and changing attitudes toward dysmenorrhea. Am J Med 84(Suppl 5A):23–29, 1988.
7. Ekstrom P, Juchnicka E, Laudanski T, Akerlund M: Effect of an oral contraceptive in primary dysmenorrhea—changes in uterine activity and reactivity to agonists. Contraception 40:30–47, 1989.
8. Emans SJH, Coldstein DP: Pediatric and Adolescent Gynecology, 3rd ed. Boston, Little, Brown, 1990, pp 291–299.
9. Lichten EM, Bombare J: Surgical treatment of primary dysmenorrhea with laparoscopic uterine nerve ablation. J Reprod Med 32:37–41, 1987.
10. Pasquale SA, Rathauser R, Doese HM: A double-blind, placebo-controlled study comparing three single-dose regimens of piroxicam with ibuprofen in patients with primary dysmenorrhea. Am J Med 84(Suppl 5A):30–34, 1988.
11. Scholst IN, Carlon AT: Pral contraceptives and dysmenorrhea. J Adolesc Health Care 8:121–128, 1987.
12. Shapiro SS: Treatment of dysmenorrhea and premenstrual syndrome with nonsteroidal anti-inflammatory drugs. Drugs 36:475–490, 1988.

5. ABNORMAL UTERINE BLEEDING

Lyman B. Spaulding, M.D., Ph.D.

1. Define abnormal uterine bleeding.

Any bleeding that does not conform in frequency, duration or amount to that of the normal cyclic withdrawal bleeding in women of reproductive age.

2. What are the causes?

Complication of pregnancy (threatened abortion, ectopic pregnancy, placental previa or abruption

Anatomic lesions (malignancy, cervical endometrial polyps, uterine leiomyomata, adenomyosis)

Steroid hormone breakthrough bleeding (oral contraceptives, hormone replacement therapy, depot medroxyprogesterone acetate)

Coagulation disorders (thrombocytopenia, von Willebrand's disease, leukemia, idiopathic thrombocytopenia purpura)

Systemic diseases (hypothyroidism, renal or liver failure)

Infection (endometritis, cervicitis, salpingitis)

Factitious bleeding (self-induced genital injuries)

Dysfunctional uterine bleeding

3. What are the characteristics of the normal menstrual cycle?

The normal physiologic menstrual cycle has a length of 28 ± 7 days, a duration of 5 ± 2 days, and a flow of 60 ± 20 ml.

4. How do the major ovarian hormones orchestrate the normal monthly menses?

The initial portion of the cycle (menstruation) is characterized by withdrawal of estrogen and progesterone support by the failing corpus luteum, leading to breakdown and shedding of two-thirds of the endometrium. Platelet plugs, vasoconstriction, and myometrial contraction function to establish hemostasis. Many of these functions appear to be mediated by prostaglandins (PGE_2, $PGF_{2\alpha}$, prostacycline, and thromboxane). During the midphase (proliferative), estrogen dominates and stimulates the basalis layer of the endometrium to heal the area of shedding. After ovulation (secretory), progesterone stimulates growth and maturation in the endometrium and antagonizes the action of estrogen. If the corpus luteum does not receive a signal from human chorionic gonadotropin (HCG) in placental tissue, it regresses and hormonal support is once again withdrawn.

5. What terms are used to describe abnormal uterine bleeding?

Menorrhagia or **hypermenorrhea:** excessive uterine bleeding in both amount and flow at regular intervals.

Hypomenorrhea: decreased menstrual flow at regular intervals.

Metrorrhagia: uterine bleeding at irregular intervals.

Menometrorrhagia: frequent, irregular, excessive, and prolonged episodes of uterine bleeding.

Polymenorrhea: frequent, regular episodes of uterine bleeding at intervals of < 18 days.

Oligomenorrhea: infrequent, irregular bleeding episodes at intervals of > 45 days.

Intermenstrual bleeding: episodes of uterine bleeding between regular menstrual periods.

6. What is dysfunctional uterine bleeding?

Abnormal bleeding in the absence of organic pathology or systemic disease. It is almost always anovulatory and a diagnosis of exclusion.

7. What is the most common cause of abnormal uterine bleeding?

Dysfunctional uterine bleeding (DUB) is by far the most common cause of abnormal bleeding. Ninety percent of DUB is anovulatory in nature, common at the extremes of reproductive years, and in most cases due to estrogen breakthrough bleeding. Anovulation is associated with the lack of progesterone maturation on the proliferating endometrium, which is required for normal monthly cycles.

8. What portion of dysfunctional uterine bleeding is ovulatory in nature?

Approximately 10% of DUB is ovulatory and manifests as any one or more of the terms in question 5. Mechanisms involved in ovulatory DUB include decreased estrogen production at midcycle, corpus luteum insufficiency and prolonged corpus luteum activity (Halban's disease).

9. How does anovulation cause excessive bleeding?

The lack of progesterone allows asynchronous, excessive endometrial proliferation. This tissue layer lacks mature structural rigidity, is fragile, and, when sloughing occurs, opens multiple vascular channels. The hemostatic mechanism of normal shedding appears to be altered in this estrogen-dominant environment.

10. Why must DUB be a diagnosis of exclusion?

Although DUB is rarely life-threatening, many other disorders that may be warrant consideration. Common mimics of DUB include uterine tumors; malignancy of the cervix, uterus, and tubes; blood dyscrasias; thyroid disease; and inflammatory disease of the vagina, cervix, and uterus.

11. What medical conditions are associated with anovulation?

Polycystic ovarian disease	Psychotropic drug ingestion
Obesity	Pituitary tumors
Hyperandrogenism	Hypothalamic dysfunction due to exercise
Adrenal disease	Weight gain or loss
Thyroid disease	Stress

12. What findings on physical exam, coupled with abnormal bleeding, may suggest anovulation?

Hirsutism and acne (increased testosterone production)	Bruises (coagulopathy, liver disease)
Galactorrhea (pituitary tumor or psychotropic drugs)	Obesity (polycystic ovarian disease)
Thyroid enlargement	Hyperpigmentation (polycystic ovarian disease, adrenal disease)

13. What laboratory tests should be ordered during the work-up of abnormal bleeding?

Essential laboratory tests include a complete blood count, coagulation profile, liver panel, and levels of thyroid-stimulating hormone and prolactin, which screen for the most common medical causes of bleeding. If hyperandrogenism or chronic anovulation is suspected, assessment of testosterone, dehydroepiandrosterone sulfate, 17-hydroxyprogesterone, follicle-stimulating hormone, and luteinizing hormone should be considered.

14. Should all patients undergo endometrial biopsy?

Sampling of the endometrium should be used selectively, depending on the patient's age and presenting complaint. Because of the difficulty in doing an office endometrial biopsy in a young menarchal woman, hormone therapy should be considered the first line of treatment. If bleeding does not respond to hormone manipulation, a careful dilatation and curettage under anesthesia may be diagnostic and, along with hormones, therapeutic. For reproductive-age, perimenopausal, and menopausal women, the newer Pipelle endometrial curette offers minimal discomfort with adequate diagnostic ability. Any biopsy reported as complex hyperplasia with or without atypia should initiate a formal dilation and curettage under anesthesia, because complex hyperplasia may be a precursor to adenocarcinoma of the uterus.

15. What is the role of hysteroscopy in abnormal bleeding?

Hysteroscopy is not cost-effective for every patient with abnormal uterine bleeding. For patients failing medical therapy and patients suspected of having an underlying anatomic cause (submucous myoma, endometrial polyp), hysteroscopy with selected biopsies of the endometrium or anatomical abnormalities is quite useful.

16. What options are available for the management of abnormal bleeding due to anovulation?

Treatment must be individualized and based on the patient's age and desire for future pregnancy. In adolescents, medroxyprogesterone acetate, 10 mg daily for the first 12 days of each month, or a low-dose oral contraceptive, given for 21 days each month, produces effective control. Acute menorrhagia in an adolescent may be the first presenting manifestation of a primary coagulation disorder and requires a hematologic work-up. Intravenous conjugated estrogen, 25 mg every 4 hours for 3 or 4 times, almost always controls acute episodes. Cyclic withdrawal bleeding can then be induced with medroxyprogesterone acetate or oral contraceptives. Progesterone in oil, 100 mg intramuscularly at 4-week intervals, is also effective in lieu of oral medication. In reproductive-age women who do not desire pregnancy, treatment as described for adolescents is most effective. Depot medroxyprogesterone acetate, 150 mg intramuscularly every 3 months, provides contraception as well as prevents bothersome bleeding. Nonsteroidal antiinflammatory drugs such as naprosyn sodium, mefenamic acid, and ibuprofen are effective in reducing menorrhagia by up to 50%. For women desiring pregnancy, clomiphene citrate or exogenous gonadotropins stimulate ovulation with the potential for conception. Once a premalignant or malignant state has been excluded, cyclic medroxyprogesterone acetate or low-dose (35 μg or less) oral contraceptives (nonsmokers only) are effective therapy in perimenopausal women. When true menopause occurs (ovarian failure), hormone replacement therapy with continuous or cycle administration is the treatment of choice.

17. What treatment options are available for patients who continue to bleed after medical therapy?

Until a few years ago, hysterectomy was the last resort for abnormal bleeding unresponsive to conservative therapy. Operative hysteroscopy using either photovaporization (laser) or electrocoagulation/resection of the basilis layer of the endometrium, has now added another option before hysterectomy.

18. How is endometrial ablation accomplished?

Patients who have failed medical therapy and who do not desire future pregnancy are prepared for ablation with a gonadotropin-releasing hormone agonist (GnRHa). This agonist causes the downregulation and desensitization of pituitary GnRH receptors. Without these receptors, follicle-stimulating hormone and luteinizing hormone are no longer released to stimulate estrogen production by the ovaries. A reversible state of ovarian failure ensues, i.e., menopause. Without estrogen stimulation the lining of the uterus becomes atrophic and readily susceptible to hystero-scopic destruction. Using a variety of liquid distending media and a bare laser fiber, a cutting loop, or roller ball electrode, one can destroy the basalis layer of the endometrium. Total destruc-tion leads to no regeneration and thus amenorrhea. Partial destruction results in hypomenorrhea.

19. How successful is endometrial ablation?

Approximately 85% of women with abnormal bleeding respond favorably to ablation. This response is related to age (greater number of failures in women < 35 years old) and presence or absence of benign uterine pathology (polyps, myomas, or adenomyosis).

20. What complications are associated with endometrial ablation?

Although uncommon, fluid overload, thought to occur when venous sinuses are flooded with the distending media, is the number one serious complication of endometrial ablation. Because of the increased intravascular volume, hyponatremia may develop, and if not recognized, cardio-vascular collapse and death may ensue. Strict quantification of distention media is mandatory, and the procedure must be terminated if the patient has absorbed 1,500 ml. Uterine perforation, the next most common complication, has the potential for small bowel damage. Thus, laparo-scopic visualization of the uterus is recommended in first learning this new technique. Finally, heavy bleeding may be encountered when vessels are severed. A 30-ml Foley catheter placed within the uterine cavity for 4–8 hours almost always controls this bleeding.

21. What alternatives are left for the patient who fails medical therapy as well as ablation?

Surgical removal of the uterus is the final therapeutic step. The type of hysterectomy de-pends on the patient's age, prior surgery, and associated medical problems.

BIBLIOGRAPHY

1. Aikins JA, Singh G, Mikuta JJ: Evaluation and significance of abnormal vaginal bleeding. Postgrad Obstet Gynecol 14(14):1–6, 1994.
2. American College of Obstetricians and Gynecologists: Dysfunctional Uterine Bleeding. ACOG Tech Bull 134, 1989.
3. American College of Obstetricians and Gynecologists: Hysterscopy. ACOG Tech Bull 191, 1994.
4. Brooks PG (ed): Operative hysteroscopy. Clin Obstet Gynecol 35:209–314, 1992.
5. Claessens EA, Cowell CA: Acute adolescent menorrhagia. Am J Obstet Gynecol 139:277–280, 1981.
6. Kempers RD: Dysfunctional uterine bleeding. In Speroff L, Simpson JL, Sciarra JJ (eds): Gynecology and Obstetrics, vol 5. Philadelphia, J.B. Lippincott, 1994, pp 1–11.
7. Lewis BV, Magos AL: Endometrial Ablation. New York, Churchill Livingstone, 1993.
8. Shaw RW (ed): Treating the patient with menorrhagia. Br J Obstet Gynecol 101(Suppl 11):1–22, 1994.
9. Speroff L, Glass RH, Kase NG: Clinical Gynecologic Endocrinology and Infertility, 5th ed. Baltimore, Williams & Wilkins, 1994.
10. Valle RF: Assessing new treatments for dysfunctional uterine bleeding. Contemp Obstet Gynecol 39(4):43–60, 1994.
11. Wortman M, Daggett A: Hysteroscopic endometrial resection: A new technique for the treatment of men-orrhagia. Obstet Gynecol 83:295–298, 1994.

6. THE PAPANICOLAOU SMEAR

Bruce Drummond, M.D., and Don McClure, M.D.

1. Why is the Papanicolaou (Pap) smear a good screening test for cervical cancer?

The Pap smear is easily performed in the office setting, noninvasive, and relatively inexpensive. During the past 40 years, the Pap smear has reduced the mortality from cervical cancer by 70%. The Pap smear prevents cervical cancer by detecting and allowing treatment in the precancerous state as well as the cancerous state of cervical neoplasia.

2. Why is the Pap smear effective despite a high false-negative rate?

The false-negative rate is the number of patients who have abnormal cervical cells and a negative test. Under optimal circumstances, it is estimated to be 5%. Some studies have claimed that the false-negative rate is as high as 15%. The sensitivity of the smear (the ability of the test to single out intraepithelial lesions) is low because of the high false-negative rate. However, the Pap smear is still effective. Low-grade cervical intraepithelial lesions progress slowly to invasive cervical cancer. The natural history of the disease has been reported to be between 8 and 30 years. When frequent serial examinations are performed, it is possible to detect and treat abnormal cytology before invasive cervical cancer develops.

3. With what frequency should Pap smears be repeated?

The American College of Obstetricians and Gynecologists (ACOG) recommends that "all women who are or have been sexually active, or have reached the age of 18 years of age, should have an annual cervical smear and pelvic examination. After a woman has had three or more consecutive, satisfactory, normal annual examinations, the cervical smear could be performed less frequently at the discretion of her physician."

There has been considerable debate about the frequency of tests. The Canadian Task Force Report in 1976 and the American Cancer Society Report in 1980 recommended a Pap smear every 3 years after two negative yearly smears. High-risk women should be screened yearly. In 1980, the U.S. Preventive Services Task Force recommended 1–3 years, depending on the presence of risk factors.

More frequent Pap tests are favored by many obstetricians and gynecologists for maintaining good patient follow-up and maximizing other health benefits associated with frequent clinic visits. Recommendations vary, but in general women without a uterus should have a Pap smear every 3 years if their hysterectomy was not done for preinvasive disease. ACOG still advised yearly Pap smears for most women.

4. What is the significance of the presence of endocervical cells on a Pap test?

The presence of endocervical cells on a Pap test is regarded as evidence of adequate sampling of the transformation zone. A smear lacking endocervical cells is classified under the Bethesda system as "satisfactory, but limited by." For a patient with no known risk factors who previously has had three consecutive annual normal Pap smears and whose current smear has no abnormalities, a physician may exercise discretion and defer for 12 months. Studies in which these smears have been repeated immediately indicate that finding significant lesions is rare.

5. What are the major risk factors for preinvasive lesions?

Early intercourse	Low socioeconomic status
Multiple sexual partners	Immunocompromised state
Early pregnancy	Nicotine abuse
Human papillomavirus (HPV) infection	Use of oral contraceptives

6. If a woman has been treated for a preinvasive lesion, how frequently should she have a Pap smear? How frequently should she be followed with the history of an invasive lesion?

For preinvasive lesions, smears should be done at 3–4 month intervals for the first year, then annually. For invasive lesions, examinations should be done more frequently, starting at intervals of every 3–4 months for 2 years, then every 6 months for 5 years after diagnosis.

7. What should the patient be told to optimize the Pap smear?

The patient should be instructed not to have intercourse, douche, or use tampons for 24 hours before the exam. She should reschedule if she is having menses or has taken intravaginal antibiotics within the past week. Care must be taken in counseling patients who are bleeding, because this is also the most common symptom of cervical cancer. Patients who cancel Pap smear appointments for "menses" should be questioned carefully about bleeding before they are rescheduled.

8. How can the physician optimize the results?

The smear should be done before lubricant or acetic acid is applied to the cervix during bimanual and colposcopic exams. Bacterial cultures should be taken afterward to lessen the possibility that blood will interfere with reading the smear. To sample the cervix correctly, a wooden spatula is rotated 360° over the cervix at the squamocolumnar junction, and a cyto-brush is rotated to collect endocervical cells. The cells are smeared over a single slide and immediately fixed with 95% ethyl alcohol to reduce drying artifact. Proper technique has been shown to reduce the high false-negative rate. The cytopathologist must be informed of any unusual patient history or clinical findings. Selecting a good cytology lab that has a high correlation between cytology reports and regional cervical intraepithelial neoplasm (CIN) rates is important. Dysplastic cells are less cohesive than normal cells; thus, cleaning off or wiping the cervix before obtaining the smear may result in fewer cells and a less than optimal smear.

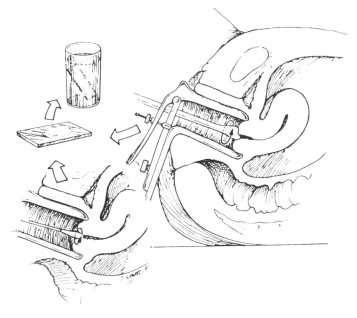

Papanicolaou smear. The transformation zone and the squamocolumnar junction of the cervix are scraped in a circular motion using the Ayre spatula. A second specimen from the endocervix is obtained using a small brush. This sample is fixed immediately on a separate slide, then submitted to the pathologist. (From Clarke-Pearson DL, Dawood MY (eds): Green's Gynecology: Essentials of Clinical Practice, 4th ed. Boston, Little, Brown, 1990, p 16, with permission.)

9. How are the cytologic readings reported from the Pap smear?

In 1988, the National Institutes of Health sponsored a consensus panel that developed the Bethesda System (TBS) to standardize the classification cytologic findings. TBS was revised in 1991. The system addressed the need for terminology that correlates well with histopathologic terminology. The format of the report includes an evaluation of specimen adequacy, general categorization, and descriptive diagnosis. Descriptive diagnoses include benign cellular changes, epithelial cell abnormalities, squamous cells, atypical squamous cells of undetermined significance (CIN I), low-grade squamous intraepithelial lesion (CIN II), and high-grade squamous intraepithelial lesion (CIN III).

10. What is the natural history of CINs?

Summary of the Natural History of Cervical Intraepithelial Neoplasia

	PATIENTS (N)	REGRESSION (%)	PERSISTENCE (%)	PROGRESSION TO CIS (%)	PROGRESSION TO INVASION (%)
CIN I	4504	57	32	11	1
CIN II	2247	43	35	22	5
CIN III	767	32	< 56	—	> 12

CIN, cervical intraepithelial neoplasia; CIS, carcinoma in situ.
From Östör AG: Natural history of cervical intraepithelial neoplasia: A critical review. Int J Gynecol Pathol 12:186, 1996, with permission.

11. What makes a specimen adequate?

1. Patient identification so that the laboratory may refer to prior exams.
2. Pertinent clinical information—uncertain cytologic findings may receive more attention if significant history is included.
3. Technical interpretability—drying artifact and blood may interfere with reading the smear.
4. Cellular composition and sampling of the transformation zone—squamous and endocervical cells must be present.

12. What are the cellular changes seen with HPV infection?

Based on strict criteria, the cellular changes of squamous cells are characterized by cytoplasmic vacuolization and nuclear enlargement, irregularity, and hyperchromasia. This is called koilocytosis, a descriptive term no longer used in TBS.

13. Why are HPV and CIN I cellular changes included in the same category of low-grade squamous intraepithelial lesion (LSIL) in TBS?

HPV effect and CIN I cellular changes overlap. Reproducibility among cytopathologists suggest koilocytosis and CIN should be included in the same category. Longitudinal studies have shown similar rates of progression between Pap smears with koilocytosis vs. CIN I. Because one cannot distinguish between HPV and CIN I on the basis of morphology, molecular biology, or clinical behavior, TBS includes them in the same category.

14. Why are moderate dysplasia and severe dysplasia combined into the same category of high-grade squamous intraepithelial neoplasia (HSIL)?

All high-grade lesions need colposcopy, and treatment is based on the extent of the lesion, not the grade. Therefore, there is no screening advantage to distinguish moderate or severe dysplasia on the basis of cytology. The reproducibility of moderate and severe dysplasia as a diagnosis is poor; but the reproducibility and natural history of the lesions is similar when they are grouped into HGSIL lesions.

15. What is ASCUS? How should a patient with ASCUS be managed?

Atypical squamous cells of undetermined significance (ASCUS) is a cytologic diagnosis based on cellular changes that exceed those attributable to benign or reactive processes but lack the criteria for squamous intraepithelial lesion (SIL). The significance of ASCUS varies among laboratories, depending on whether they have few or many cases of intraepithelial lesions included in this category. ASCUS rates of 3–5% are reasonable. A significant proportion (20–30%) of patients with ASCUS have dysplasia.

ACOG recommends that patients who are reliable should be followed by cytology alone at intervals 3–6 months. Two reports with ASCUS are an indication for colposcopy. If patient compliance is an issue, initial colposcopy should be performed.

Atypical glandular cells of undetermined significance (AGUS) are much less common than ASCUS (0.3% vs. 5%). Follow-up is no less important and in selected cases may require endometrial and endocervical sampling. The specificity of AGUS varies widely. Some investigators have felt that AGUS should be qualified to favor either AGUS, most likely reactive, or AGUS, most likely neoplastic. In follow-up studies of AGUS smears considered abnormal enough to favor neoplasia, glandular neoplasia has been confirmed on follow-up biopsy in 27–83%. On the other hand, biopsy follow-up of AGUS smears in which atypical glandular cells were felt likely reactive revealed neoplasia in less than 5% of the cases. A significant percentage of AGUS cases may actually be an indicator of a squamous precursor lesion.

16. What does the ACOG recommend for Papanicolaou results of LSIL and HSIL?

About 60% of LSILs regress spontaneously so that the patient may be followed and retested in 4–6 months after initial colposcopy has ruled out high-grade lesions. Patients with HSIL should undergo colposcopy and directed biopsy by an experienced colposcopist. Therapy should be based on histologic results of directed biopsies and ECC.

17. In determining where to send Pap smears, what questions should the cytopathologist be asked?

1. What is the pathologist's ASCUS/dysplasia ratio? An acceptable ratio is 2.0–3.0. Cytopathology labs that have lower ratios may miss important lesions that should be reported as ASCUS rather than normal. High ratios tend to reduce the significance of ASCUS. This may lead the gynecologist to perform unnecessary procedures on a patient group with low incidence of disease.

2. How do the number of normal, atypical, suspicious, and unsatisfactory results compare with regional and national averages? Ask the number of screeners, their level of training, and the number of smears they are required to read per day to ensure that each smear gets adequate attention.

18. What is the role of adjunctive techniques in diagnostic gynecologic cytology?

Divergent technologies have been approved by the Food and Drug Administration, each of which has advantages and disadvantages. PAPNET (Neuromedical Systems, Inc.) has developed a system targeting selected negative Pap smears for review. PAPNET searches for suspicious cells on negative smears, isolating 128 cell images of potentially significant cells to be reviewed by a trained cytologist. AutoPap (NeoPath, Inc.) is licensed to rescreen all negative Pap smears with a predetermined threshold for review. This system enriches the subset of manually screened negative smears for rescreening. The ThinPrep (Cytyc) collects cells in a fluid medium, maximizing cell preservation and minimizing background artifact to enhance the quality of the smear available for manual screening. All of the techniques reduce the false-negative rate, but it is too early to predict the evolution of adjunctive Pap smear techniques.

BIBLIOGRAPHY

1. American Cancer Society (ACS): ACS report on the cancer-related health checkup. CA 30:215–223, 1980.
2. American College of Obstetricians and Gynecologists (ACOG): Cervical cytology: Evaluation and management of abnormalities. ACOG Tech Bull 183, 1993.
3. Hoskins WJ, et al: Principles and Practice of Gynecologic Oncology. Philadelphia, J.B. Lippincott, 1992.

4. Kurman RJ, Henson DE, Herbst AL, et al: Interim guidelines for management of abnormal cervical cytology. JAMA 271:1866, 1994.
5. Koss LG, Lin E, Schreiber K, et al: Evaluation of the PAPNET cytologic screening system for quality control of cervical smears. Am J Clin Pathol 101:220, 1994.
6. National Cancer Institute Workshop: The revised Bethesda system for reporting cervical/vaginal cytologic diagnoses: Report of 1991 Bethesda Workshop. Acta Cytol 36:273, 1991.
7. The Bethesda system for reporting cervical/vaginal cytologic diagnoses. Acta Cytol 37:115–123, 1993.

7. BARTHOLIN'S GLAND CYST AND ABSCESS

Matthew B. Cort, M.D.

1. What is the Bartholin's gland?

The Bartholin's or vulvar vaginal glands are two glandular structures located within the vulvar tissue on both sides of the fourchette. They secrete mucus and drain into the posterior introitus. Normally they are small and not palpable unless swollen by infection, fluid, or tumor.

2. What is a Bartholin's cyst or abscess?

A Bartholin's cyst is due to the obstruction of the duct, usually near its opening, with subsequent swelling due to the build-up of mucus secretions. It is the most important vulvar cyst in clinical practice. Most cysts are unilateral and unilocular. In an infected cyst, the contents become purulent; this constitutes a Bartholin's abscess.

3. What is the cause?

The underlying cause, including whether the cyst or abscess came first, is often difficult to determine. In the past it was thought that gonococcal infection was the predominant cause. More recent studies indicate the presence of gonorrhea in 10–50% of Bartholin's abscesses. Other causative organisms include *Escherichia coli*, *Proteus* sp., and vaginal flora, usually anaerobes. Most Bartholin's abscesses contain mixed bacterial organisms.

Noninfectious causes include: (1) congenital stenosis or atresia; (2) mechanical trauma, including poorly placed sutures from episiotomy or posterior colporrhaphy repair, which may even ligate the duct; and (3) inspissated mucus.

4. What are the symptoms of Bartholin's cysts and abscesses?

Cysts that are small are often asymptomatic. They may be noticed on self-examination or by the physician during a routine check-up. Larger cysts tend to cause discomfort, usually associated with walking, sitting, or sexual intercourse.

Abscesses usually cause pain and tenderness, often intense. Abscesses often develop rapidly over a few days and may rupture spontaneously.

5. What are the clinical characteristics of Bartholin's cysts and abscesses?

Cysts are usually unilateral, 1–5 cm, nontender, round to ovoid in shape, and located in the posterior labia.

Abscesses are usually erythematous and tender and may be caused by infection with *Neisseria gonorrhoeae*.

6. What is the treatment for Bartholin's cysts?

Small, asymptomatic cysts can usually be left alone. A symptomatic or recurrent cyst usually requires surgery, catheterization with a Word catheter, marsupialization, or laser vaporization of the cyst wall.

7. What is a Word catheter?

A Word catheter is a single-lumen catheter with a 1-inch stem and an inflatable balloon tip. A small incision is made at the introitus (not on the skin). The balloon tip is inserted into the cyst and insufflated with 2–4 ml of water. The catheter is left in place 3–6 weeks. The balloon is then deflated, the catheter is removed, and a permanent ostium secondary to epithelialization remains.

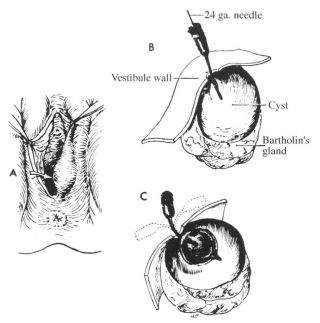

Inflatable bulb-tipped catheter used in the treatment of Bartholin's duct cysts and abscesses. *A*, An *arrow* indicates the location for a stab wound in a cyst or abscess. *B*, Insertion of the catheter in the stab wound. *C*, Inserted catheter inflated with 2–4 ml of water. (From Word B: New instrument for office treatment of cyst and abscess of Bartholin's gland. JAMA 190:777, © 1964, American Medical Association, with permission.)

8. What is marsupialization?

A vertical incision is made in the vaginal mucosa over the cyst outside the hymenal ring. The cyst wall is sutured to the vaginal mucosa medially and to the skin of the introitus laterally.

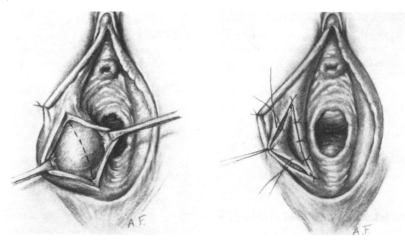

A, Incision for marsupialization. *B*, Marsupialization. (From Tancer ML, Rosenberg M, Fernandez D: Cysts of the vulvovaginal (Bartholin's) gland. Obstet Gynecol 7:609, 1956, with permission.)

9. What is the treatment for a Bartholin's abscess?

Treatment of a Bartholin's abscess is incision and drainage. A Word catheter can be placed to maintain patency. Marsupialization can also be performed in the acute stage but has a higher failure rate due to the difficulty of identifying the cyst wall lining and subsequent closure of the opening.

10. What are the risks and indications for Bartholin's gland excision?

Gland excision is not generally recommended because it is associated with significant complications, including hemorrhage, hematoma, cellulitis, incomplete removal with subsequent recurrence, and painful scar formation. One author said that this can be "the bloodiest little operation in gynecology." However, excision is indicated for persistent or recurrent abscesses or cysts. In the postmenopausal woman a new Bartholin's gland "cyst" may represent a malignant tumor and also needs to be excised.

BIBLIOGRAPHY

1. Aghajanian A, Bernstein L, Grimes DA: Bartholin's duct abscess and cyst: A case-control study. South Med J 87:26–29, 1994.
2. Anderson PG, Christensen S, Detlefsen GU, Kern-Hansen P: Treatment of Bartholin's abscess. Marsupialization versus incision, curettage and suture under antibiotic cover: A randomized study with 6 month's follow-up. Acta Obstet Gynecol Scand 71:59–62, 1992.
3. Bleker OP, Smalbraak DJ, Schutte MF: Bartholin's abscess: The role of *Chlamydia trachomatis.* Genitourin Med 66:24–25, 1990.
4. Brook I: Aerobic and anaerobic microbiology of Bartholin's abscess. Surg Gynecol Obstet 169:32–34, 1989.
5. Cho JY, Ahn MO, Cha KS: Window operation: An alternative treatment method of Bartholin gland cysts and abscesses. Obstet Gynecol 76(5 Pt 1):886–888, 1990.
6. Davis GD: Management of Bartholin duct cysts with carbon dioxide laser. Obstet Gynecol 65:279, 1985.
7. Kaufman RH, et al: Benign Diseases of the Vulva and Vagina, 4th ed. St. Louis, Mosby, 1994.
8. Mattingly RF, Thompson JD: TeLinde's Operative Gynecology, 7th ed. Philadelphia, J.B. Lippincott, 1992.
9. Word B: New instrument for office treatment of cysts and abscesses of Bartholin's gland. JAMA 190:777, 1964.

8. BENIGN LESIONS OF THE VULVA AND VAGINA

E. *Stewart Taylor,* M.D.

1. Describe solid benign tumors that occur on the vulva.

Nevi. Nevi are pigmented lesions composed of clusters of nevus cells. These lesions should be treated with wide local excision, especially if located in areas of chronic irritation or if undergoing a color change.

Leiomyomas. Leiomyomas may occur on the vulva, arising from smooth muscle in erectile vulvar structures or remnants of the round ligament.

Fibromas and lipomas. Fibromas are similar to leiomyomas but of mesodermal origin. Lipomas develop in the adipose tissue of the vulva. Treatment for fibromas and lipomas is wide local excision.

Glomus tumors. Glomus tumors occur in the dermis and are painful solid vulvar tumors.

Hidroadenomas. Hidroadenomas are benign sweat gland tumors arising from the labia minora or majora. They are small firm tumors with a pointed center. Although they are benign lesions, the microscopic picture may be mistaken for adenocarcinoma. Simple surgical excision is necessary for diagnosis and cure.

2. Which lesions on the vulva are caused by sexually transmitted infectious agents? Describe their clinical appearance and treatment.

Condylomata accuminata. These lesions may be few or numerous and may involve the perineum, vulva, vagina, and cervix. The condylomata are caused by one or many of the known human papillomaviruses. If a specific organism is causing a vaginal discharge, it should be treated. Condylomata accuminata can be removed with repeated applications of podophyllin, cautery, cryosurgery, or laser. Unfortunately, none of these treatments is entirely curative. Recurrences are frequent. If a woman is pregnant, podophyllin should be avoided for fear of fetal damage. After several years, some of these lesions may be followed by squamous cell carcinoma of the vulva, but this sequence is rare.

Syphilis of the vulva. *Primary chancre* of the vulva is rare. Most primary lesions of syphilis in women occur in the vagina or on the cervix. The primary lesion of syphilis, when on the vulva, may be found on the labia minora or majora. The lesion is typically a painless ulcer, 1–2 cm in diameter, with firm, raised edges that give a craterlike appearance. The primary lesion of syphilis appears 3–4 weeks after the sexual exposure causing the disease. At first, the primary lesion is only a small fissure but later becomes a cratered ulcer from which the spirochete can be recovered for dark-field identification. Bilateral lymphadenopathy often accompanies a chancre. If the primary lesion is unrecognized or untreated, the chancre will heal and the patient will develop later stages of syphilitic infection. The *secondary lesions* of syphilis appear as moist, grayish patches on the perineum and are called condylomata lata. Dark-field examination of scrapings from these lesions yields spirochetes. Penicillin is the specific treatment for syphilis. *Later stages* of syphilis may consist of ulcerative and necrotic lesions of the vulva. Like all chronic granulomatous lesions of the vulva, they may later become squamous carcinoma.

Granuloma inguinale. This sexually transmitted disease is caused by the Donovan bacillus. The disease starts as a small papule on the vulva and spreads in a serpiginous manner until the entire vulvoperineal area is a mass of chronic granulomatous tissue. The disease spreads to the lymph nodes of the groin. Symptoms are vulvar itching, burning, pain, and discharge. A hematoxylin and eosin stain of scrapings from the lesion demonstrates Donovan bodies. Tetracycline is an excellent drug for treatment of granuloma inguinale.

Lymphogranuloma venereum. This venereal disease is caused by the lymphogranuloma venereum virus. The primary lesion on the vulva appears 3 or 4 days after exposure to an infected sexual partner. Two or three weeks later, marked inguinal adenitis appears. All of the regional lymph nodes of the pelvis become involved. As a result, multiple fissures of the perineum and rectum may develop. Rectal and vaginal strictures may develop later. The disease is not limited to the pelvis. Meningitis, pleurisy, peritonitis, and arthritis may be caused by the virus. Treatment is not highly effective, but tetracycline is the drug recommended.

Chancroid. Chancroid is a venereal disease characterized by the presence of a soft chancre. This disease is caused by Ducrey's bacillus. Chancroid appears as a soft chancre following a small papule or pustule, 2–4 days after exposure to an infected sexual partner. Inguinal adenitis with suppuration may follow. Tetracycline and broad-spectrum antibiotics are effective treatments.

3. Which cystic lesions occur on the vulva and in the vagina?

Vulva	Vagina
Sebaceous cysts	Inclusion cysts
Inclusion cysts	Gartner's duct cysts
Bartholin's gland cysts	Endometriosis
	Adenosis

4. What is lichen sclerosus et atrophicus? How can it be treated? Is it a premalignant lesion?

Lichen sclerosus et atrophicus (LS&A) is a slowly developing, chronic, localized lesion of unknown etiology. It may occur at any age, but most patients are age 50 years or older. It is a chronic lesion that may appear anywhere on the skin but primarily affects the vulva and perineum. Favorite sites, other than the vulva and perineum, are the neck, axillae, shoulders, and forearms. The lesions undergo remissions and exacerbations and occasionally disappear entirely. Inspection of the vulva reveals an ivory white, smooth surface. The patient complains of vulvar itching and burning. The diagnosis can be proved by vulval biopsy, which shows a dense, subepidermal zone of homogenized collagen beneath which is found a collection of lymphocytes. Keratotic plugging of follicles and dense parakeratosis are seen.

5. What is vestibular adenitis? How is it treated?

Vestibular adenitis is a debatable lesion. From time to time, it is considered the cause of perineal pain and dyspareunia. The typical history given by the patient is acquired dyspareunia of a severe nature. Usually the patient has been treated for months for a wide variety of vaginal infections with no relief. When the diagnosis is finally made, there must be an absence of all indications of a vaginal infection. A cotton-tipped applicator is touched to the vulvovaginal ring to test for areas of tenderness. If red tender areas are found at the posterior forchette of the vestibule, a diagnosis of vestibular adenitis can be made.

Initial treatment should be medical; 1% hydrocortisone ointment should be applied locally twice daily. Sexual rest for 2 weeks is recommended. Dibucaine (nupercaine) ointment should be applied to the tender areas before intercourse is reinitiated. If the patient's symptoms persist after 2 or 3 months of conservative treatment, local excision of the areas of adenosis should be performed. It will be 6 months before the patient is cured, and, in some instances, the syndrome recurs.

6. Which lesions in the vagina are a result of abnormal development? How are they treated?

Imperforate hymen. Imperforate hymen may lead to hematocolpos, hematotrachelos, hematometrium, and hematosalpinx. Imperforate hymen is usually not recognized until puberty when external manifestations of maturity occur. Inspection of the introitus reveals an imperforate hymen with a bulging fluid mass in the vagina. The treatment is quite simple; it consists of a cruciate incision of the imperforate hymen.

Septate vagina. Septate vagina may be complete or incomplete with a soft tissue septum running from the introitus to the cervix. Many patients have two cervices, one on each side of the septum. If the septum (whether complete or incomplete) gives no symptoms, it can be left alone. If it causes dyspareunia, it can be surgically removed.

Transverse vaginal septum. This rare congenital defect consists of a septum dividing the vagina into upper and lower compartments. A small opening in the septum permits menstrual flow. Pregnancy can occur. Delivery may require a cesarean section; excision of the septum permits vaginal delivery in some cases.

7. What lesions of the urethra occur as vaginal masses? How are they treated?

Urethral diverticulum. A diverticulum may appear on the vaginal side of the urethra and bulge into the vagina as a small cystic pouch. If the diverticulum becomes infected or abscessed, considerable pain and dysuria result. The most common symptom of a urethral diverticulum is dribbling of urine after voiding. It may be difficult to make the diagnosis of urethral diverticulum from physical examination alone. Even cystoscopy may fail to reveal the lesion. Special radiographic techniques that fill the urethra with radiopaque contrast solution may be necessary to establish the diagnosis of urethral diverticulum. If the diverticulum causes no symptoms, it need not be removed.

Suburethral abscess. An abscess may present in the vagina in the diverticulum or in a periurethral gland. Such an abscess should be drained from the vaginal side.

Urethral caruncle. This lesion may be of the chronic granulomatous variety or hemangiomatous. It appears as a small red lesion protruding from the edges of the urethra. It must be differentiated from cancer and from prolapse of the urethral mucosa. Patients may be asymptomatic or have local pain or minimal bleeding from the surface of the lesion. If the patient has no symptoms, the condition requires no treatment. If treatment is necessary, the lesion can be removed with cautery or laser, using local anesthesia.

8. Why does a vulvar hematoma often need to be evacuated?

A severe direct blow or picket-fence perforation of the vulval area may be complicated by a subcutaneous hematoma, which may dissect widely beneath the fascia of the perineum and vulva. It is often necessary to evacuate the hematoma surgically. It may not be possible to isolate and ligate the bleeding point or points. After the hematoma is drained, it may be necessary to pack the excavated area to control bleeding.

BIBLIOGRAPHY

1. Buttram VL: Mullerian anomalies and their management. Fertil Steril 40:159, 1983.
2. Chapel TA: The signs and symptoms of secondary syphilis. Sex Transm Dis 7:161, 1980.
3. Davis GD: The management of vulvar vestibulitis syndrome with the carbon dioxide laser. J Gynecol Surg 5:87, 1989.
4. Friedrich EG: The vulvar vestibule. J Reprod Med 28:773, 1983.
5. Greenblatt RB: Management of Chancroid, Granuloma Inguinale, Lymphogranuloma Venereum in General Practice. Washington, DC, U.S. Dept. of Health, Education and Welfare, USPH No. 225, 1953.
6. Huddock VV, Dupayne N, McGeary JA: Traumatic vulvar hematomas. Am J Obstet Gynecol 70:1064, 1955.
7. Janooski NA, Ames S: Lichen sclerosus et atrophicus of the vulva: A poorly understood disease entity. Obstet Gynecol 22:697, 1963.
8. Kaufman RH, Friedrich E (eds): Benign Diseases of the Vulva and Vagina, 3rd ed. Chicago, Year Book, 1989.
9. McKay M: Vulvodynia. Diagnostic patterns. Dermatol Clin 10:423–433, 1992.
10. Ridley CM: Lichen Sclerosus. Dermatol Clin 10(20):309, 1992.
11. Rock B: Pigmented lesions of the vulva. Dermatol Clin 10:361, 1992.
12. Vince JO, Martin NJ: Transverse vaginal septum, McKusick-Kaufman syndrome. An J Med Genet 32:174, 1989.
13. Woodworth H, Dockerty MD, Wilson RB, et al: Papillary hidradenoma of the vulva: A clinical pathological study of 691 cases. An J Obstet Gynecol 110:501, 1971.

9. LEIOMYOMATOUS UTERUS

Kathleen Doyle, M.D.

1. What is a leiomyoma?

A leiomyoma is a benign tumor of muscle cell origin that usually also contains varying amounts of fibrous tissue. Other names for these tumors include myoma, fibroid, and fibromyoma.

2. How common are leiomyoma?

Leiomyomas are the most common pelvic tumors, with the highest incidence in the fifth decade of life. They are thought to occur in as many as 1 of 4 white women and 1 of 2 black women. Leiomyomas are the most common indication for hysterectomy in the United States.

3. What is the etiology of leiomyomas?

The etiology of leiomyomas is incompletely understood. Each myoma is monoclonal and results from a single muscle cell, whose origin is unclear.

4. Do leiomyomas develop or grow in response to increased estrogen levels?

Myomas appear to be sensitive to estrogen, because they grow during childbearing years and regress with menopause. They also shrink when treated with analogs of gonadotropin-releasing hormone (GnRH), which induce a menopause-like state. However, there is no evidence that myomas grow in response to oral contraceptive pills, and many myomas do not enlarge during pregnancy. Estrogen receptors are higher in myoma than in surrounding myometrium.

5. **Where in the uterus are myomas located?**
   Subserosal: just beneath the serosa
   Intramural: in the uterine wall
   Submucosal: just below the endometrium
   These are the 3 most common type of leiomyomas. Although submucosal myomas account for only 5–10% of myomas, they are thought to be the most symptomatic clinically, especially through excessive bleeding. Leiomyomas also may grow laterally into the broad ligament, where they may mimic a solid ovarian mass on pelvic exam or ultrasound. Parasitic leiomyomas are pedunculated myomas that wander into the peritoneal cavity and attach to another organ (i.e., the omentum) and parasitize its blood supply. These myomas are rare.

6. **What are the symptoms associated with leiomyoma?**
   1. **Bleeding.** About 30% of women with fibroids complain of abnormal bleeding. The most common type of bleeding is menometrorrhagia, although intermenstrual bleeding also may occur. Such bleeding may lead to acute or chronic anemia.
   2. **Pressure.** An anterior myoma may cause symptoms of pressure on the bladder, such as frequency and urgency. Posterior fibroids, especially those arising in the lower uterine segment, may cause pain or pressure on defecation or, in severe cases, constipation secondary to obstruction.
   3. **Pain.** One of three women with fibroids complains of pelvic pain, with acquired dysmenorrhea the most common complaint. Acute pain may occur with vascular compromise, as in acute degeneration.

7. **Can leiomyomas impair fertility?**
   A leiomyoma can impair fertility by occlusion of the cervical canal, distortion of the fallopian tubes, or change or distortion of the endometrium that impairs implantation. Leiomyomas may also complicate pregnancy by causing spontaneous abortion, preterm labor, or, rarely, dystocia via obstruction.

8. **Are leiomyomas ever malignant?**
   Leiomyosarcomas, which represent 0.3–0.7% of all myomas, are highly malignant tumors, whose origin is unclear. It is not known whether myomas undergo malignant degeneration into sarcomas or whether sarcomas arise spontaneously in myomatous uteri.

9. **When do myomas require treatment?**
   There are three main indications for treatment:
   1. Bleeding that causes anemia or impairment of the woman's lifestyle.
   2. Pressure that causes significant discomfort.
   3. Rapid growth of a myoma or any growth in a postmenopausal woman. Growth of either kind may indicate a sarcoma. Note that size alone is not an indication for treatment.

10. **What treatments are available for symptomatic leiomyomas?**
    Both surgical and medical treatments are available for symptomatic leiomyomas. Therapy depends on the desired goals, including whether preservation of fertility is desired.

11. **What surgical treatments are available for leiomyomas?**
    Surgical options include definitive treatment with hysterectomy, conservative treatment with myomectomy, or therapy with hysteroscopic destruction or removal of submucosal leiomyomas.

12. **What are the indications for myomectomy?**
    If the patient wants to preserve her fertility and has indications for surgical treatment, myomectomy is indicated. It is important to emphasize to the patient that she may require a hysterectomy because of bleeding. The enlarged uterus may be a result of adenomyosis rather than a single myoma; thus, conservative surgery may not be possible. More often myomas are removed via the hysteroscope.

13. What medical treatments are available for symptomatic leiomyomas?

Medical therapy for leiomyomas includes Depo-provera, danazol, GnRH analogs, and most recently, RU-486. Since the discovery that GnRH analogs (such as Depo-Lupron) shrink myomas up to 50%, they are the most commonly used drugs for treatment. RU-486 also has been shown to shrink myomas to the same extent. Both drugs have only a temporary effect, and most myomas grow back to their original size within 4 months of discontinuing treatment. GnRH analogs (and in the future possibly RU-486) have been important in preparing a woman for surgery, because it may be possible to remove a smaller uterus vaginally and anemia secondary to heavy bleeding can be corrected before surgery. Research is ongoing in treating perimenopausal women with GnRH analogs and giving them "add-back" hormone replacement therapy to avoid surgery before menopause.

14. What is the cause of uterine leiomyomas?

There are two main theories: (1) the cell of origin is from persistent embryonic cell nests, and (2) the cell of origin is from the smooth muscle of blood vessels.

15. Why do leiomyomas cause abnormal bleeding?

Some submucous myomas cause bleeding due to ulceration of endometrium over the area of the myoma. This, however, is rare. More likely, myomas cause changes in the venous drainage pattern and vascular alteration of the endometrial surface. The bleeding is not due to an increased endometrial surface area.

16. What is the differential diagnosis for an irregular pelvic mass that is thought to be caused by a myoma?

The differential diagnosis includes adenomyosis, pregnancy, and possible ovarian neoplasm.

17. What is intravenous leiomyomatosis?

Intravenous leiomyomatosis is a rare condition in which smooth muscle cells invade the venous channels of the pelvis. The tumor cells are benign but may grow by direct extension and rarely extend out of the pelvis via the venous system. Rare reports exist of tumors extending into the right heart via the vena cava.

BIBLIOGRAPHY

1. Barbieri RL, et al: RU-486 uses in gynecology. ACOG Update 19(9), 1993.
2. Droegemueller W: Benign gynecologic lesions. In Droegemuller W, et al (eds): Comprehensive Gynecology. St. Louis, Mosby, 1992.
3. Gambone JC, et al: Indications for hysterectomies. ACOG Update 19(10), 1993.
4. Polan ML, et al: GnRH in gynecology. ACOG Update 19(7), 1993.

10. PELVIC RELAXATION

Tim Sorrells, M.D.

1. What is pelvic relaxation?

Pelvic relaxation is the weakening of the supporting structures of the female pelvis, which causes varying degrees and combinations of prolapse of the urethra (urethrocele), bladder (cystocele), rectum (rectocele), uterus (uterine prolapse) and posterior vaginal wall hernia (enterocele).

2. What causes pelvic relaxation? When does it occur?

Pelvic relaxation is usually considered to be caused by childbirth. Frequently a genetic factor is involved, and indeed sometimes it occurs in the absence of childbirth. A recent study of collagen synthesis suggests that women with urinary stress incontinence have altered connective tissue metabolism. Chronic and repetitive increases in intraabdominal pressure increase the risk of developing pelvic organ prolapse. Although it can occur at almost any time, it is most commonly seen during and after menopause because of loss of hormonal support and generalized weakening of supporting tissues that occurs with age.

3. What is the pelvic floor or diaphragm?

The pelvic floor is made up of the pubococcygeus subdivisions of the levator ani, which include the pubococcygeus proper, pubovaginalis, and puborectalis muscles.

4. What supports the vagina and uterus?

The uterosacral and cardinal ligaments and endopelvic fascia.

5. How is relaxation graded?

Relaxation is graded in degrees. If the structure in question is prolapsed but not to the introitus, the prolapse is considered first degree. For example, first-degree cystocele is prolapse of the bladder but not to the introitus. A second degree prolapse is to the introitus and a third-degree prolapse is through the introitus.

6. In what position should relaxation be evaluated?

Although a good assessment can frequently be made in the dorsolithotomy position, to evaluate the extent of the descent optimally, the patient must be standing and asked to bear down or do the Valsalva maneuver. Patients should be examined before, during, and after a maximum Valsalva effort in the lithotomy, sitting, and standing positions.

7. What is cystocele?

Cystocele is a protrusion of the bladder into the vagina and beyond. It appears as a protrusion of the anterior vaginal wall.

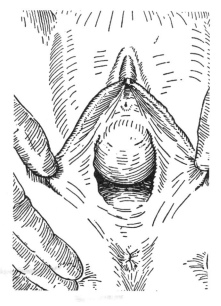

Cystocele, the protrusion of the urinary bladder through the vaginal wall, is often present because of the close proximity of the bladder to the vagina. (From Parsons L, Sommers SC (eds): Gynecology, 2nd ed. Philadelphia, W.B. Saunders, 1978, with permission.)

8. What causes cystocele?

Cystocele usually results from childbirth trauma to the urogenital diaphragm and pubococcygeus muscles. However, genetic predisposition and host factors, such as general health status, nutritional status, and hormonal status, also play a role.

9. What are the symptoms of cystocele?

The patient complains of a bulge or lump in the vagina or protruding from the introitus. This can be painful or merely cause mild pelvic pressure. It may be associated with urinary symptoms of incontinence, frequency, and dysuria.

10. What is the treatment for cystocele?

The mere presence of cystocele on exam does not require treatment. However, if the patient is symptomatic, the first line of treatment, especially in milder cases, is Kagel exercises, which contract the pubococcygeus muscles isometrically to achieve increased strength and bulk. Estrogen replacement therapy often improves minor degrees of pelvic relaxation. If this fails to correct symptoms or if symptoms are severe, surgical treatment in the form of an anterior colporrhaphy (anterior repair) may be indicated. Patients with potential genuine stress incontinence (determined after urodynamic evaluation) need concomitant urethropexy.

11. What is uterine prolapse? What is procendentia?

Uterine prolapse is relaxation of the cardinal and uterosacral ligaments, which allows descent of the cervix and uterus into the vagina and beyond. Procedentia is prolapse of the uterus to the second degree or greater; i.e., the cervix is at the introitus or beyond.

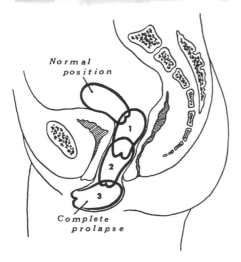

Normal position

Complete prolapse

Prolapse of the uterus is any descent of the uterus below its normal position in the pelvis. In first-degree prolapse, the uterus has descended to the point where the cervix is at the vaginal opening. When the cervix protrudes through the vaginal opening, a second-degree prolapse is present. In complete or third-degree prolapse, the entire uterus descends outside the vagina. This is rare. (From Parsons L, Sommers SC (eds): Gynecology, 2nd ed. Philadelphia, W.B. Saunders, 1978, with permission.)

12. What causes uterine prolapse?

Childbirth trauma, with the predisposing factors discussed earlier, weaken the uterosacral and cardinal ligaments.

13. What are the symptoms of uterine prolapse?

The patient complains of a bulge or lump in the vagina, which may be painful. Sometimes she complains only of pelvic pressure. On occasion uterine prolapse interferes with coitus

14. What is the treatment for uterine prolapse?

Only symptomatic prolapse warrants treatment. The usual treatment is hysterectomy; when this is not an option, pessaries are often successful.

15. What is rectocele?

Rectocele is the herniation of the rectum into the posterior vagina. It appears as a protrusion of the posterior vaginal wall into the vagina and beyond (see figure, top of next page).

16. What causes rectocele?

The primary cause is childbirth trauma along with the same predisposing factors. In addition, increased abdominal pressure from heavy lifting and straining may contribute; rarely, sexual injuries are implicated.

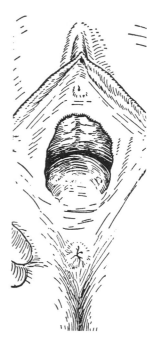

Rectocele, the hernial protrusion of part of the rectum into the vagina, is a frequent complication of prolapse because of laxity of pelvic floor structures. (From Parsons L, Sommers SC (eds): Gynecology, 2nd ed. Philadelphia, W.B. Saunders, 1978, with permission.)

17. What are the symptoms of rectocele?

The patient complains of a bulge or lump in the introitus or beyond. At times, she reports pelvic pressure or pain. Manual aid to defecation is not uncommon; rarely, the patient has difficulty with coitus.

18. What is the treatment for rectocele?

The main treatment is posterior colporrhaphy (posterior repair), although at times the patient improves with Kagel exercises. When surgery is not an option, rectocele may be managed with a pessary.

19. What is vault prolapse?

Vault prolapse is the prolapse of the vaginal cuff in the hysterectomized patient. It is caused by failure of the uterosacral ligaments to support the vagina and appears as a protrusion of the top of the vagina into the vagina and beyond.

20. What are the symptoms of vault prolapse?

The patient complains of a bulge or lump in her vagina or beyond that may be associated with pelvic pressure or pain.

21. What is the treatment for vault prolapse?

Treatment is indicated only if the patient is symptomatic. Vault prolapse is usually treated surgically, with either a vaginal sacrospinous suspension (Nichols procedure) or an abdominal sacral colpoplexy suspension with a graft (usually Gortex).

22. What is colpocliesis? When is it indicated?

Colpocliesis is the surgical obliteration of the vagina. It is indicated in the elderly woman with symptomatic prolapse who no longer desires to retain sexual function. Variations include the rarely done Lefort and Manchester procedure, in which the uterus is left in place.

23. What are pessaries?

Pessaries are devices, usually made of lucite or rubber, that are designed to be placed into the vagina to return pelvic structures to their normal position and hold them there. The popular varieties are the ring, cube, and Smith-Hodge pessaries, which are most useful when surgery is not elected or contraindicated.

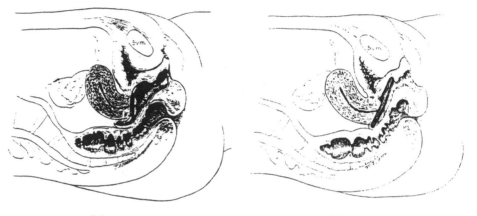

Cube pessary.   Ring pessary.

BIBLIOGRAPHY

1. American College of Obstetricians and Gynecologists: Pelvic Organ Prolapse. ACOG Tech Bull 214, 1995.
2. Cruikshank SM: Sacrospinous fixation—should this be performed at the time of vaginal hysterectomy? Am J Obstet Gynecol 164:1072, 1991.
3. Fakoner C, Gunvor E, Malmatiom A, et al: Decreased collagen synthesis in stress incontinent women. Obstet Gynecol 583, 1994.
4. Lasif CF: Abdominalsacral colpoplexy with use of synthetic mesh. Acta Obstet Gynecol Scand 72:214–217, 1993.
5. McCall ML: Posterior culdeplasty: Surgical correction of enterocele during vaginal hysterectomy, a preliminary report. Obstet Gynecol 10:592, 1857.
6. Moschowitz AV: The pathogenesis, anatomy and cure of prolapse of the rectum. Surg Gynecol Obstet 15:7, 1912.
7. Nichols DH, Randall CL: Vaginal Surgery, 3rd ed. Baltimore, Williams & Wilkins, 1989.
8. Young SB, Zyestra S: Managing vaginal vault prolapse with sacrospinous fixation. Contemp Obstet Gynecol 40:64, 1995.

11. URINARY STRESS INCONTINENCE

Dan Eicher, M.D., and Debra Gussman, M.D.

1. What is incontinence?

Incontinence is a sign or symptom of involuntary urine loss. A myriad of etiologies can be responsible for incontinence. Two common causes of incontinence that gynecologists are asked to diagnose and treat are genuine stress incontinence and detrusor dyssynergia.

Causes of Incontinence

I. Local Causes
   1. Infection: bacterial or chlamydial or TB
   2. Bladder stones
   3. Bladder tumors
   4. Fistulas following surgery or radiation
   5. Ectopic ureters
   6. Radiation or post-infection fibrosis
   7. Interstitial cystitis
   8. Pelvic mass compressing bladder
 	
II. Neurologic Causes
   1. Stroke
   2. Multiple sclerosis
   3. Parkinsonism
   4. Senile dementia
   5. Meningomyelocele
   6. Spinal injury
	III. Pharmacologic Causes
	   1. Parasympathomimetic
	   2. Diuretics
	   3. Antidepressants
	   4. Phenothiazines
	
	IV. Medical Causes
	   1. Hypothyroidism
	   2. Estrogen deficiency
	   3. Diabetes
	   4. Depression
	
	V. Detrusor Dyssynergia
	
	VI. Stress Incontinence

2. What is genuine stress incontinence (GSI)?

Stress incontinence is the involuntary loss of urine during physical activity. GSI is incontinence caused by the loss of the normal anatomic angle between the bladder and the urethra. The angle loss allows the pressure inside the bladder to exceed the intraurethral pressure. The result is an immediate loss of urine. GSI accounts for 75–80% of all cases of incontinence. Common causes of GSI include vaginal delivery, instrumented deliveries, and delivery of large infants. GSI is often associated with other pelvic relaxation problems, such as cystocele, rectocele, and uterine prolapse.

3. What is detrusor dyssynergia (DD)?

DD is also referred to as unstable bladder or urge incontinence. DD can be caused by uninhibited bladder contractions (motor urge incontinence) or strong sensory input from the bladder secondary to inflammation, tumors, or lack of estrogen (sensory urge incontinence). The patient has a sudden inability to control her bladder, followed by a delayed loss of urine.

In some patients, DD is due to an upper motor neuron disease, such as multiple sclerosis. DD also may be seen after pelvic surgery. The exact mechanism is unknown but is believed to be secondary to partial denervation of the bladder. DD is often confused with GSI.

4. What aspects of the patient's history are important in differentiating GSI and DD?

With GSI, the patient often complains of loss of urine with physical activity, such as coughing, sneezing, climbing stairs, laughing, bouncing, and intercourse. Urine loss is instantaneous and often described as a "squirt" of urine. In DD, women complain of urgency after physical activity or while at rest. The urge is then followed by a large loss of urine.

Voiding logs can be helpful in the history. The patient keeps track of the number of times per day that she urinates, oral intake, urine output, and timing of any involuntary urine loss. In taking a history, a careful review of systems should be undertaken to rule out the other causes of incontinence listed in question 1.

5. What are the significant physical findings?

The physical exam is performed to rule out other causes of incontinence. A pelvic exam often reveals evidence of pelvic relaxation, such as cystocele, rectocele, or uterine prolapse. A pelvic mass also may be found. If the patient has GSI, it is often possible to demonstrate incontinence when the patient coughs. In postmenopausal women, attention should be paid to the estrogen status of the vagina and bladder, because estrogen deficiency contributes significantly to incontinence. Gynecologists should be reminded that a neurologic examination is essential in evaluating urinary stress incontinence.

6. What laboratory tests are helpful in evaluating incontinence?

The laboratory is useful to rule out other causes of incontinence. Urinalysis and urine culture help to diagnose urinary tract infection or underlying renal disease, such as stones or tumors. Blood work may be necessary to rule out diabetes, syphilis, or other systemic diseases.

7. What are the most helpful tests in differentiating between GSI and DD?

Postvoid residual is an easy initial test to obtain. After the patient voids, there should be less than 10 ml of urine in the bladder. Postvoid residual is measured by ultrasound or catheterizing the patient. Catheterization also provides a good opportunity to obtain urine for culture. A patient with an elevated postvoid residual may have an underlying neurologic disorder (neurogenic bladder).

A **cystometrogram** should be performed on all incontinent patients. This test involves filling the bladder to measure volume-pressure relationships. As the bladder is filled to its normal capacity of 300–500 ml, the pressure inside the bladder should remain at < 15 cm H_2O. The patient usually experiences the first urge to void at 150–200 ml. In patients with GSI, the cystometrogram is normal. Patients with DD often have reduced bladder capacity (< 300 ml) and bladder contractions. The bladder contractions are demonstrated by a pressure increase of 15 cm H_2O above baseline.

Cystoscopy should be performed to rule out inflammation, tumors or anatomic deformities.

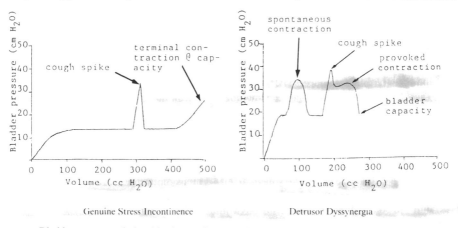

Bladder pressure relationships in genuine stress incontinence and detrusor dyssynergia.

8. What tests are less helpful in differentiating between GSI and DD?

The Q-tip test is a test of urethral motility. A sterile Q-tip swab is placed in the urethra to a depth of 3 cm to evaluate the angle between the urethra and bladder. When the patient coughs, the angle of the Q-tip changes by > 35°. This is considered to be evidence of poor bladder neck support, but it is not a reliable test; all patients with GSI do not have a positive test (see table below).

The **Marshall test** assesses pelvic support. The tips of a Kelly clamp are placed on each side of the urethra to restore the urethra to its normal anatomic position. If incontinence is corrected, the test is believed to be positive for GSI, and the patient is judged a good candidate for surgical correction. Current studies show that the Marshall test causes obstruction of the urethra and that it is not helpful in differentiating between GSI and DD.

Tests to Differentiate GSI from DD

	GENUINE STRESS INCONTINENCE	DETRUSOR DYSSYNERGIA
History	Immediate loss with Valsalva maneuver. No symptoms of bladder irritation.	Delayed urine loss. Symptoms of bladder irritation.
Voiding diary	Patient voids < 6 times per day Amounts > 250 cc per void	Patient voids > 6 times per day Amounts < 250 cc per void
Urine culture	Negative	Positive or negative
Q-tip test	> 35° change	≤ 35° change
Pelvic examination	Possible cystocele, rectocele or uterine prolapse	Normal
Marshall's test	Incontinence resolves with elevation of urethrovesical angle.	Incontinence does not resolve with angle elevation.
Cystoscopy	No evidence of inflammation. Bladder neck funnels when the patient coughs.	May or may not be evidence of inflammation. Bladder neck does not funnel.
Continuous cystometrics	Capacity is 300–500 cc H_2O Pressure < 15 cm H_2O Negative for contractions	Capacity < 300 cc H_2O Pressure > 15 cm H_2O Positive for contractions
Urethral pressure profile	Normal	Abnormal

9. What are indications for more extensive testing with multichannel urodynamics?

Approximately 10% of patients with urinary incontinence require more extensive testing. Multichannel urodynamics can be used to confirm the type of incontinence in a patient with mixed incontinence symptoms or a patient for whom prior continence procedures have failed. The presence of detrusor instability in a woman with a suggestive history but negative simple cystometry should be further evaluated. Intrinsic sphincter dysfunction can be diagnosed, or voiding mechanism can be determined to attempt to predict which patients may experience post-operative urinary retention. These urological tests can simultaneously record urethral, vesical, and intraabdominal pressures as well as electromyographic activity of the pelvic musculature.

10. What medical treatments are available for genuine stress incontinence?

No good medical treatment exists for GSI. Postmenopausal women should receive adequate estrogen replacement, which may eliminate or improve incontinence in addition to its other benefits. Other noninvasive methods that may be helpful in controlling minimal symptoms include Kegal exercises, behavior modification, bladder retraining, and biofeedback.

11. What medical treatments are available for detrusor dyssynergia?

Bladder contractions are caused by stimulation of the parasympathetic nervous system, which is mainly accomplished through the release of acetylcholine. Therefore, anticholinergics are often successful in controlling DD. Examples include probanthine, ditropan, and imipramine. Imipramine is advantageous in treating mixed stress incontinence and detrusor instability because of its combined alpha-adrenergic and anticholinergic properties. Muscle relaxants and bladder training also improve symptoms.

Treatment of Detrusor Dyssynergia

I. Drugs to enhance urine storage
   A. Anticholinergics
      1. Propantheline (Pro-Banthine)
      2. Oxybutynin (Ditropan)
      3. Imipramine (Tofranil)
   B. Beta-sympathomimetics
      1. Salbutamol
      2. Orciprenaline
   C. Prostaglandin synthetase inhibitors
      1. Indomethacin
   D. Calcium antagonists
   E. Musculotrophic drugs
      1. Flavoxate (Urispas)
   F. Dopamine receptor stimulants
      1. Bromocriptine (Parlodel)

II. Bladder drill or bladder retraining techniques
III. Psychotherapy
IV. Biofeedback
V. Electronic suppression
VI. Surgery
   A. Sacral denervation
   B. Vesicle denervation

12. Which surgical repairs are best for GSI?

Surgical management of genuine stress incontinence can be divided into (1) procedures that restore the anatomic support of the proximal urethra and the urethrovesical junction in women with hypermobility and normal intrinsic urethral sphincter and (2) procedures designed to compensate for a poorly functioning urethral sphincter. Over the past century, a large number of different surgical repairs have been used to correct GSI. No one method has proved preferable.

Many different types of repairs are used today, including abdominal approaches, such as the Marshall-Marchetti-Krantz procedure and the Burch procedure. Vaginal approaches include the Pereyra, Raz, and Stamey procedures. Abdominal and vaginal procedures use different techniques to resuspend the urethrovesical angle in its normal anatomic position. When primary surgical procedures fail, a sling is often placed under the urethra to lift it. Experimental techniques include artificial sphincters and Teflon injection to elevate the bladder neck.

13. What are the surgical outcomes?

The traditional vaginal approach to stress incontinence has been the Kelly plication, but recent studies have suggested that it does not provide adequate long-term support of the urethrovesical junction. The cure rate for stress incontinence following anterior colporrhaphy is only 40–70%.

Treatment of stress urinary incontinence resulting from hypermobility of the urethrovesical junction is best performed with the Marshall-Marchetti-Krantz or Burch procedure, both of which have an overall success rate of 78%. Surgical failures often result from inadequate preoperative evaluation of the cause of incontinence.

14. Intrinsic urethral sphincter dysfunction can be treated by which methods?

Intrinsic urethral sphincter dysfunction can be treated by the use of a suburethral sling procedure, periurethral bulking injections (with GAX-collagen or Teflon paste), or placement of an artificial urinary sphincter. These operations are associated with a high risk of postoperative urinary retention.

BIBLIOGRAPHY

1. American College of Obstetricians and Gynecologists: Urinary Incontinence. ACOG Tech Bull 213, 1995.
2. DeLancey JOL: Anatomy and mechanics of structures around the vesical neck: How vesical neck position might affect its closure. Neurourol Urodynam 7:161, 1988.
3. Nichols DH, Randall CL: Operation for urinary stress incontinence. In Nichols DH, Randall CT (eds): Vaginal Surgery, 3rd ed. Baltimore, Williams & Wilkins, 1989.

4. Pereyra AJ: A simplified surgical procedure for the correction of stress incontinence in women. West J Surg 67:223, 1959.
5. Stenchever MA: Gynecologic urology. In Droegemueller W, et al (eds): Comprehensive Gynecology. St. Louis, Mosby, 1992.
6. Valaitis SR, Stanton SL: Surgery for genuine stress incontinence. Contemp Obstet Gynecol 40(10):65, 1995.

12. ADNEXAL MASS

Mary Bowman, M.D., and Sally E. Berga, Ph.D., M.D.

1. Why must adnexal masses be diagnosed and evaluated?

Adnexal masses must be diagnosed and evaluated because of possible malignancy. Annual gynecologic examinations play a critical role because adnexal masses frequently are asymptomatic. Women with symptomatic adnexal masses usually present with complaints of pain, tenderness, dyspareunia, and nausea or vomiting. Presently no biochemical markers are useful in screening for ovarian neoplasms. Although the vast majority of adnexal masses are found to be benign neoplasms or functional cysts, it is necessary to consider worst-case scenarios carefully because of the high morbidity and mortality rates of ovarian cancer.

2. What is the differential diagnosis for adnexal masses?

Physiologic/functional
  Follicular cysts
  Corpus luteum cyst, mature
    corpus lutea
  Theca lutein cyst, luteoma
    of pregnancy
Nonfunctional
  Ectopic pregnancy
  Endometrioma
  Germinal inclusion cyst
    (remnants of Wolffian ducts)
  Inflammatory cyst
  Polycystic ovary
  Paraovarian or paratubal cyst
Mechanical
  Ovarian or tubal torsion
  Hydrosalpingx
  Hematosalpingx
  Tuboovarian abscess
Nonadnexal
  Diverticulitis
  Appendiceal abscess
  Pelvic kidney
  Leiomyomata
  Lymphoma
  Gastrointestinal tumors
Neoplastic-benign
  Mature cystic teratoma
  Fibroma

Neoplastic-benign (*cont.*)
  Brenner tumor
  Adenofibroma, cystadenofibroma
  Serous cystadenoma
  Mucinous cystadenoma
Malignancies (World Health Organization
  classification)
  Epithelial
    Serous cystadenocarcinoma
    Mucinous cystadenocarcinoma
    Endometrial
    Clear cell
    Brenner
    Mixed
  Sex cord
    Granulosa cell
    Gynandroblastoma
    Androblastoma
    Unclassified
  Germ cell
    Dysgerminoma
    Lipid cell
    Endodermal sinus
    Mixed
    Embryonal
    Gonadoblastoma
    Choriocarcinoma
    Immative teratoma

3. What patient characteristics are important to consider in creating a differential diagnosis?

Age is an important factor. Although 80% of all ovarian tumors are benign, the majority of malignant tumors occur in women older than 45 years. Only germ cell tumors are more common in children and young women, and 95% of these are mature cystic teratomas. Physiologic cysts should not occur in prepubertal or postmenopausal women except in extremely rare instances. Nulliparity is associated with increased risk for ovarian malignancy. Current hormonal contraceptive use makes physiologic cysts unlikely, and long-term use of oral contraceptives decreases the lifetime risk of ovarian carcinoma. Menstrual irregularities are more common with physiologic cysts.

Weight loss, chronic abdominal distention, or urinary and gastrointestinal tract complaints are more likely associated with ovarian malignancy. However, most adnexal masses are asymptomatic. Ascites is associated generally with ovarian malignancy but may be associated with benign tumors. Meigs' syndrome, the association of ovarian tumor, ascites, and hydrothorax, was classically described with benign fibromas. Bilateral adnexal masses are more likely to represent malignancy.

4. What characteristics of adnexal masses help to distinguish malignant and benign masses?

Size (in centimeters). Smaller masses are more likely to be benign, whereas larger masses are more likely to be malignant. Very large masses are more likely to be low-grade or borderline (low malignant potential). Mucinous tumors often grow to be very large and are usually benign.

Consistency (cystic, solid or complex). Benign masses are more likely to be simple cysts. Malignant masses are more likely to be solid or complex.

Morphology (smooth, nodular, vague or sharp borders). Benign masses are usually smooth with distinct borders. Malignant masses are usually nodular with vague borders, surface excrescences intracystic papillae, and surface peritoneal studding.

Mobility. Benign masses are usually mobile. Malignant masses are more likely to be non-mobile or adherent to other pelvic structures.

Unilateral vs. bilateral. Benign masses are more likely to be unilateral; bilaterality is more common in malignancy.

Hemorrhagic or necrotic areas. Malignant masses are likely to have necrotic and/or hemorrhagic areas. Hemorrhagic corpus luteum or endometriomas are exceptions.

Ascites. Ascites is usually associated with malignancies.

5. Name three types of functional cysts.

Follicular, corpus luteum, and theca lutein cysts (in order of frequency).

6. When are physiologic cysts most likely to occur?

Functional cysts are most common in the reproductive years between puberty and menopause. Women using contraceptive methods that suppress ovulation are not likely to have physiologic cysts. Now that ultrasound exams are being done in postmenopausal women, cysts have been documented in this population; 50% regress spontaneously.

7. What problems are associated with corpus luteum cysts?

Persistent corpus luteum cysts may cause diffuse abdominal or pelvic pain, tenderness, mild leukocytosis, and fever. They may be confused with appendicitis, ovarian torsion, or pelvic inflammatory disease. Endocrine effects due to progesterone secretion may lead to abnormal uterine bleeding. Intraperitoneal bleeding can occur with ruptured corpus luteum cysts, which infrequently lead to significant hematoperitoneum.

8. Describe the typical physical characteristics and symptoms of follicular cysts.

The average size of a follicular cyst is 2 cm, but the size may vary from a few millimeters to 8 cm. It is a single, simple cyst that is translucent, thin-walled, and filled with clear to straw-colored watery fluid. Pathologic examination reveals a simple cyst lined by granulosa cells within the ovarian stroma. Follicular cysts are often asymptomatic but may cause dull pain or heavy sensation in the pelvis. They are rarely associated with intraperitoneal hemorrhage or abnormal uterine bleeding. Follicular cysts are more easily ruptured but are rarely associated with hemorrhage.

9. How are follicular cysts created?

The process is poorly understood but is thought to result from failed rupture of the dominant follicle or failed atresia of secondary follicles.

10. How do follicular cysts associated with polycystic ovary (PCO) syndrome differ from other follicular cysts?

Follicular cysts in PCO syndrome are usually small, numerous, hormone-producing, and bilateral. They result from follicular hyperplasia of both granulosa and theca interna cells. Mild ovarian enlargement occurs with thickening of the tunica albuginea. These cysts produce estrogen and androgens, leading to clinical signs and symptoms. Anovulation and abnormal uterine bleeding are common. Patients are at increased risk for endometrial adenocarcinoma related to constant exposure of the endometrium to estrogen without production of progesterone.

11. Why do theca lutein cysts develop?

Theca lutein cysts develop with prolonged or excessive stimulation of the ovaries by gonadotropins. They may occur in molar pregnancies, multiple gestations, or pregnancies with large placentas (diabetes). They also occur in women treated with exogenous gonadotropins for ovulation induction. Gonadotropins produce luteinization of cells in mature, immature, and atretic follicles. Ovaries are bilaterally enlarged and can reach 20–30 cm in size. Theca lutein cysts are usually asymptomatic and resolve spontaneously.

12. How should physiologic cysts be managed?

Observation is the management of choice with physiologic cysts. Most cysts resolve spontaneously over 1–2 months. Ovulation suppression with hormones is common to remove the gonadotropin influence and to prevent formation of additional functional cysts. Oral contraceptives do not facilitate regression of the cyst. Indications for operative evaluation for functional cysts include large cystic masses (> 8 cm), failure to resolve with conservative therapy, severe symptoms, and intraperitoneal hemorrhage. Laparoscopy and conservative surgery with cystotomy or cystectomy are the treatments of choice.

Theca lutein cysts may become very large (≥ 8–10 cm) and regress more slowly. Theca lutein cysts should not be removed at cesarean section and may regress slowly as the levels of human chorionic gonadotropin (HCG) decrease. Hemorrhage with theca lutein cysts may be difficult to control.

13. What is an endometrioma?

Endometriomas are endometrial implants on the ovary. They may be small (1–5 mm) or large (up to 10 cm) multiloculated hemorrhagic cysts. They are frequently bilateral. Patients are usually asymptomatic but may have pelvic pain, dysmenorrhea, dyspareunia, or infertility.

14. How are endometriomas managed?

Endometriomas are usually managed operatively because of the complex nature of the adnexal mass, need to rule out malignancies, and poor response to medical management. Laparoscopic cystotomy is the preferred surgical treatment.

15. How is ectopic pregnancy distinguished from a hemorrhagic corpus luteum of pregnancy?

Ectopic pregnancy is diagnosed or presumed in patients who have inappropriately rising titers of beta-HCG and no evidence of intrauterine pregnancy. Patients often have vaginal bleeding or spotting, unilateral lower quadrant pain, pelvic mass, and tenderness on exam. If the ectopic pregnancy has caused rupture of the cornua or tube, the patient also may be hemodynamically unstable, but pain is generally improved. Laparoscopy may be required to distinguish the two if hemoperitoneum is present.

16. Is ultrasound useful in the management of adnexal masses?

High-resolution transvaginal ultrasound is a valuable tool in evaluating an adnexal mass. The size, consistency, complexity, bilaterality, location, and relationship to other pelvic organs can be determined by ultrasonography. The presence of ascites can be documented by ultrasonography. Follow-up studies can be used to document changes with time (resolution or changes in complexity and size). A transvaginal sonography scoring system to help predict ovarian malignancy was described in 1991. Using objective characteristics, this system was able to distinguish between ovarian malignancies and benign disease. The system was designed to be highly sensitive, and most false-positive scores were mature cystic teratomas. Color flow imaging with transvaginal ultrasonography may further improve the high rate of false-positive results. This procedure detects intraovarian vascular changes. It is believed that the neovascularization and changes in impedance of blood flow may be useful in discriminating benign from malignant masses.

17. What other diagnostic tests are useful to evaluate the adnexal mass?

Initial studies should include **laboratory tests** for infection, pregnancy (to rule out ectopic pregnancies), tuboovarian abscesses, and nongynecologic infections as sources for the mass.

CA125 is a tumor marker that has been widely used to evaluate adnexal masses. CA125 is markedly elevated in most epithelial, nonmucinous ovarian malignancies, but it also may be elevated with other malignancies and benign conditions, such as menstruation, leiomyomas, pregnancy, pelvic infection, endometriosis, and hepatitis. In addition, false-negative CA125 tests may occur in as many as 50% of patients with early-stage ovarian malignancies. An elevated CA125 in a patient with a pelvic mass is useful in that one can arrange for a gynecologic oncologist to be available at the time of exploration.

Computerized tomography (CT) can help to delineate the nature of a complex pelvic mass. Information about involvement of the uterus, omentum, and abdominal and pelvic lymph nodes can also be obtained.

18. What is the role of laparoscopy in the management of adnexal masses?

The role of laparoscopy has been rapidly expanding. Recent studies show that the majority of adnexal masses can be managed with diagnostic laparoscopy and pelviscopy. The advantages of laparoscopic therapy are reduced morbidity, fewer adhesions, faster recovery, and greater patient acceptance. The disadvantages are failure to diagnose early ovarian cancers and intraoperative spillage of malignant cells with possible worsening of prognosis. Careful selection of patients based on risk factors and adnexal mass characteristics minimizes the risk of inappropriate management of ovarian malignancies at the time of laparoscopy. Recent data also show that intraperitoneal spillage does not worsen the prognosis if definitive surgery is performed immediately. The liberal use of biopsy and frozen section and the experience of the surgeons are important to appropriate laparoscopic management of masses.

Endometriomas, mature cystic teratomas, and benign-appearing masses in postmenopausal women have been managed successfully with pelviscopy. Pelviscopic procedures include salpingectomy, salpingostomy, cystectomy, opening and biopsying of cyst wall, oophorectomy, and salpingooophorectomy.

19. What are the possible causes of torsion?

Ovarian enlargement due to a benign cystic mass is the most common cause of adnexal torsion. Approximately 50% of torsions demonstrate an ovarian mass at the time of surgery. Mature cystic teratomas are the most common tumors leading to torsion, but paraovarian cysts, other benign solid tumors, and serous cysts are also common.

Ovarian torsion occurs twice as often with the right adnexa than with the left adnexa, suggesting anatomic differences. Torsion of an adnexal mass poses additional risks from infarction.

The twisted cyst may be grossly ischemic. Debate persists about concern for embolus if the cyst is untwisted.

20. What considerations are important in the management of adnexal torsion?

Clinical features of adnexal torsion are pain, nausea and vomiting, adnexal mass, leukocytosis, and low-grade fever. These findings also may occur with many other conditions, including hemorrhagic corpus luteum cyst, tuboovarian abscess, hydrosalpingx, appendicitis, endometriomas, and ectopic pregnancy. In the classic study of adnexal torsion almost one-half of presumed torsions were other conditions (listed above in order of frequency).

One-third of adnexal torsions were diagnosed initially as another condition. One study found that 2% of torsions involved ovarian malignancies. Thus the surgeon should be prepared for definitive therapy at the time of surgery. Laparoscopy is the ideal first approach to adnexal torsion. Diagnostic laparoscopy can be used to rule out the many conditions confused with torsion. Adnexectomy is the accepted method of management of adnexal torsion. Most cases of adnexal torsion can be managed with pelviscopy.

21. Must adnexectomy always be performed?

Removal of the torsed adnexa has been the standard therapy. Reasons for adnexectomy include delays in diagnosis resulting in necrosis, inability to distinguish by inspection between necrosis and strangulation, and fear of thromboembolic disease from the ovarian veins.

Most cases of adnexal torsion occur in women of reproductive age, and preservation of ovarian function and fertility are important issues. Recent studies suggest that conservative treatment with untwisting of structures and cystectomy can be performed. No resulting thromboembolic complications have been observed. One recent study examined the use of intravascular fluorescein to distinguish between viable and nonviable tissue.

BIBLIOGRAPHY

1. Bider D, Masiach S, Outlitzky M, et al: Clinical, surgical and pathologic findings of adnexal torsion in pregnant and nonpregnant women. Surg Gynecol Obstet 173:363, 1991.
2. Bourne T, Campbell S, Steer C, et al: Transvaginal colour flow imaging: A possible new screening technique for ovarian cancer. BMJ 299:1367, 1989.
3. Bromley B, Goodman H, Benacerraf B: Comparison between sonographic, morphologic and Doppler waveform for the diagnosis of ovarian malignancy. Obstet Gynecol 83:434, 1994.
4. Curtain JP: Management of the adnexal mass. Gynecol Oncol 55:542, 1994.
5. Finkler NJ, Benacerraf B, Lavin PT, et al: Comparison of serum Ca125, clinical impression, and ultrasound in the preoperative evaluation of ovarian masses. Obstet Gynecol 72:659, 1988.
6. Parker WH: The case for laparoscopic management of the adnexal mass. Clin Obstet Gynecol 38:362, 1995.

13. ECTOPIC PREGNANCY

Ty B. Erickson, M.D.

1. What is an ectopic pregnancy?

An ectopic pregnancy is one that develops at any site other than the endometrium.

2. What is the incidence of ectopic pregnancy?

The true incidence is difficult to determine because of the varied populations studied, but it ranges from 1 of 64 to 1 of 241 pregnancies, with an average of approximately 10 per 1000 pregnancies. There has been a fourfold increase over the past 20 years. In 1989, 34 deaths occurred from ectopic pregnancies with a fatality rate of 3.8 per 10,000 cases. Ectopic pregnancy continues to be the most common cause of maternal death in the first half of pregnancy and the second most common overall.

3. Why has the incidence increased over the past 20 years?

The increase is due to a combination of increasing salpingitis and better antibiotics, which allow tubal patency. The resultant tube is patent but has luminal damage.

4. What is the cause of ectopic pregnancy?

The major cause of ectopic pregnancy is salpingitis. The incidence of histologic evidence of prior salpingitis is 40%. Any mechanism that causes abnormal tubal motility, so that the blastocyst remains in the tube at the time of implantation, will also cause an ectopic gestation. Examples include infection, exposure to diethylstilbestrol (DES), prior tubal surgery, smoking at the time of conception. Failure of tubal sterilization methods has been reported to account for 3% of ectopic pregnancies. Chromosomal and structural anomalies of the conceptus may predispose to ectopic pregnancy.

5. Where do the majority of ectopic pregnancies occur?

Of ectopic pregnancies, 97.7% occur in the fallopian tube, 1.4% are abdominal, and < 1% are ovarian or cervical. The majority of tubal pregnancies occur in the ampulla, 12% in the isthmus, and 5% in the fimbriated end.

6. What are Spiegelberg's criteria for identification of an ovarian pregnancy?
1. The tube, including fimbria ovarica, must be intact.
2. The gestational sac must occupy normal ovarian position.
3. The sac must be connected to the uterus by the uteroovarian ligament.
4. Ovarian tissue must be identified histologically in the wall of the gestational sac.

7. What is the incidence of an intrauterine pregnancy with an ectopic pregnancy (heterotopic pregnancy)?

The classic estimate is 1 of 30,000, but a more likely estimate is 1 of 4000–15,000. Newer ovulation induction methods and in vitro techniques probably will increase the incidence.

8. Does the risk of ectopic pregnancy vary according to contraceptive methods?
Yes.

Contraceptive method	Risk of ectopic pregnancy (%)
None	1
Oral contraceptives	1
Diaphragm	1
Intrauterine device (IUD)	5
Progestasert IUD	15

9. What is the likelihood that a woman with one ectopic pregnancy will have a subsequent ectopic pregnancy?

Recurrence risk varies from 7–15%.

10. What are risk factors for an ectopic pregnancy?
Tubal surgery (reconstructive or tubal ligation, particularly if done by coagulation)
History of pelvic inflammatory disease
Previous ectopic pregnancy
IUD use
Progestin-only oral contraceptives
DES exposure

11. What is the differential diagnosis of an ectopic pregnancy?

Threatened or incomplete abortion	Dysfunctional uterine bleeding
Gestational trophoblastic disease	Adnexal torsion
Ruptured corpus luteal cyst	Degenerative uterine leiomyomata
Salpingitis	Endometriosis
Appendicitis	

Up to one-third of patients with ectopic pregnancy will be seen once before the diagnosis is confirmed; delayed diagnosis increased morbidity substantially.

12. What are the most common symptoms of an ectopic pregnancy?

Over 90% of patients have abdominal pain; however, only 35% report totally missing a period, although careful history reveals some abnormality with the preceding cycle. Abnormal bleeding at the time of presentation is not uncommon.

13. Why do some patients have shoulder pain?

Shoulder pain is referred from diaphragmatic irritation due to hemoperitoneum and occurs in up to 25% of patients.

14. What are the most common signs?

Patients are usually afebrile, and orthostasis is not commonly seen unless massive hemoperitoneum is present. Abdominal tenderness is seen in over 90% of patients. A palpable pelvic mass is not helpful, because it is present in only 50% of patients, 20% of whom have the ectopic pregnancy on the side contralateral to the mass. Uterine size is normal in 70% of patients.

15. What is the role of human chorionic gonadotropin (HCG) titers in the diagnosis and management of ectopic pregnancy?

HCG, a glycoprotein produced by trophoblastic tissue, can be measured in the serum within 8–12 days after fertilization. Two reference standards are used by various labs to report the titers. The first is the International Reference Preparation (IRP), which is identical to the third international standard of the World Health Organization. The second is the Second International Standard (SIS), which approximates one-half the value of the IRP. The IRP is most commonly used. During the first 6–7 weeks the serum HCG values approximately double every 48 hours in 90% of intrauterine pregnancies. A subnormal rise < 66% is seen in 85% of nonviable pregnancies, and a rise of < 20% is 100% predictive of a nonviable pregnancy. Following titers in the stable patient is helpful in early gestations to rule out ectopic pregnancies.

16. When is ultrasound helpful in the diagnosis of ectopic pregnancy?

Ultrasound is definitive if cardiac activity is identified either in the tube or uterus. In conjunction with HCG titers, it is also helpful in confirming intrauterine pregnancy. Newer endovaginal probes allow earlier detection of pregnancy location at least 1 week before transabdominal scans. A discriminatory zone, using HCG titers with ultrasound, has been identified at a level of 6500 mIU/ml (IRP), at which transabdominal ultrasound should identify an intrauterine gestational sac, or 2000 mIU/ml (IRP) if endovaginal ultrasound is available. Specific findings using endovaginal probes for ectopic pregnancy include a tubal ring (1–3 cm mass with a 2–4-mm concentric echogenic rim surrounding a hypoechoic center) in 68% of tubal pregnancies. The probe also allows better evaluation of the pseudosac, fluid in the cul-de-sac, and character of pelvic masses.

Each medical center should establish criteria for evaluating possible ectopic pregnancies with combined modalities of ultrasound and HCG values, including which reference standards are to be used. The criteria must take into consideration the quality of ultrasound equipment and personnel.

17. What is the role of culdocentesis in the diagnosis of ectopic pregnancy?

With the advent of accurate serum HCG values and endovaginal probe ultrasound, culdocentesis is less frequently needed. It still has a role for the patient with a positive pregnancy test and fluid in the culdesac in whom a definitive intrauterine sac is not identified or when titers are not available.

18. Why is the blood obtained by culdocentesis nonclotting?

The nonclotting blood results from lysis of blood that has clotted previously. The hematocrit of the nonclotting blood should exceed 15% to be significant.

19. What is the role of progesterone levels in the diagnosis of ectopic pregnancies?

Serum progesterone levels are not dependent on gestational age; therefore, a single value gives a snapshot view of pregnancy viability. In 98% of viable pregnancies values exceed 10 ng/ml, and in 98% of ectopic pregnancies not associated with ovulation induction values are less than 20 ng/ml. A single level < 15 ng/ml is highly suggestive of a nonviable pregnancy but does not distinguish between pending miscarriage and ectopic pregnancy. Unfortunately, because of differences in populations, assay kits, and overlap in the 10–20 ng/ml range, the clinical use of serum progesterone levels is limited.

20. What role does laparoscopy have in the diagnosis of tubal pregnancy?

If a patient has a subnormal rise in HCG titers or an abnormal ultrasound, frozen-section dilatation and curettage may be performed; if the result is negative, the laparoscope will allow visualization of the tube. However, false-negative rates approach 4% and may be higher if surgery is performed early in the pregnancy.

21. What about expectant management of ectopic pregnancies?

If patients are hospitalized for observation, with surgery only for hemorrhage, 57% of ectopic pregnancies spontaneously resolve; however, 60% of patients have length of stays exceeding 4 weeks, which is not practical.

22. What surgical options are available?

Traditionally a laparotomy with partial salpingectomy of the ipsilateral side has been performed. Recently the trend has been toward preservation of the tube. Fimbrial evacuation by digital expression is not advocated because of the high failure rate with persistent trophoblast (> 25%). Linear salpingostomy, either by laparotomy or, more recently, laparoscopy, is the method of choice, even with tubes dilated as much as 4 cm. There is, however, a 10% risk of persistent trophoblast, and titers should be followed until they reach nondetectable levels. The recurrent ectopic rate is not increased by this technique, and subsequent fertility is equal and possibly slightly better.

23. What is the role of methotrexate (MTX) in treating ectopic pregnancy?

As managed care has increased, the economics of treating ectopic pregnancy nonsurgically has become attractive. Clinical studies have demonstrated success with varying treatment regimens in ectopic pregnancy: multidose MTX with citrovorum rescue or single-dose protocols have been advocated. MTX also has been reported to be successful in treating interstitial, abdominal, and cervical pregnancies, which have substantial surgical risk. Perhaps the most commonly used technique is to give a single intramuscular dose, 50 mg/m^2, without citrovorum. Success rates approach 95%, with the remainder requiring either a second dose or surgical intervention. Tubal patency after treatment approaches 80%. The absence of randomized trials makes outcome analysis of medical and surgical treatments difficult; therefore, methotrexate therapy must still be considered experimental, with extensive requirements of informed consent.

24. How does MTX work?

MTX acts as a folic acid antagonist and interferes with DNA synthesis and cellular multiplication. It has been used in treating gestational trophoblastic disease (GTN) for years with excellent results.

25. What risks are associated with MTX treatment?

The traditional complications of stomatitis, dermatitis, pleuritis, and altered liver function have been reported. Additionally, 60% of patients experience increased pelvic pain during the days after treatment.

26. Are other pharmacologic treatments available?

Actinomycin-D, a more potent chemotherapeutic agent than MTX, has been used success-fully in treating a limited number of ectopic pregnancies, especially in advanced gestations (HCG levels > 10,000 mIU/ml), in which MTX has a higher failure rate. Potassium chloride (KCl) in-jected into the fetal heart in advanced ectopic pregnancy has been reported to induce asystole, and may have a role in treating heterotopic pregnancy. Antiprogestin (RU486) therapy has not been successful in treating ectopic pregnancy and requires substantial further testing.

27. What about subsequent fertility after an ectopic pregnancy?

The intrauterine pregnancy rate for patients with previous full-term pregnancies approaches 80%. The rate is about 40% if the patient is nulliparous. Patients with ruptured ectopic pregnancies have improved rates compared with ruptured ectopic pregnancies (65% vs. 82%, respectively).

BIBLIOGRAPHY

1. Balasch J, Barri P: Treatment of ectopic pregnancy: The new gynaecological dilemma. Hum Reprod 9:547, 1994.
2. Fleischer A, Pennell R, McKee M, et al: Ectopic pregnancy: Features at transvaginal sonography. Radiology 174:377, 1990.
3. Kadar N, Caldwell B, Romero R: A method of screening for ectopic pregnancy and its indications. Obstet Gynecol 58:162, 1981.
4. Parker J, Thompson D: Persistent ectopic pregnancy after conservative management successful treatment with single-dose intramuscular methotrexate. Aust N Z J Obstet Gynaecol 34:99, 1994.
5. Stabile I, Grudzinskas J: Ectopic pregnancy: A review of incidence, etiology and diagnostic aspects. Obstet Gynecol Surv 45:335, 1990.
6. Stovall TG, Ling FW: Single dose Methotrexate: An expanded clinical trial. Am J Obstet Gynecol 168:1759, 1993.
7. Tulandi T: Medical and surgical treatment of ectopic pregnancy. Curr Opin Obstet Gynecol 6:149, 1994.
8. Vermesh M, Silva P, et al: Management of unruptured ectopic gestation by linear salpingostomy: A prospective randomized clinical trial of laparoscopy versus laparotomy. Obstet Gynecol 73(Pt 1): 400, 1989.

14. ENDOMETRIOSIS

Kenneth Faber, M.D.

1. What is endometriosis?

Endometriosis is the presence of tissue that is morphologically similar to endometrium in lo-cations other than the endometrial cavity. Microscopic confirmation includes the presence of en-dometrial glands and stroma and also may include fibrosis and hemorrhage.

2. What is the incidence of endometriosis?

Accurate assessment of the incidence of endometriosis within the general population is diffi-cult because laparoscopy or laparotomy is required for diagnosis. Endometriosis is found in 5–28% of all laparoscopies, including those for tubal ligation. Patients with either pelvic pain or infertility have an increased incidence, as do first-degree family members of women with en-dometriosis.

3. What are the most common locations for endometriosis?

The most common sites are the anterior and posterior cul-de-sac; 65% of patients with en-dometriosis have ovarian involvement. Other frequently involved sites include pelvic peritoneum; uterosacral, round, and broad ligaments; and fallopian tubes.

4. List infrequent sites of endometriosis.

Lung   Kidney
Nasal mucosa   Legs
Umbilicus   Episiotomy scars
Bladder

5. What are the three theories about the pathogenesis of endometriosis?

1. **Implantation.** Retrograde menstruation carries fragments of müllerian mucosa, arising in the uterus or tube, into the peritoneal cavity. The following evidence supports this theory: (1) endometrial cells in menstrual fluid are capable of implanting on peritoneal surfaces; (2) endometriosis is most often seen in dependent sites in the pelvis; and (3) patients with functioning uterus and outlet obstruction are at great risk for endometriosis.

2. **Lymphatic-vascular metastasis.** Endometrium is transported via lymphatic channels and the vascular system. This theory explains occurrences at distant sites such as the umbilicus, eye, and lung.

3. **Coelomic metaplasia.** The peritoneal mesothelium, müllerian epithelium, and germinal epithelium of the ovary may be derived from a common embryonic tissue. This theory suggests that endometriosis develops from metaplasia of cells lining the pelvic peritoneum. There is no proof that the peritoneum undergoes spontaneous or induced metaplasia to form endometriosis.

6. What are the more common presenting symptoms of endometriosis?

Endometriosis may present in various ways. Classical symptoms include:
1. Pain
   • 25–80% of patients with pelvic pain or dysmenorrhea have endometriosis. The pelvic pain is believed to be related to sequential swelling and extravasation of blood into surrounding tissues.
   • Disease severity does not predict the degree of pain.
   • Endometrial lesions are associated with increased tissue and peritoneal fluid levels of prostaglandin (PGF2 and PGE2).
   • Prostaglandin synthetase inhibitors are better than placebo in treating pain associated with endometriosis.
2. Infertility (30–40% of women with endometriosis)
   • Mild disease coexists with delayed fertility, and severe disease predicts delayed fertility.
   • Treatment of mild endometriosis with medication or surgery has not been shown to increase pregnancy rate.
   • Treatment of anatomic distortion with severe endometriosis may improve pregnancy rate.
3. Dyspareunia (especially with cul-de-sac disease)
4. Dyschezia (also related to disease in the cul-de-sac)
5. Abnormal uterine bleeding (frequent)

7. What are the most common physical findings in patients with endometriosis?

Physical exam of patients with endometriosis may be unrevealing, and physical findings (when present) are quite variable. The most common findings include:
   • Diffuse abdominal or pelvic pain of variable location
   • Nodular thickening and tenderness along the uterosacral ligaments, on the posterior surface of the uterus, and in the posterior cul-de-sac
   • Variable degrees of induration and fixation of contiguous structures
   • Fixed, retroverted uterus
   • Scarring and narrowing of posterior vaginal fornix
   • Adnexal enlargement and tenderness (often asymmetric)

8. How does one diagnose endometriosis?

The diagnosis is made by laparoscopy with visualization of the lesion, confirmed by biopsy of affected areas. The biopsy must reveal both endometrial stroma and glands.

9. What does endometriosis look like?
- Powder-burn appearance
- Hemorrhagic or flame-shaped lesion
- Fibrotic or scarified peritoneum
- Cystic or vesicular
- Ovarian cysts (chocolate cyst)

10. How is endometriosis staged?

The American Society of Reproductive Medicine staging system is based on the depth, location, and size of endometriotic implants; presence or absence of cul-de-sac obliteration; and extent and quality of adhesions.

11. What causes delayed conception in patients with infertility?

1. Anatomic distortion can prevent fertilization.

2. Immune factors also play a role in delayed conception. Antiendometrial antibodies may be either cause or consequence of endometriosis. Activation of peritoneal macrophages results in increased inflammatory environment and decreased survival of gametes.

12. Explain the theoretical basis of pharmacologic suppression of endometriosis.

Ectopic endometrium, like normal endometrial tissue, responds to hormonal regulation. The objective in treatment of endometriosis is to cause atrophy or inactivity of the endometrial implants. This objective can be attempted by simulating the normal physiologic states of endometrial inactivity or atrophy, i.e., postmenopause or pregnancy.

13. List four hormonal regimens used to suppress endometriosis. Explain the mechanism of action.

1. **Oral contraceptives.** Combination estrogen-progestin pills have been used to induce a pseudopregnancy state. The endometriotic implants initially undergo a decidual reaction, eventually undergo necrosis, and then are absorbed.

2. **Danazol.** Danazol, an orally active synthetic derivative of 17-alpha-ethinyl testosterone, is the most effective approved drug for suppression of endometriosis. There is evidence for effects on the hypothalamus, pituitary, ovary, and endometrium as well as on endometriotic lesions. Plasma levels of luteinizing hormone and follicle-stimulating hormone, especially mid-cycle surges, are suppressed, probably through suppression of the release of gonadotropins from the pituitary. In addition, danazol directly inhibits multiple enzymes involved in steroidogenesis. Finally, the drug interacts with other cytosolic hormone receptors, explaining in part the androgenic, progestational, glucocorticoid, and estrogenic activities of danazol.

3. **Progestins.** Medroxyprogesterone (Depo-Provera) has been used with success in the treatment of endometriosis for patients in whom preparations containing estrogen are contraindicated. Progestins produce endometrial atrophy, and breakthrough bleeding may be a problem. Medroxyprogesterone acts as a potent gonadotropin inhibitor.

4. **Agonists of gonadotropin-releasing hormone (GnRH-a).** Clinical trials using agonists of luteinizing hormone-releasing hormone suggest that estrogen (after a brief, temporary increase) is reduced to levels lower than those achieved with danazol and comparable to those found in oophorectomized women. Amenorrhea, relief of pain, and resolution of active disease have been documented in a high percentage of patients. GnRH agonists are approved for treatment of pain only in patients with endometriosis; no evidence suggests that they improve fertility.

14. When is surgical therapy preferable to medical therapy for endometriosis?

Surgery is required for patients with acute rupture of a large endometrioma, blockage of a ureter, or compromise of bowel function. Laparoscopic ablation of endometriotic lesions may improve pain. Other surgical procedures used to alleviate pain include presacral neurectomy and uterosacral nerve ablation.

15. Does any evidence suggest that laser is better than electrosurgery or scissors in treating endometriosis?

No. The most frequently used lasers in the treatment of endometriosis are carbon dioxide, argon Nd:Yag, and, more recently, KtP-532. Proponents of laser surgery believe that it is superior because lasers allow precise tissue destruction, minimize damage to the surrounding tissues, promote tissue healing without adhesion formation, and allow a relatively bloodless surgical field. These are all theories; no data suggest that laser is better than traditional surgical techniques.

BIBLIOGRAPHY

1. American Fertility Society: Revised American Fertility Society classification of endometriosis. Fertil Steril 43:35, 1985.
2. Bergqvist IA: Hormonal regulation of endometriosis and the rationales and effects of gonadotrophin-releasing hormone agonist treatment: A review. Hum Reprod 10:446, 1995.
3. Dmolski WP, Radwanska E: Current concepts on pathology, histogenesis and etiology of endometriosis. Acta Obstet Gynecol Scand (Suppl) 123:61, 1984.
4. Haney AF: Endometriosis, macrophages, and adhesion. Prog Clin Biol Res 381:19, 1993.
5. Olive DL, Haney AF: Endometriosis-associated infertility: A critical review of therapeutic options. Obstet Gynecol Surv 41:538, 1986.
6. Olive DL, Haney AF, Weinberg JB: The nature of intraperitoneal exudate associated with infertility: Peritoneal fluid and serum lysozyme activity. Fertil Steril 48:802, 1986.
7. Revelli A, Modotti M, Ansaldi C, Massobrio M: Recurrent endometriosis: A review of biological and clinical aspects. Obstet Gynecol Surv 50:747, 1995.
8. Schenken RS: Endometriosis classification for infertility. Acta Obstet Gynecol Scand Suppl 159:414, 1994.

15. SPONTANEOUS ABORTION

Jean Abbott, M.D., and Stacy Mellum, M.D.

1. What percentage of pregnancies end in miscarriages?

The miscarriage rate is about 15–20% overall. Total embryonic loss is probably much higher. When levels of human chorionic gonadotropin (HCG) were measured in women attempting to conceive, 22% miscarried before pregnancy was clinically apparent. Thus the total embryonic loss rate was up to 31%.

2. What is the incidence of vaginal bleeding in the first trimester of pregnancy?

Approximately 20% of women bleed during the first trimester of pregnancy. The main differential diagnosis is between threatened miscarriage and ectopic pregnancy (which usually, but not always, is accompanied by some degree of pain). Bleeding also may be caused by vaginal lesions, endometrial infection, increased friability of cervical tissue, or molar pregnancy.

3. What is the risk of miscarriage in patients with first-trimester vaginal bleeding?

Approximately one-half to two-thirds of women who bleed from the uterus in the first trimester will miscarry. There is also a greater risk for subsequent preterm delivery and low-birth-weight infants.

4. Which prognostic factors assist the physician in advising the patient with a threatened miscarriage?

If fetal heart activity is detected by ultrasound, there is only a 10% incidence of miscarriage in the patient with first-trimester vaginal bleeding. With transvaginal sonography (TVS), fetal heart activity should be detected at 5 weeks. The absence of activity after the expected gestational age is associated with a high incidence of intrauterine fetal demise.

5. How is intrauterine fetal demise diagnosed in the first trimester?

A formal ultrasound demonstrating absence of fetal heart activity with a gestational sac larger than 1.2 cm indicates failure of normal fetal growth, although the threshold for seeing the fetal heart accurately varies with sonographic equipment and skill of the sonographer. In addition, declining serial quantitative levels of HCG indicate fetal demise.

6. What is a missed abortion?

Missed abortion is a term formerly used to denote a pregnancy that fails to enlarge over 4–6 weeks, as determined by physical exam. Because ultrasonography and serial quantitative HCG levels detect intrauterine fetal demise over a shorter time, the term is largely obsolete. Most fetal deaths occur 1–2 weeks before symptoms appear, and almost all progress to spontaneous miscarriage within 1–2 weeks (although frequently the miscarriage is incomplete).

7. How should the patient be instructed if she presents with a threatened miscarriage?

Patients should be instructed to avoid activities that are likely to introduce infection into the uterus: tampon use, sexual intercourse, and douching. No evidence suggests that bed rest is helpful, and the patient should be reassured that she has not caused the miscarriage and will not negatively influence fetal outcome by continued moderate activities. Likewise, no evidence suggests that trauma to the maternal abdomen or falls cause first-trimester spontaneous miscarriages.

8. What clues allow the clinician to suspect an ectopic pregnancy in the patient who presents with vaginal bleeding?

The presence of any degree of cramping or abdominal pain or any signs of blood loss out of proportion to vaginal bleeding should alert the physician to the possibility of ectopic pregnancy. Occasionally ectopic pregnancies present with painless vaginal bleeding. Thus, in the patient with pain or risk factors for ectopic pregnancy, an ultrasound should be performed as early as possible to locate the pregnancy. An intrauterine pregnancy can be visualized by vaginal ultrasound if the HCG level is > 2000 mIU/ml and by abdominal ultrasound if the HCG level is > 6000. Abnormal pregnancies are also associated with low serum levels of progesterones. A progesterone level < 5 ng/ml is nearly 100% predictive of an abnormal gestation, although it does not distinguish between an ectopic and an anembryonic gestation. Levels > 15 ng/ml are reassuring; however, there is some overlap between normal and abnormal gestation.

9. What is the risk of a combined intrauterine and ectopic pregnancy?

The risk of a combined or heterotrophic pregnancy is approximately 1 of 3,000 pregnancies. Recently this risk has been rising and is now estimated to be as high as 1 of 100 pregnancies in patients who take fertility drugs.

10. What is the utility of quantitative HCG measurement in the patient with threatened miscarriage?

Quantitative HCG levels should double every 2–3 days in a normal viable intrauterine pregnancy for the first 7–8 weeks after the last menstrual period (LMP). In patients with abnormal gestation (either intra- or extrauterine), levels tend to rise more slowly, plateau, or actually decline. Disappearing HCG levels indicate completion of the miscarriage. After a completed miscarriage, either spontaneously or induced, HCG levels decline but may take 1–2 weeks to disappear.

11. When should dilatation and curettage (D&C) be performed in the patient with vaginal bleeding in pregnancy?

D&C is reasonable management in patients with documented fetal demise, patients with an open cervical os (incomplete miscarriage), and patients with passage of products of conception that are believed to be incomplete.

12. Are there any patients who do not require D&C with spontaneous miscarriage?

In the patient who has passed tissue in which villi have been identified, D&C may be avoided if the uterus is contracted, the cervix is closed, the patient has stopped cramping, and bleeding is minimal. Ultrasound can be used to assess for an empty uterus when it is unclear whether tissue has been passed. Measurement of serial HCG levels or a repeat pregnancy test in 1–2 weeks is required to ensure that miscarriage has indeed occurred, unless the villi have been identified by pathologic exam.

13. How can the physician identify whether the patient has indeed miscarried?

If gross fetal parts are seen on visual inspection, the patient can be presumed to have an intrauterine pregnancy that has miscarried. In the absence of identifiable fetal parts, villi should be identified before the diagnosis of spontaneous abortion is certain. If the tissue is suspended in saline, placental villi that frond often can be differentiated from an organized clot or endometrial shedding. Endometrial tissue may be passed even by patients with ectopic pregnancies; thus tissue obtained by D&C or spontaneous passage always should be sent to the pathologist for identification.

14. Which patients with miscarriage should get RhoGAM?

Any Rh-negative patient who experiences spontaneous miscarriage or ectopic pregnancy at less than 12 weeks of gestation should receive MICRhoGAM (50 µg). After 12 weeks of gestation, a full dose (300 µg) of RhoGAM should be administered to all patients with spontaneous abortion or ectopic pregnancy. Although data are lacking in regard to Rh sensitization in women with threatened abortions, it is recommended RhoGAM be given when the patient is first seen.

15. Describe the management of patients who have undergone D&C for miscarriage.

The patient should be observed until medication used during the D&C has worn off. On discharge the patient should take methylergonovene (Methergine) for 1–2 days, and doxycycline, 100 mg twice daily, for 7 days. The patient should be advised to abstain from sex, tampons, and other vaginal contaminants for 2 weeks. The current recommendation is that the patient use birth control 2–3 months before attempting to become pregnant.

16. What grief process is experienced by patients with spontaneous abortion?

Patients with spontaneous miscarriage experience a significant grief reaction. The process is often more difficult because the pregnancy has not been acknowledged, rituals surrounding fetal death do not occur, and friends who might provide support may be unaware of the pregnancy. The physician should advise the patient that her feelings are normal and should requestion the patient about her progress in working through the grief process at the follow-up visit in 6 weeks.

17. What is the most generally accepted definition of recurrent pregnancy loss (RPL)?

RPL is classically defined as three or more consecutive spontaneous abortions.

18. What is the chance of a live birth after two consecutive miscarriages? Three consecutive miscarriages?

After two consecutive miscarriages the chance of a live birth is about 70–75%. After three losses with no previous live births, there is a 50–65% chance of live birth. After three losses with a previous live birth, there is a 70% chance of a subsequent live birth.

19. How often is an identifiable cause for recurrent pregnancy loss found?

An identifiable cause is found in 50–60% of cases.

20. What is a differential diagnosis for RPL?

Genetic causes
Anatomic abnormalities of the uterus

Endocrine disorders
  • Uncontrolled diabetes
  • Hypothyroidism (questionable contributor)
Autoimmune
  • Lupus anticoagulant
  • Antiphospholipid antibody
Alloimmunity
Environmental factors (smoking, alcohol)
Infectious causes (*Ureaplasma urealyticum* and *Mycoplasma hominis* have been
  investigated)

21. When should evaluation of recurrent pregnancy loss begin?

Generally after three consecutive losses. Evaluation may begin after two losses, depending on the patient's age and concern. Diagnostic evaluation should be performed after a woman has had a second-trimester loss because it is more likely to be of uterine origin.

22. When should karyotypic evaluation of a couple be performed in evaluation of RPL?

Karyotyping of a couple can be done after one loss if a previous delivery revealed a translocation. Otherwise, genetic causes of RPL are found in only 3–8% of couples. Therefore, due to the low yield and expense, karyotyping should be deferred until two or three losses, again depending on the patient's age and concern.

23. What are common correctable anatomic abnormalities of the uterus?

Of women with RPL, 12–15% have uterine abnormalities, of which a septate uterus is the most commonly reported. More than 80% of pregnancies after hysteroscopic removal of septa have resulted in a term birth or pregnancy extending beyond 20 weeks. Other common abnormalities include uterine fibroids, intrauterine adhesions (Ashermans' syndrome), and incompetent cervix.

Anatomic evaluation is begun with physical exam, followed by hysterosalpingogram. This protocol detects most common abnormalities, including leiomyomata, intrauterine adhesions (Asherman's syndrome), and unicornuate and bicornuate uterus.

24. What is luteal phase defect (LPD)? How is it diagnosed?

LPD is attributed to deficient secretion of progesterone by the corpus luteum; thus the endometrium is not properly stimulated. Diagnosis can be obtained by measurement of serum progesterone levels 1 week after ovulation. Levels > 15 ng/ml are considered reassuring, whereas levels < 10 ng/ml strongly suggest LPD. Endometrial biopsy performed 7 days after ovulation for 2 cycles and revealing a 3-day lag in maturity had been the gold standard. However, this method is painful and expensive, and subjective interpretation has raised questions about its efficacy.

25. Does treatment of LPD influence outcome?

LPD is treated by progesterone replacement (25–50 mg vaginal suppositories twice daily; progesterone injections, 12.5 mg, once daily, or clomid). No well-controlled studies provide convincing information that this regimen works, but no data suggest that it causes harm either.

26. What is alloimmunity?

Fetal antigens cause the mother to reject the fetus immunologically. It is hypothesized that the antigens stimulate a maternal response in which blocking factors are secreted to prevent immunologic rejection. Lack of this antigenic stimulation may result in a lack of blocking factors, with subsequent rejection of the fetus. This disorder is theorized to arise in couples who share similar HLA antigens; thus blocking response is not adequately stimulated by the fetus. Data related to this theory are conflicting.

27. How is alloimmunity treated?

Attempts have been made to enhance maternal response by injection of paternal lymphocytes into the mother. Studies to date have had conflicting results.

28. What is the proposed pathophysiologic mechanism of antiphospholipid antibody (anticardiolipin) and lupus anticoagulant in RPL?

Antiphospholipid and lupus antibodies block prostacyclin formation (a potent vasodilator and inhibitor of platelet aggregation), which results in unbalanced thromboxane excess and thus leads to vasoconstriction and thrombosis.

29. How are antiphospholipid and lupus antibodies detected?

Lupus anticoagulant in vivo causes thrombosis. In vitro, however, it prolongs the activated partial thromboplastic time (APTT). If the test is prolonged, an equal amount of normal plasma is added to the patient's plasma, and the APTT is repeated. If it is still prolonged, the presence of lupus anticoagulant is likely; it can be confirmed by correcting the APTT with the addition of phospholipid.

Anticardiolipin antibodies can be detected by specific solid-phase or enzyme-linked immunoassays.

30. How are these antibodies treated?

Treatment consists of low-dose aspirin (75–80 mg) combined with either heparin (initial dose, 10,000 subcutaneously every 12 hr) or corticosteroids (prednisone, 20–60 mg). Treatment regimens are still experimental. Generally, the smallest dose of heparin or steroid that corrects APTT is preferred.

BIBLIOGRAPHY

1. deCrespigny L: Early diagnosis of pregnancy failure with transvaginal ultrasound. Am J Obstet Gynecol 159:408–409, 1988.
2. Jain KA, Hamper UM, Sanders RC: Comparison of transvaginal and transabdominal sonography in the detection of early pregnancy and its complication. AJR 151:1139–1143, 1988.
3. Gelder MS, Boots LR, Younger JB: Use of a single random serum progesterone value as a diagnostic aid for ectopic pregnancy. Fertil Steril 55:497–500, 1991.
4. Leach RE, Ory SJ: Modern management of ectopic pregnancy. J Reprod Med 34:324–338, 1989.
5. Lindahl B, Ahlgren M: Identification of chorionic villi in abortion specimens. Obstet Gynecol 67:79–81, 1986.
6. Mars RP, Kletsky OA, Howard WF, et al: Disappearance of human chorionic gonadotropin and resumption of ovulation following abortion. Am J Obstet Gynecol 135:731, 1979.
7. Mishell D Jr: Recurrent abortion. J Reprod Med 38:250–259, 1993.
8. Ordi-Ros J, Perez-Peman P, Monasterio J: Clinical and therapeutic aspects associated to phospholipid binding antibodies (lupus anticoagulant and anticardiolipin antibodies). Haemostasis 24(3):165, 1994.
9. Pridjian G, Moawad Ah: Missed abortion: Still appropriate terminology? Am J Obstet Gynecol 161: 261–262, 1989.
10. Simpson JL, Mills JL, Holmes LB, et al: Low fetal loss rates after ultrasound-probed viability in early pregnancy. JAMA 258:2555–2557, 1987.
11. Stoval TG, Ling FW, Carson SA, Buster JE: Serum progesterone and uterine curettage in differential diagnosis of ectopic pregnancy. Fertil Steril 57:457–567, 1992.

16. INDUCED ABORTION

Dell Bernstein, M.D.,

1. What are the four major methods by which a physician can terminate a pregnancy?

1. Evacuation by vaginal route, using either suction dilatation and curettage or dilatation and extraction
2. Stimulation of uterine contractions by intrauterine installation of hypertonic saline, urea, or prostaglandin
3. Abdominal hysterotomy
4. Medical: antiprogestogens, prostaglandins, and methotrexate

2. What method of pregnancy termination is most commonly used for first-trimester termination? Why?

Suction curettage is presently the primary method of pregnancy termination in the first trimester. Vacuum aspiration is simple and safe. Complication rates are in the range of 0.8–7.3 per 100 abortions. In early pregnancy, fewer complications are associated with vacuum aspiration than with dilatation and curettage, but after 10 weeks' gestation the complication rates of vacuum aspiration vs. dilatation and curettage increase.

The introduction of newer medical methods of abortion induction may eventually replace suction curettage as the primary method of pregnancy termination.

3. How does the method of vaginal evacuation vary in relation to the weeks of gestation?

To 10 weeks. Use suction curettage with a smaller cannula and hand suction.

> 10 weeks. Use suction curettage after initial dilatation with laminaria. Use larger suction curettes and a suction machine that can generate more constant and higher levels of suction.

13–16 weeks. Use dilatation and evacuation as the method of choice. Cervical dilatation is obtained, using multiple laminaria. (The timeframe may be shortened with the new lamicel artificial laminaria, which achieves maximal expansion over a few hours but may fracture or shorten.) Special instruments are used to evacuate the fetus, followed by suction and/or sharp curettage.

17–24 weeks. Dilatation and evacuation or amnio-infusion procedures may be used. More recently, prostaglandin suppositories have been used to induce abortion. The dilatation and evacuation procedure has been shown to be safer than amnio-infusion techniques in the hands of an experienced operator.

4. What is a menstrual extraction? What is the failure rate of this procedure?

Menstrual extraction refers to an early pregnancy termination (i.e., 5–7 weeks' gestation). Prior to sensitive pregnancy tests, this was the time after a missed period but before a positive pregnancy test. The failure rate for this procedure is 0.26%. Menstrual extraction has a higher failure rate in terms of continued pregnancy than abortion by suction curettage in later stages of pregnancy.

5. How can one be certain that products of conception were obtained?

1. Perform a float test to look for placental tissue. Tissue is floated in a clear plastic dish over a light source to identify the characteristic seaweed, cottonball, or powder-puff pattern of villi.
2. If none is visualized, follow the patient with serial B-HCGs and ultrasounds, as needed.

6. What methods of medical termination of first-trimester pregnancies are available?

Mifepristone (RU-486) has been shown to be useful in early pregnancies. Experimental studies in the U.S. showed that a single 600-mg oral dose of mifepristone had an overall efficacy of

78–97%. Because RU-486 is still not available in the U.S. for pregnancy termination, misoprostil and methotrexate have been used, with 95% efficacy up to 9 weeks' gestation. RU-488 should be available soon in the U.S.

7. What is the mechanism of action of mifepristone?

The mechanism is not known, but it is thought to relate to both endometrial and myometrial effects. The drug is a synthetic 19-norsteroid with antiprogesterone activity. Its competitive inhibition of endometrial progesterone receptors leads to sloughing of the endometrium. RU-486 also stimulates prostaglandin production by the myometrium.

8. What is the difference in blood loss with surgical vs. medical termination of pregnancy?

Surgical termination has a significantly lower blood loss, but the majority of patients lost less than 300 ml and did not require transfusion.

9. Which agents have been used for amniotic instillation for second-trimester terminations?

Hypertonic saline (20–23%), prostaglandin F2α, urea and, rarely, ethacridine lactate.

10. What serious complications may occur with instillation of hypertonic saline?

Hyperosmolar coma
Hypernatremia
Diffuse intravascular coagulation

11. What is the preferred method of second-trimester terminations?

Intraamniotic infusions have been replaced with dilatation and extraction or vaginal prostins for second-trimester terminations because of the high incidence of complications with intraamniotic instillations. Up to 20 weeks' gestation, dilatation and evacuation are safer than vaginal prostin in experienced hands. After 20 weeks the optimal technique is debatable. Induction of fetal death with fetal injection of digoxin or hyperosmolar urea, followed by rupture of membranes and induction of labor, allows safe pregnancy terminations for fetal anomalies and death.

12. How should patients requesting pregnancy termination be screened and counseled?

Routine history, physical exam, documented positive pregnancy test, and, possibly, ultrasound determination of gestation age should be obtained initially. Counseling should include discussion of the patient's feelings about the pregnancy, plans for future birth control, and information about the procedure itself. Risks to be discussed include:
Missing an early gestation
Perforation
Bleeding
Retained products, requiring further surgery
Infection

13. Which laboratory tests are necessary before termination of pregnancy?

1. Rh determination so RhoGAM is given when appropriate
2. Baseline hematocrit
3. Pregnancy test
Other tests for sexually transmitted diseases and Papanicolaou smears depend on individual patients.

14. Which medications are recommended after termination of pregnancy?

Studies have shown that postabortal infections, although low, can be reduced even more with the use of prophylactic antibiotics. Tetracycline is recommended for 5–7 days after the procedure. Methergine is often used in later gestations to decrease risk of hemorrhage. Some form of adequate analgesic (often a nonsteroidal antiinflammatory medication) is also indicated.

15. What methods of anesthesia, analgesia, or sedation are safe for office procedures?

General anesthesia may be considered in patients with extreme anxiety, psychotic disorder, or mental retardation, but the added risk of general anesthesia is usually unwarranted. **Paracervical block** is the most commonly used form of anesthesia. **Sedatives**, with or without narcotics, may be given intravenously or orally before the procedure.

16. How is a paracervical block given?

1. Place the single-toothed tenaculum vertically at 6 o'clock after a small amount of lidocaine is injected just under the mucosa. This allows easy access to the uterosacral ligaments, which will be outlined with gentle traction on the cervix.

2. Inject 2 ml of the anesthetic agent just under the mucosa at 1-3-5 o'clock on the patient's right and 7-9-11 o'clock on the patient's left. Most important in a paracervical block is the anatomic point of injection; inject at the point the cervix reflects onto the vaginal mucosa, that is, in the fornix.

17. What are the potential complications of a cervical block?

Risks of paracervical blocks include direct intravascular injection, which results in seizures or cardio-respiratory arrest.

18. What can be done if it is difficult to dilate the cervix?

If difficulty is encountered in passing a dilator, try rotating or angling the instrument so that its tip can seek the internal os. Replacement of the tenaculum to the anterior lip of the cervix also may change the endocervical angle. Pretreatment with lamineria and/or prostaglandins may reduce the need for rapid mechanical dilatation.

19. What type of suction cannulas are used?

Questions are always asked as to which is better—plastic or metal, curved or straight. The answers vary. Plastic cannulas are disposable but have the disadvantage of a thick wall, whereas metal cannulas have a larger inside diameter for the same outside diameter. In addition, disposable cannulas are more expensive—an important point in areas where health care resources are scarce. Some physicians believe that if the fundus is acutely ante- or retroflexed, a curved cannula is best. Still, the procedure is much easier and causes infinitely less discomfort to the patient if the cannula is straight.

20. How is the size of the cannula determined?

The size of a plastic cannula should be determined by gestational age (i.e., no. 8 for 8-week gestation). Studies suggest a rigid one-hole cannula is preferable to a flexible cannula after 8–10 weeks' gestation.

21. Does artificially dilating the cervix impair future ability to carry a pregnancy?

No, not if it is done atraumatically. The use of laminaria has decreased the incidence of difficult dilatation.

22. What is the major cause of mortality associated with pregnancy terminations?

General anesthesia.

23. Does induced abortion cause sterility or pregnancy complications?

No. Studies have shown similar pregnancy rates for patients who have previous abortions compared with matched controls. Women with three or more induced abortions had a higher pregnancy complication rate. Pregnancy complications, such as bleeding in first and third trimesters, premature rupture of membranes, abruptio placentae, low birth weight, or short gestation, occurred more often in women with a history of two or more induced abortions. A history of one or more prior induced abortions do not appear to increase substantially the risk of adverse late outcomes of subsequent pregnancies.

24. How does the number of pregnancy terminations performed today compare with the number performed before legalization?

There is no way to know how many illegal pregnancy terminations were performed, but the incidence of patients hospitalized for incomplete and septic pregnancy terminations has decreased markedly. About 1.3 million legal pregnancy terminations are performed in the U.S. annually.

25. Did the 1973 U.S. Supreme Court decision in *Roe v. Wade* result in any change in maternal mortality?

Yes. The maternal mortality from illegally induced abortions was 39% in 1972 whereas the rate was 6% in 1974.

26. Have the laws concerning pregnancy terminations changed since 1973?

Subsequent to *Roe v. Wade*, court decisions have significantly narrowed a woman's constitutional right to pregnancy termination (e.g., *Webster v. Reproductive Health Service*, 1989). In addition, some states have limited or prohibited the use of public funds for pregnancy terminations for the medically indigent.

27. Has the attitude of residents training in obstetrics and gynecology also changed?

Presently, fewer residents are willing to be involved in pregnancy termination procedures than in the 1970s and early 1980s. In addition, residents who are willing to be involved in pregnancy termination procedures are often unable to do so because of the lack of public funding for the medically indigent. The American Board of Obstetricians requires experience.

28. How have changes in law and resident attitude affected the risk of pregnancy termination?

Extensive training in abortion procedures is required to preserve the low mortality and morbidity rates. Such training is often not obtained by residents because the change in laws and the change in resident attitudes.

29. Are the majority of Americans in favor of or against the availability of pregnancy termination procedures?

Many studies have shown that the majority of the general population (> 70%) believes that pregnancy termination procedures should be available to women. A vociferous minority has led to the recent limitations placed on availability of pregnancy termination procedures by courts and state legislatures.

BIBLIOGRAPHY

1. Castadot RG: Pregnancy termination: Techniques, risks, and complications and their management. Fertil Steril 45:5, 1986.
2. Chan YF, Ho PC, Ma HK: Blood loss in termination of early pregnancy by vacuum aspiration and by combination of mifeprestone and gemeprost. Contraception 47:85, 1993.
3. Edstrom K: Techniques of induced abortion, their health implications and service aspects: A review of the literature. WHO Bull 57:48, 1979.
4. Grimes DA, Bernstein L, Lacarra M, et al: Predictors of failed attempted abortion with the antiprogestin mifepristone (RU 486). Am J Obstet Gynecol 162:910, 1990.
5. Hausknecht RU: Methotrexate and misoprostol to term early pregnancy. N Engl J Med 333:537, 1995.
6. Hern WM, et al: Outpatient abortion for fetal anomaly and fetal death from 15–34 menstrual weeks' gestation: Techniques and clinical management. Obstet Gynecol 81:301, 1993.
7. Linn S, et al: The relationship between induced abortion and outcome of subsequent pregnancies. Am J Obstet Gynecol 146:136, 1983.
8. Stubblefield PG: Surgical techniques of uterine evacuation in first- and second-trimester abortion. Clin Obstet Gynaecol 13:53, 1986.

17. CONTRACEPTION

Lynn A. Barta, M.D.

1. What methods of contraception are currently available to women in the United States?
- Abstinence, withdrawal, and rhythm
- Sterilization
- Hormonal contraceptives
    - Oral contraceptives
    - Depot medroxyprogesterone acetate (DMPA, Depo-Provera)
    - Norplant
- Intrauterine device (IUD)
- Barrier methods
    - Diaphragm
    - Cervical cap
    - Condoms (male and female)
- Spermicides

2. What is the failure rate for each method?

Sterilization	0.3/100 women-years
Combination oral contraceptives	0.16–0.30/100 women-years
Norplant	0.8/100 women-years
Depo-Provera	0.0–0.7/100 women-years
IUD	1.2–3/100 women-years
Diaphragm	2/100 women-years
Condoms	3.5–4/100 women-years
Spermicides	12/100 women-years
Withdrawal and rhythm	6.5–15 women-years

3. Which is the most popular method? Which is the most effective?
Tubal ligation is the most frequently chosen and most effective method in the United States. In terms of reversible methods, oral contraceptives remain the most popular and effective choice. Eighty-five percent of women of childbearing age can safely take oral contraceptives.

4. What is the mechanism of action of oral contraceptives?
- Estrogen effects–prevent ovulation by inhibiting secretion of follicle-stimulating hormone (FSH) via pituitary hypothalamic effects.
- Progestin effects—prevent ovulation by inhibiting secretion of luteinizing hormone via pituitary and hypothalamic effects and alter cervical mucus by the formation of thick, viscid, scanty mucus, thereby making it impervious to sperm transport.
- Altered motility of the uterus and fallopian tubes
- Alteration of endometrium by decreasing glycogen production

5. What are the metabolic effects of oral contraceptives?
Combination oral contraceptives have a possible effect on cardiovascular disease, lipoprotein profile, and carbohydrate metabolism. They also have been shown to influence the incidence of hypertension and gallbladder disease. Most studies of these effects used high-dose pills (> 50 µg of the estrogen component), which are no longer in use. The low-dose pills (< 50 µg of the estrogen component) currently in use are believed to have few, if any, metabolic effects.

6. What is the association of oral contraceptives with cardiovascular disease?
A significantly increased risk of ischemic heart disease occurs in all oral contraceptive users over the age of 35 who smoke. A significant increase also occurs in patients of any age with additional risk factors, including vascular disease, hypertension, diabetes mellitus, and hypercholesterolemia. In the absence of significant risk factors, there appears to be no additional risk of ischemic heart disease.

7. How do oral contraceptives affect lipoproteins?

The estrogenic component of oral contraceptives stimulates an increase in high-density lipoprotein (HDL) cholesterol. The progestin component decreases the level of HDL cholesterol and increases low-density lipoprotein (LDL) cholesterol. The newer progestins (norgestimate and desogestrel) are less androgenic than other commonly used synthetic progestins and may increase HDL cholesterol more than other pills.

8. Can diabetic women use oral contraceptives?

In the past, impaired glucose tolerance was noted in women using high-dose pills. This progestin effect is dose-related. No clinically significant changes in glucose tolerance have been noted with the current low-dose pills. This seems to be true in healthy women as well as diabetic women and women with a previous history of gestational diabetes. Especially in view of the risks of pregnancy in diabetic women, it is believed that diabetics with well-controlled disease and no history of cardiovascular, renal, or thromboembolic disease can safely use low-dose pills with close surveillance.

9. Can hypertensive women use oral contraceptives?

Five percent of high-dose oral contraceptive users were initially observed to develop hypertension after starting the pills. There has been no increased incidence of clinically significant hypertension in users of low-dose pills. The use of low-dose oral contraceptives is acceptable in well-controlled hypertensives.

10. What are the absolute contraindications to oral contraceptive use?

- History or presence of thrombophlebitis, thromboembolic disease, or cerebral vascular disease
- Significantly impaired liver functions
- Known or suspected cancer of the breast
- Undiagnosed abnormal vaginal bleeding
- Known or suspected pregnancy
- Smokers over the age of 35

11. What is the association of oral contraceptives with cancer?

Endometrial cancer. Use of oral contraceptives decreases the risk by approximately 50%, with the greatest effect seen after 3 or more years of use. Protection persists for more than 15 years after discontinuation of the pill. The benefit is seen with the use of any low-dose, monophasic pill. Nulliparous women enjoy the greatest reduction in risk.

Ovarian cancer. The risk of epithelial ovarian cancer is decreased by approximately 40% overall (or approximately 11% per year of use) for all pill users. The protection is first noted 3–6 months after beginning oral contraceptive use and reaches an 80% reduction in risk after 10 or more years of pill use. It continues for 10–15 years after discontinuation.

Breast cancer. No increase in the incidence of breast cancer is associated with use of any current pill formulation, and there is no increased association with long-term use. There may be a slightly increased risk of breast cancer in women < 35 years of age who use pills for 4 or more years. However, there seems to be a slight decrease in risk in women more than 45 years old. Because of the age-adjusted incidence of breast cancer, the overall effect may actually be a decreased incidence of disease.

12. What are the noncontraceptive benefits of oral contraceptives?

The noncontraceptive benefits of oral contraceptives are numerous and significant. Use is associated with a decreased risk of endometrial and ovarian cancer and a decreased incidence of benign breast disease as well as pelvic inflammatory disease (PID) and ectopic pregnancy. There is an improvement in menses-related complaints, including menorrhagia and dysmenorrhea, and symptoms of endometriosis are occasionally improved with continuous low-dose pills. Additional benefits may include improvement in the symptoms of rheumatoid arthritis, increase in bone density, protection against atherosclerosis, and a small decrease in the incidence of functional ovarian cysts.

13. What other hormonal contraceptives are available? What is their mechanism of action?
In the early 1990s, two long-acting progestin compounds were introduced for the purpose of contraception. In 1991 levonorgestrel implant (Norplant) was approved for use in the U.S., and in 1992 injectable depot medroxyprogesterone acetate (DMPA, or Depo-Provera) was approved.

Norplant consists of six soft plastic implants, each filled with 36 mg of levonorgestrel. Plasma levonorgestrel levels are considerably lower with Norplant than with low-dose levonorgestrel combination oral contraceptives. These levels remain sufficient for effective contraception for 5 years after insertion. The mechanism of action includes ovulation inhibition along with luteal insufficiency and impaired oocyte maturation when ovulatory activity occurs. There is also the contribution of hostile cervical mucus produced by the progestin.

Depo-Provera is an aqueous suspension of microcrystals for injection. Active levels persist for 3–4 months after a 150-mg injection. The primary mechanism of action is ovulation inhibition.

14. How effective are the long-acting hormonal contraceptives?
Norplant carries an annual pregnancy rate of 0.8/100 users during 5 years of use. However, the pregnancy rate gradually increases over time. The failure rate may be higher in women weighing more than 70 kg.

Depo-Provera carries a failure rate of 0.3/100 women-years (0.0–0.7/100 women-years). This rate does not vary with patient weight.

15. What potential problems and side effects are attributed to long-acting hormonal contraception?
Menstrual side effects are the most common side effects of both methods and are the most common reason for discontinuation of both. Almost all women using Depo-Provera experience irregular bleeding and spotting initially, and approximately 50% report amenorrhea after 1 year of use. Headaches are the most frequent nonmenstrual complaint that leads to discontinuation of both methods. Other side effects include bloating, mood swings, and hair loss. After discontinuation of Norplant, return of fertility is rapid. It may be delayed for up to 18 months after discontinuation of Depo-Provera.

16. What is the effect of hormonal contraception on pregnancy?
The use of oral contraceptives, Norplant, and Depo-Provera in early pregnancy does not increase the risk of congenital anomalies or early pregnancy loss.

17. What is the "morning after pill"? How is it administered?
The morning after pill (emergency postcoital contraception) consists of high doses of estrogenic agents or combination estrogen-progestin agents that may exert unfavorable influences on both the endometrium and corpus luteum. The recommended regimens include:

Conjugated estrogens	15 mg orally twice daily for 5 days
	50 mg intravenously for 2 days
Ethinyl estradiol	2.5 mg orally twice daily for 5 days
Ovral	2 pills twice daily for 1 day
Loovral	4 pills twice daily for 1 day

The failure rates range from 0.1% with ethinyl estradiol to 2% with oral contraceptives. Treatment should be initiated as soon as possible after exposure and must be given within 72 hours. The most common side effect is nausea and vomiting, experienced by 15–30% of women. If pregnancy occurs despite this treatment, pregnancy termination should be considered.

18. Which patients are the best candidates for contraception with an intrauterine device?
The IUD is best suited for older, parous women who are not ready for a permanent method of contraception. The woman should be involved in a mutually monogamous, stable relationship and have no history of PID or ectopic pregnancy.

Absolute contraindications to IUD insertion include confirmed or suspected pregnancy, known or suspected pelvic malignancy, undiagnosed vaginal bleeding, acute or chronic pelvic infection, high risk behaviors for sexually transmitted diseases, and hyperbilirubinemia secondary to Wilson disease (for copper-containing devices only).

19. What is the mechanism of action of the IUD?
1. Interference with sperm transport from the cervix to the fallopian tube
2. Inhibition of sperm capacitation and survival
3. Endometrial changes that inhibit implantation

20. What are the major risks associated with IUD use?
Pelvic infection
Displaced string
Uterine perforation

21. What types of IUDs are available in the U.S.?
Currently only two different IUDs are available in the U.S. Progestasert is a steroid hormone-releasing device that must be replaced every 12 months. The Paragard (Copper T380A) is a copper IUD currently approved for use and replacement every 10 years.

22. What is the role of barrier methods of contraception?
Barrier methods may prove to be highly satisfactory for motivated, educated women. The **diaphragm** is effective when used in conjunction with spermicidal cream or jelly. It must be properly sized and fitted. Interference with spontaneity is cited as a disadvantage. **Cervical caps** must also be fitted in the office and may be worn for longer periods of time than the diaphragm. They may irritate and erode the cervix. **Condoms** ideally should be used with a spermicide to be at all effective. They are the only means of preventing transmission of sexually transmitted diseases, including HIV. This must be stressed to every patient during counseling about contraception.

23. What is the role of permanent sterilization as a contraceptive method?
Tubal ligation is the most frequently used method of contraception in the U.S. today. It is also highly effective for women desiring permanent sterilization (failure rate of 1/300). The risks associated with tubal ligation are method-related and include the risk of anesthesia, infection, and bleeding.

BIBLIOGRAPHY

1. American College of Obstetricians and Gynecologists: Sterilization. ACOG Tech Bull 113, 1988.
2. American College of Obstetricians and Gynecologists: The Intrauterine Device. ACOG Tech Bull 164, 1992.
3. American College of Obstetricians and Gynecologists: Hormonal Contraception. ACOG Tech Bull 198, 1994.
4. Centers for Disease Control: Oral contraceptive use and the risk of breast cancer. N Engl J Med 315:405, 1986.
5. Centers for Disease Control: Combination oral contraceptive use and the risk of endometrial cancer. JAMA 257:796, 1987.
6. Centers for Disease Control: The reduction of risk of ovarian carcinoma associated with oral contraceptive use. N Engl J Med 316:650, 1987.
7. Croxatto HB: Norplant: Levonorgestral-releasing contraceptive implant. Ann Med 25:155, 1993.
8. Speroff L, Glass RH, Kase NG: Clinical Gynecologic Endocrinology and Infertility, 5th ed. Baltimore, Williams & Wilkins, 1994.

18. PREMENSTRUAL SYNDROME (PMS)

Richard Allen, M.D.

1. What is premenstrual syndrome (PMS)?

The first published description was in 1931, and the syndrome was given the name PMS by Dalton in 1953. Speroff defines it as "a constellation of symptoms that occurs in a cycling pattern, always in the same phase of the menstrual cycle, interfering with work or lifestyle and followed by a period entirely free of symptoms."

2. What symptoms are associated with PMS?

Symptoms may be both physical and emotional. Physical symptoms include weight gain, breast swelling and tenderness, skin changes such as acne, hot flashes, diarrhea or constipation, headache, craving of sweets, and pelvic pain. Emotional symptoms include irritability, insomnia, depression, confusion or forgetfulness, anxiety, fatigue, and a feeling of being "out of control."

3. Do we know what causes PMS?

The short answer is no, but we do know that PMS is real. Numerous theories have been postulated, virtually all of which have to do with various hormonal alterations: ovarian hormones (estrogen and progesterone), fluids and electrolytes (prolactin, aldosterone, renin/angiotensin, and vasopressin), neurotransmitters (monoamines, acetylcholine), and other hormones (endorphins, androgens, glucocorticoids, melatonin, and insulin). It is likely that there is no single cause.

4. What is the theory behind progesterone as a cause and treatment for PMS?

This theory was first proposed by Dalton in England as a defense in a murder trial! It was postulated that a decrease in progesterone levels, perhaps with an inadequate luteal phase, triggered depression and other emotional symptoms. If that were so, then treatment with progesterone (usually given as a natural intravaginal suppository) would "cure" PMS. Unfortunately, this treatment works only in a small group of patients, and the benefits may even be due to a placebo effect. In fact, progesterone actually worsens symptoms in most patients. Progesterone increases monoamine oxidase levels in the plasma during the luteal phase. One theory relates levels of monoamine oxidase (MAO) to depression as a result of deficiency in catecholamines.

5. What role do endorphins have in cause and treatment?

Endorphins are elevated in the luteal phase of the menstrual cycle and inhibit catecholamines with menses, leading to irritability and tension. Endorphins increase with exercise and in turn raise serotonin levels, which reduces stress and improves sleep. There is still much to be learned about endorphins, but exercise is recommended as helpful in many respects.

6. What is the role of an aldosterone antagonist?

The physical symptoms of fluid retention (i.e., weight gain and breast tenderness) and some of the emotional symptoms are related to elevations in renin/angiotensin and aldosterone. Therefore, a specific antagonist, such as spironolactone, would be a treatment of choice. Spironolactone also has antiandrogenic effects and offers excellent symptomatic relief to many women.

7. Will changes in diet help?

Carbohydrate craving, especially for chocolate and sweets, is a common symptom. This is thought to be related to serotonin levels. By ingesting sugars the body attempts to increase serotonin, which in turn increases levels of L-tryptophan in the brain. In normal metabolism, serotonin levels rise and fall throughout the day. A rise in serotonin accompanies the ingestion of protein, which then lowers serotonin to begin a new cycle. In PMS, serotonin levels do not reach a level high enough to trigger protein ingestion, even after ingestion of carbohydrates. Therefore, the patient with PMS continues to crave and overeat carbohydrates. Thus, a healthy diet that is low in fat, salt, and sugar but more moderate in proteins and complex carbohydrates (whole grains, vegetables, and fruit) is most beneficial to the patient with PMS. Vitamin and mineral supplements have been studied without definitive results.

8. What role do vitamin and mineral supplements play?

Vitamins, particularly B6 in dosages of 200–800 mg/day, reduces serum estrogen levels and increases progesterone levels. Others, such as vitamin E, calcium, and magnesium (500 mg/day), may raise serotonin levels and help to relieve symptoms of anxiety, fluid retention, and insomnia.

9. Do prostaglandins help?

Prostaglandin PGE1 may be low in some types of PMS, particularly those associated with alterations in carbohydrate metabolism. Prostaglandins also contribute to dysmenorrhea; thus an inhibitor is beneficial in such cases.

10. Can sterilization contribute to PMS?

No. At least two recent comprehensive studies have shown no correlation with tubal sterilization.

11. How is PMS treated?

First, the physician must reassure the patient that her symptoms are real and can be treated. She should then be encouraged to chart her symptoms for several cycles to see if it is indeed premenstrual. While she is doing so, the importance of a healthy diet, exercise, and sleep should be stressed. A plan of management should be formulated with the patient, depending on her symptoms and their specific treatments. Specific simple medical treatments, such as spironolactone and prostaglandin inhibitors, can then be prescribed. Progesterone therapy should be reserved for a small subgroup that does not respond to the above. If the patient also needs contraception, birth control pills are beneficial.

Women with severe depressive disorders that require medication, such as lithium, MAO inhibitors, and tranquilizers, probably should be referred for appropriate psychiatric counseling. Double-blind, placebo-controlled studies have shown marked reduction of PMS symptoms in patients receiving the serotonin reuptake inhibitor fluoxetine at a dosage of 20 mg/day throughout the menstrual cycle. Recent research has shown that other SSRIs (i.e., sertraline) may be helpful.

The vast majority of women who are troubled with PMS affliction can be helped.

12. What therapy is suggested for the breast tenderness associated with PMS?

Bromocriptine, 5 mg/day during the luteal phase.

13. What is the theory relating a yeast-free diet to improvement of PMS symptoms?

1. Researchers in candidiasis have found an estrogen-binding protein in *Candida albicans*.

2. Defects in cellular immunity and resultant immunosuppression may be the result of suppressor substances generated by macrophages, induction of *Candida*-specific suppressor T-lymphocytes, and/or accumulation of *Candida* carbohydrates.

3. Some women with candidiasis appear to have an interleukin-2 defect in lymphocyte proliferation, which places them at risk for autoimmune disease and alterations in hormones.

4. Kroker outlines the broader role for *Candida* sp. in causing chronic illness from tissue sensitivity to the organism and/or its byproducts rather than direct tissue invasion by the organism itself.

A defective immune response causes psychoneuroendocrine dysfunction. Eliminating exogenous and endogenous *Candida* sp., plus addressing food, chemical, and inhalant allergies, currently provides good relief from PMS symptoms.

Treatment Options for PMS

SYMPTOM	TREATMENT
Affective, behavioral symptoms	Alprazolam, agonists of gonadotropin-releasing hormone, SSRIs
Anxiety	Alprazolam, buspirone, fluoxetine, sertraline
Breast swelling and tenderness	Bromocriptine
Edema, bloating	Spironolactone, danazol
Tension, depression	Antiprostaglandins
Irritability	Danazol
Headache	Alprazolam, progesterone

BIBLIOGRAPHY

1. American College of Obstetricians and Gynecologists: Premenstrual Syndrome. ACOG Committee Opinion 155, 1995.
2. Brandenburg S, Tuynman Qua H, Verheij R, Pepplinkhuizen L: Treatment of premenstrual syndrome with fluoxetine: An open study. Int Clin Psychopharmacol 8:315, 1993.
3. Frank RT: The hormonal causes of premenstrual tension. Arch Neurol Psychiatry 26:1052, 1931.
4. Freeman E, Rickles K, Sondheimer S, Polanski M: Ineffectiveness of progesterone suppository treatment for premenstrual syndrome. JAMA 264:349, 1990.
5. Freeman E, et al: Treatment of severe PMS. JAMA 274:51, 1995.
6. Ginsburg KA: Some practical approaches to treating PMS. Contemp Obstet Gynecol 40:24, 1995.
7. Green R, Dalton K: The premenstrual syndrome. BMJ 1:1007, 1953.

19. ACUTE AND CHRONIC PELVIC PAIN

Corinne Dix, M.D.

1. What is the definition of chronic pelvic pain in women?

Chronic pelvic pain in women may be defined as nonspecific pelvic pain of more than 6 months' duration that is not relieved by narcotic analgesics. It is a nonspecific term that involves pain associated with laparoscopically evident pathology, occult somatic pathology, and nonsomatic disorders.

2. How common is chronic pelvic pain in women?

Chronic pelvic pain prompts up to 10% of outpatient gynecology consultations and is responsible for approximately 10–35% of laparoscopies and 12% of hysterectomies performed in the U.S. There are no reliable data about disability and lost work days attributable to chronic pelvic pain, but the total direct and indirect cost in the U.S. may be conservatively estimated to exceed two billion dollars annually.

3. What is the major difference between acute and chronic pelvic pain?

Acute pain is of short duration and generally is associated with tissue damage appropriate to the degree of symptoms. Chronic pelvic pain often has an indefinite beginning, and the structural damage alone usually is not enough to account for the degree of pain that the patient reports.

4. What is the innervation of the individual pelvic organs?

The innervation of the lower abdominal wall and anterior aspect of the vulva, including the clitoris and urethra, is by mixed somatic nerves that originate in the ventral branches of the first and second spinal lumbar segments. The dorsal rami derived from L1 and L2 innervate the lower back, often a region of referred gynecologic pain. The perineum, anus, and lower vagina are innervated by somatic branches of the pudendal nerve, which is derived from the second and fourth sacral root ganglia. Painful visceral stimuli from the upper vagina, cervix, uterine corpus, medial fallopian tubes, broad ligament, upper bladder, cecum, appendix, and terminal large bowel travel in thoracolumbar sympathetics via the vaginal, uterine, and hypogastric plexus and to the lumbar and lower thoracic sympathetic chain. The impulses next pass through the white rami communicans associated with T11, T12, and L1 and then through the dorsal roots of these nerves, after which they enter the spinal cord at T11, T12, and L1.

At least a portion of the vagina, however, is embryologically derived from the urogenital sinus, as are the bladder and rectum. Therefore, there are likely sacral afferents in addition to thoracolumbar afferents.

The afferent pathway from the ovary, upper ureter, and outer two-thirds of the fallopian tube enters the main sympathetic chain at the fourth lumbar sympathetic ganglion and ascends with the sympathetic chain to enter the spinal cord at the level of the ninth and tenth thoracic segments.

5. What is the differential diagnosis of chronic pelvic pain?

Gynecologic causes	Orthopedic musculo-	Gastrointestinal causes
Pelvic inflammatory	skeletal causes	Irritable bowel syndrome
disease	Osteitis pubis	Constipation
Endometriosis	Stress fracture of pelvis	Inflammatory bowel disease
Pelvic adhesions	Abdominal wall pain	Dietary intolerance
Pelvic relaxation	**Urinary tract causes**	
Pelvic congestion	Interstitial cystitis	
Ovarian cysts	Urethral syndrome	
Mittelschmerz	Bladder spasms	

6. What are the most common causes of acute pain related to the reproductive organs?

1. **Mittelschmerz** is a dull pressure or aching sensation during midcycle in either the right or left lower quadrant secondary to ovulation, distention of the ovarian capsule, or mild bleeding associated with the process of ovulation.

2. **Functional ovarian cysts.** *Follicular cysts* result from failure of egg release from a mature follicle during ovulation. Symptoms include an aching sensation in the right or left lower quadrant. Findings include an enlarged cystic ovary on exam or ultrasound and clear cervical mucus with spinnbarkheit and ferning pattern on microscopic examination. Clinical course may include spontaneous resolution, torsion with pain, rupture with pain, and rupture with hemorrhage possibly requiring surgical evaluation. *Corpus luteum cysts* may persist in the center of the corpus luteum. The lutein cysts may be functional or nonfunctional; therefore, menstruation may be delayed. Cyst persistence is rare except in cases of pregnancy. Complications include torsion, rupture, and hemorrhage.

3. **Intrauterine pregnancy** may cause abdominal pain by possible stretching of the visceral peritoneum by the enlarging uterus, early uterine contractions, stretching of the ovarian capsule from the corpus luteum cyst, rupture of the corpus luteum, and threatened miscarriage. The diagnosis of pregnancy is based on historical information of amenorrhea, nausea, breast tenderness, fatigue, and urinary frequency and on the physical findings of a softening isthmus and enlarging fundus.

4. **Ectopic pregnancy** may cause pelvic pain before and after rupture secondary to stretching of the hollow viscus of the fallopian tube or peritoneal irritation from a hemoperitoneum. Ectopic pregnancies occur in 1 of 110 gestations. Location of the gestation may be tubal, cervical, ovarian, intramural, or abdominal.

5. **Pelvic infections** are a common cause of both acute and chronic pelvic pain. The infection commonly involves the fallopian tubes and ovaries, parametrial and pelvic wall tissue, uterus, and other organs of the pelvic and abdominal cavity.

6. **Uterine tumors.** Leiomyomatas or leiomyosarcomas may cause pain secondary to torsion necrosis, stretching of the visceral peritoneum of the uterus, or pressure against surrounding intraabdominal structures.

7. **Adnexal neoplasia** may cause abdominal or pelvic pain when associated with hemorrhage, necrosis, torsion, or rupture. Symptoms may include gradual onset of abdominal pain, intermittent or acute severe pain, abdominal distention, nausea, vomiting, anorexia, or unilateral lower extremity edema.

8. **Torsion** may involve a normal or cystic ovary, tube, or uterine mass. Symptoms may be constant and severe or intermittent. Associated symptoms include nausea, vomiting, diaphoresis, and severe pelvic pain. Venous blood flow ceases first, resulting in enlargement. Arterial obstruction causes necrosis. The patient most commonly presents with an acute abdomen requiring immediate surgical exploration.

9. **Endometriosis** is the presence of endometriotic implants on the peritoneal surfaces of the intraabdominal structures, resulting in hemorrhage and pelvic adhesion development. The pain is characteristically present several days before the period and ends with menstruation; however, it may be constant throughout the cycle. Dyspareunia and infertility are also common presenting complaints.

10. **Dysmenorrhea** is lower abdominal pain or pelvic pain associated with the immediate premenstrual phase and menstruation.

7. What diseases of the urinary tract cause pelvic pain?

1. **Urinary tract infection, cystitis, and pyelonephritis** may present with lower abdominal and/or right flank pain, dysuria, hematuria, and frequency of urination. The patient is usually febrile. White blood cells and bacteria are noted on urinalysis. Treatment is antibiotics.

2. **Ureteral obstruction** secondary to a stone, tumor, or blood clot may cause severe, sudden pain beginning in the flank and radiating into the groin and ipsilateral labia. Symptoms include restlessness, sweats, nausea, vomiting, frequency of urination, and colicky pain. Findings include hematuria, flank tenderness, and tachycardia.

3. **Perinephric abscess** is usually unilateral and caused most commonly by staphylococci. Symptoms include flank tenderness, more pronounced than in pyelonephritis, and fever.

4. **Interstitial cystitis and urethral syndrome**—frequency, urgency, and dysuria in absence of bacteriuria.

8. What are the most common gastrointestinal causes of pelvic and lower abdominal pain?

1. **Appendicitis** is the most common surgical condition in the abdomen, although it is less common in women than in men. Pain is secondary to luminal distention and necrosis. The symptoms vary, depending on the anatomic location of the appendix and the status of the infection. A dull aching is initially reported in the periumbilical area, advancing to a more severe pain at McBurney's point. Right hip extension may cause an increase in pain.

2. **Diverticulitis** is most commonly seen in elderly women and may present with peritonitis similar to appendicitis or with a pelvic mass. Pain may be acute and severe, or there may be a history of chronic bouts of pain.

3. **Bowel obstructions** secondary to postoperative adhesion, neoplastic lesions, hernias, foreign bodies, gallstones, parasites, enteritis, or traumatic hematoma of the bowel wall may cause colicky abdominal pain with associated distention, dehydration, hypovolemia, vomiting, and constipation.

4. **Strangulated hernias** and hernias in general are commonly symptomatic. Pain occurs when the intraperitoneal contents are trapped in the hernia sac and the blood supply is compromised. The most common forms associated with abdominal pain are inguinal, femoral, umbilical, and obturator hernias. Presenting symptoms are obstructive. Treatment is surgical with restoration of a patent bowel lumen.

5. **Cholecystitis, cholangitis, gastroduodenal ulcers, and pancreatitis** most commonly cause upper abdominal pain but rarely are associated with lower abdominal symptoms.

6. **Irritable bowel syndrome** is usually associated with bowel spasms and diarrhea. Irritable bowel syndrome predisposes women to hysterectomy and negatively influences pain postoperatively.

9. How is levator muscle tenderness diagnosed and treated?

Gentle palpation of the relaxed levator muscles with the index finger directed posteriorly helps to diagnose spasm. Injection of the trigger area is of diagnostic and therapeutic value and may be repeated up to three times.

10. What are the causes of deep vaginal pain?

1. Tender trigger points in the paracervical region or margins of the vaginal cuff after hysterectomy. These points are reproducible. Injection with 1% procaine or 0.25% bupivacaine requires minimal penetration (3–5 mm) of vaginal mucosa to reproduce the painful sensation. The treatment may need to be repeated weekly, up to three times.

2. The second component is a deep aching sensation made worse with coitus, menses, and exam. Trigger points are hard to identify. The pain is more diffuse. Blocks result in temporary improvement, lasting only until the anesthesia wears off. Diagnostic laparoscopy is indicated to rule out pelvic adhesions and endometriosis. Laser therapy is available for fulguration of endometriosis, lysis of adhesions, and uterosacral ligament transection.

11. What test is a valuable tool in assessing abdominal wall pain from the underlying viscera?

Carnett's test, in which the rectus muscles are tensed. Abdominal wall pain worsens with tensing of the rectus abdominis muscle. Patients with visceral pain often present with a tense rectus abdominis muscle and may be curled up in a semi-Fowler position.

12. What are myofascial trigger points versus abdominal wall trigger points?

Myofascial trigger points are hyperirritable spots usually within a taut band of skeletal muscle or muscle fascia. Abdominal wall trigger points have been identified in fat or fascial planes above the aponeurosis on needle localization.

13. How are myofascial trigger points detected and treated?

The points are painful on compression (jump sign) and may give rise to characteristic referred pain (to the arm, leg, or back), tenderness, and autonomic phenomenon (tearing, coryza, visual disturbances, tinnitus). Treatment involves hyperstimulation, analgesia (such as stretch and cold spray), needling with local injection, transcutaneous electrical nerve stimulation (TENS), and acupuncture, all of which act as counterirritants that alter the central gate or threshold control and result in a prolonged response.

14. What diagnostic method can be used to distinguish visceral pathologic conditions from chronic abdominal pelvic pain of neurologic origin?

The tissue source of pain can be identified by a careful neurologic assessment with palpation of small areas of tissue; by placement of a needle into the tissues either abdominally or vaginally; or by injection of saline or anesthetic into the local tissue and reproduction of the same pain with the needle tip.

15. What is the association of sexual abuse with chronic pelvic pain?

Women with chronic pelvic pain have a high incidence of sexual abuse history (48%, compared with 6.5% of pain-free controls).

16. What has been the history of pelvic vascular congestion syndrome?

Congestion of the pelvic venous system has been suggested as a source of chronic dull, aching pain. The pain is usually worse premenstrually after standing or after orgasmic coitus. The findings were rarely documented, and laparoscopically visible varicosities were evident in a significant number of asymptomatic women undergoing tubal sterilization procedures. Psychophysiologic factors also may contribute.

Beard et al. and Reginald et al. have reported work with fluoroscopic venography and intravenous injections of dihydroergotamine. In their model, symptomatic pelvic congestion is viewed as a dynamic vascular process, similar to migraine headache, in which active, radiographically evident vascular dilatation can be observed to reverse after administration of dihydroergotamine. Of note, Beard and coworkers have reported a 60% incidence of "significant emotional disturbances" among 35 women with pelvic vascular congestion. Research in this area is still ongoing. Therapy is usually a combination of psychotherapy and elimination of the menstrual cycle.

17. What are the recommendations for treatment of chronic pelvic pain?
1. Complete and careful medical, social, and sexual history and physical examination.
2. Differentiation between somatic and visceral foci for pain, using trigger-point identification and analgesia for these foci to improve accuracy of pelvic examination.
3. Pelvic ultrasound, CT scan, MRI, and abdominal and renal radiographic procedures may be helpful adjunctive diagnostic tools.
4. Use of medication should be minimal. Analgesics should be taken continuously but limited if addicting. Antidepressants may potentiate analgesics. Anxiolytics also may potentiate analgesics but have a high addiction potential.
5. Surgical therapy should be limited to severe refractory cases, avoiding removal of normal pelvic tissues. Up to 78% success rate in surgical treatment of pain with hysterectomy, even without uterine pathology.
6. Psychological consultation as indicated based on history and response to evaluation and treatment.

18. What is the role of laparoscopy in chronic pelvic pain?
Forty percent of all laparoscopy is done for chronic pelvic pain. Although 61% of patients had diagnosable abnormalities, < 50% were helped with diagnostic and operative laparoscopies.

BIBLIOGRAPHY

1. Droegemueller W, et al (eds): Comprehensive Gynecology. St. Louis, Mosby, 1987.
2. Beard RW, Highman JH, Pearce S, et al: Diagnosis of pelvic varicosities in women with chronic pelvic pain. Lancet ii:946, 1984.
3. Howard FM: The role of laparoscopy in chronic pelvic pain: Promise and pitfalls. Obstet Gynecol Surv 48:357, 1993.
4. Lescomb GH, Ling FW: Chronic pelvic pain. Med Clin North Am 79:1411, 1995.
5. Mathias SD, Kupperman M, et al: Chronic pelvic pain: Prevalence, health-related quality of life, and economic correlates. Obstet Gynecol 87:321, 1996.
6. McDonald JS: Management of chronic pelvic pain. Obstet Gynecol Clin North Am 20:817, 1995.
7. Rapkin AJ: Neuroanatomy, neurophysiology, and neuropharmacology of pelvic pain. Clin Obstet Gynecol 119–128, 1990.
8. Reiter RC: A profile of women with chronic pelvic pain. Clin Obstet Gynecol 130–135, 1990.
9. Reiter RC, Gambone JC: Demographic and historic variables in women with idiopathic chronic pelvic pain. Obstet Gynecol 75:428, 1990.
10. Reiter RC: Occult somatic pathology in women with chronic pelvic pain. Clin Obstet Gynecol 154–159, 1990.
11. Roseff SJ, Murphy AA: Laparoscopy in the diagnosis and therapy of chronic pelvic pain. Clin Obstet Gynecol 137–143, 1990.
12. Slocumb JC: Chronic somatic myofascial, and neurogenic abdominal pelvic pain. Clin Obstet Gynecol 145–152, 1990.

20. SEXUAL DYSFUNCTION

William B. Wilson, Jr., M.D.

1. Why is a knowledge of sexuality and sexual functioning of value to the obstetrician-gynecologist?

The past three decades have led to increasing openness about sexuality, and patients are more willing to discuss sexual problems with their physicians. Many women view obstetricians and gynecologists as their primary care physicians, to whom they bring all of their health problems, including those related to sexuality. Physicians must be comfortable in responding to their concerns. Many events in a woman's life expose her to changes that cause concern about or affect her self-image and sexual health. Physicians must anticipate such feelings and discuss their emotional, physiologic and social bases. Every physician should be able to assess a patient with sexual concerns and provide either treatment (if comfortable doing so) or appropriate referral.

2. What essential knowledge about sexuality is required of all physicians?

All physicians should understand the physiology of sexual response and the phases of the sexual response cycle. They also must know the emotional, societal, and physiologic influences on sexuality associated with events in a woman's life that cause concern about her sexual health. Menarche (or its absence), sexual activity, use of contraception, surgical procedures, childbearing, and change in marital status are among these events.

3. What are the physiologic phenomena of sexual response?

The principal responses are increased muscle tone and vasocongestion, which produce changes in the genitalia, breasts, and skin. Masters and Johnson studied these changes extensively and introduced the concept of a human sexual response cycle.

4. What are the phases of the human sexual response cycle?

Masters and Johnson proposed a four-phase cycle of response in both men and women to facilitate an understanding of anatomic and physiologic changes: (1) excitement, (2) plateau, (3) orgasm, and (4) resolution. Such definitions are somewhat arbitrary, and the phases are not always clearly demarcated. In addition, they may vary considerably among different people and in one person at different times.

Kaplan believed that it was more helpful in diagnosing and treating patients to classify the phases as (1) desire, (2) arousal, and (3) orgasm. She argued that a certain energy allows an individual to initiate or respond to sexual stimulation. In light of the variability of the excitement and plateau phases described by Masters and Johnson and the increased presentation of problems of desire, this three-phase response is more widely used today.

5. What changes are seen during arousal?

The initial response in women is vaginal lubrication; this transudate results from vasocongestion in the walls of the vagina. There are no secretory glands in the vaginal walls, and the glands lining the cervix do not contribute meaningfully to lubrication of the vagina. Other changes include expansion of the upper two-thirds of the vaginal barrel, elevation of the cervix and corpus uteri, flattening and elevation of the labia majora, and increase in size of the clitoris, which results from vasocongestion.

Women characteristically display nipple erection, but full erection of both nipples may not be reached simultaneously. The surface veins become more prominent as arousal progresses, and may increase breast size.

As arousal continues, the lower third of the vagina undergoes prominent vasocongestion, described as forming the orgasmic platform. The opening narrows as a result, but the upper two-thirds show additional expansion, with increased elevation of the uterus. Vaginal lubrication often slows in comparison to earlier arousal but may be pronounced. The shaft and glans of the clitoris retract, and it may be difficult to visualize them. Areolar tumescence becomes prominent and may make nipple erection less apparent, although it is still present. Breast size continues to increase and may reach 20–25% above baseline.

The sex flush, a rash resembling measles, develops in 50–75% of women. A much smaller percentage of men display this phenomenon. It usually begins on the epigastrium and spreads over the breasts and anterior chest wall; it may appear also on the back, buttocks, extremities, and face.

In men, arousal is characteristically marked by penile erection, which also results from vasocongestion. However, psychological and physical arousal may be present without a firm erection when the man feels anxiety or fatigue. Vasocongestion also produces a smoothing of the skin ridges of the scrotum, which flattens because of thickening of the scrotal integument. The cremaster muscles shorten the spermatic cords, partially elevating the testes toward the perineum.

As arousal continues, men show a minor increase in diameter of the proximal portion of the glans with a deepening in color due to venous stasis. Testicular vasocongestion continues, and size may increase to 50–100% over baseline volume. Elevation of the testicles continues, and anterior rotation brings the posterior testicular surface into contact with the perineum. This has been called preejaculatory positioning of the testes. Small amounts of fluid may appear from the urethral meatus, presumably from Cowper's glands; live spermatozoa have been observed in this fluid.

Early in arousal the physical changes are neither constant nor always ascending in either sex, and the mechanisms of vasocongestion do not constitute a quantitative appraisal of arousal. Later, both men and women display generalized myotonia, tachycardia, tachypnea, and increased blood pressure.

6. What occurs during the orgasmic phase?

Female orgasm is marked by simultaneous rhythmic contractions of the uterus, orgasmic platform (ischiocavernosus and pubococcygeal muscles), and rectal sphincter. Contractions begin at 0.8-second intervals and then diminish in intensity, duration, and regularity. There is a total body response, with measurable changes in heart beat, respiration, peripheral muscle contractions, and electroencephalogram. The same response occurs after hysterectomy and clitoral excision.

Male orgasm begins with a series of contractions in the accessory sex organs. The contractions cause seminal fluid to pool in the prostatic urethra and are experienced as a sensation of ejaculatory inevitability. The actual expulsion of seminal fluid follows in several seconds. Rhythmic contractions of the prostate, perineal muscles, and shaft of the penis occur initially at 0.8-second intervals, as in women, but they diminish somewhat more rapidly.

Women may be multiorgasmic; men do not seem to share this capacity. Men experience a refractory period during which ejaculation cannot recur; this period varies from minutes to hours and is lengthened by age and with repeated ejaculations.

After orgasm the anatomic and physiologic changes that occurred during arousal are reversed. The orgasmic platform disappears, the uterus returns to the true pelvis, the vagina begins to decrease in length and width, and the clitoris returns to its normal position. Penile contractions reduce vasocongestion, and men experience a prompt loss of erection, followed by a second stage of detumescence as normal vascular flow slowly returns. The testes decrease in size and descend into the scrotum, which also undergoes reversal of vasocongestion.

7. What constitutes sexual dysfunction?

Masters and Johnson pioneered the investigation of sexual dysfunction. They believed that sexual function involved activation of various inborn reflexive responses that ordinarily are incorporated into a psychosocial format. The basic physiologic responses of normal sexual function may be impaired by various factors of organic or psychogenic etiology. By this definition, sexual dysfunction is marked by impaired physiologic response as opposed to problems such as alterations in behavior, feelings, or attitudes without impairment of physiologic function.

The definition has broadened over the years, and impaired physiologic response is not a requirement. A recurrent barrier during any of the stages of sexual response can establish a sexual dysfunction. Lack of desire, lack of arousal, or lack of orgasm may be presenting complaints for which the patient seeks help; but careful history taking may show that the physiologic changes can, and do, occur.

8. What are the sources of sexual dysfunction?

There are many causes of failure to achieve satisfaction in sexual interchanges. Medical factors always must be ruled out before pursuing other causes such as intrapsychic problems or relationship difficulties. Reaction to illness and some medical treatments have been the causes of some dysfunctions. Having ruled these out, one can look for misconceptions about human sexual response, performance anxiety, and relationship problems as sources.

9. What are the common dysfunctions in women?

Hypoactive sexual desire or lack of sexual desire is the most common complaint encountered today. In the past this was often seen in nonorgasmic women who, after years of failing to achieve orgasm, resigned themselves to never experiencing it and ultimately lost interest in sexual activity. Such conditioning is not as common today, and many of the desire problems result from anger or resentment toward the partner. This may be secondary to sexual failures or to difficulties in the relationship.

Orgasmic dysfunction and vaginismus were the principal dysfunction in past years. Orgasmic dysfunction is classified as primary when the woman has never achieved orgasm under any circumstances. Situational dysfunction describes a woman who has attained orgasm on one or more occasions but only under certain circumstances. A subcategory of situational anorgasmia is coital orgasmic dysfunction, in which women are orgasmic by many means but not during intercourse. Random orgasmic dysfunction describes women who experience orgasm in various activities but only infrequently. Secondary orgasmic dysfunction applies to women who were regularly orgasmic at one time but no longer experience orgasm.

Vaginismus is the involuntary constriction or spasm of the muscles surrounding the vaginal outlet and lower one-third of the vagina. It may occur in response to a real or imagined attempt at penetration. It occurs in women of any age, and the spectrum extends from unconsummated marriages to painful, but possible, intercourse. Although vaginismus may make a woman fearful of sexual activity and limit her overall responsiveness, more commonly she experiences little problem with sexual arousal. Vaginal lubrication occurs normally, noncoital activity can be pleasurable, and the orgasmic response is often intact.

10. What are the common dysfunctions in men?

The principal male dysfunctions are disorders of erection and disturbances of ejaculation. Premature ejaculation has long been considered the most common male disorder. Unfortunately, no precise definition is clinically satisfactory; but if rapid ejaculation limits a partner's ability to reach high levels of arousal or orgasm, a problem exists. When there is a pattern of ejaculation before, during, or shortly after insertion of the penis into the vagina, it is easy to diagnose severe premature ejaculation. When the problem is less severe, definitions vary greatly. Masters and Johnson make the diagnosis when the man is unable to control ejaculation long enough to satisfy his partner in 50% of coital encounters. Despite the lack of a precise definition applicable to all cases, a good history can indicate when lack of ejaculatory control is a problem.

Ejaculatory incompetence (the inability to ejaculate intravaginally) is the rarest male dysfunction. Erectile difficulty is rarely seen with this disorder, and afflicted men typically maintain a firm erection during lengthy episodes of coitus. The most common form of this disorder is primary (the man has never been able to ejaculate intravaginally), but sometimes secondary or acquired ejaculatory incompetence is seen (the loss of ability to ejaculate intravaginally after a previous history of normal intravaginal ejaculation with coitus). This disorder occurs with a variation in pattern of incompetence; some men can ejaculate with masturbation, some with noncoital partner stimulation, and others cannot ejaculate by any means. In some cases the disorder is situational, occurring with one partner but not with another.

Impotence is the inability to achieve or maintain an erection adequate for penetration or completion of coitus. It can be primary or secondary. Isolated transient episodes of inability to get or maintain an erection occur normally (usually due to fatigue, acute illness, anxiety, excessive alcohol intake, or distraction) and do not require evaluation or treatment. When impaired function becomes a persistent pattern, diagnostic and therapeutic attention is warranted.

Hypoactive sexual desire is also a prominent complaint in recent years. This problem has been described as a "Yuppie" dysfunction, implying that the pressures of employment, achieving a desired standard of living, and fatigue are contributing causes that result from the lifestyle.

11. What other dysfunctions may be encountered in practice?

One almost certainly will encounter inhibited sexual desire and, possibly, true sexual aversion. Having defined dysfunction as an altered state of physiologic response, Masters and Johnson did not consider inhibited desire and sexual aversion as dysfunctional problems. They were described as nondysfunctional disorders characterized by impeded initiatory sexual behavior or impeded sexual receptivity, representing a spectrum of intensity. True sexual aversion is infrequently encountered. It is a consistent negative reaction of phobic proportions; it applies to sexual activity or the thought of sexual activity. Afflicted people experience overwhelming, irrational anxiety at the thought of sexual contact. As with other phobias, anticipation of the activity may engender more anxiety than the actual activity; in fact, patterns of sexual arousal are apt to be largely intact.

BIBLIOGRAPHY

1. Anon JS: Behavioral Treatment of Sexual Problems. Hagerstown, MD, Harper & Row, 1976.
2. Garrera M: Sex: The Facts, the Acts and Your Feelings. New York, Crown, 1981.
3. Green R: Homosexuality—A Health Practitioner's Text, 2nd ed. Baltimore, Williams & Wilkins, 1979.
4. Kaplan HS: Disorders of Sexual Desire. New York, Simon & Schuster, 1979.
5. Kaplan HS: The Evaluation of Sexual Disorders. New York, Brunner Mazel, 1983.
6. Kolodny RC, Masters WH, Johnson VE: Textbook of Sexual Medicine. Boston, Little, Brown, 1979.
7. Lieblum SR, Rosen RC (eds): Sexual Desire Disorders. New York, Guilford Press, 1988.
8. LoPiccolo J, LoPiccolo L: Handbook of Sex Therapy. New York, Plenum Press, 1978.
9. Masters WH, Johnson VE: Human Sexual Inadequacy. Boston, Little, Brown, 1970.
10. Masters WH, Johnson VE, Kolodny RC: Masters and Johnson on Sex and Human Loving. Boston, Little, Brown, 1986.
11. Pion R, Hopkins J: The Last Sex Manual. New York, Wyden Books, 1977.
12. Rosen RC, Beck JG: Patterns of Sexual Arousal. New York, Guilford Press, 1988.
13. Zilbergeld B: The New Male Sexuality. New York, Bantam Books, 1992.

21. BREAST LUMPS

Patrick English, M.D.

1. How is the breast exam performed?

In general, be methodical and consistent. Examine the patient in the sitting and supine positions. Have the patient flex the pectoralis muscle and open the axilla.

2. If a mass is discovered, how is it best described?

Size, contour, consistency, and mobility are noted, along with attachment to skin or underlying fascia. Careful examination of the axillary and supraclavicular nodes should be part of the exam. Note nipple discharge or rashes. A simple diagram of the breasts with findings drawn in facilitates subsequent exams.

3. Why is a newly discovered breast mass important?

In the United States approximately 180,000 women will be diagnosed with breast cancer in the next year. Most will present with a palpable breast mass.

4. In regard to the mass, what aspects of the history are important to highlight?

Most newly discovered breast masses are found by the patient herself. It is important to ask when it was first found, how it has changed, whether it changes with the menstrual cycle, and whether it is painful.

5. What characteristics of a breast mass suggest malignancy?

Palpable breast cancers usually have irregular or indistinct borders and may be attached to the skin, its dermal attachments, or underlying fascia. However, these characteristics are not invariable. No physical characteristics allow one to distinguish reliably between benign and malignant lesions.

6. What are the risk factors for breast cancer?

Age, family history of breast cancer, history of breast cancer in the opposite breast, and history of lumpectomy in the same breast are among the more important risk factors. In general, in women under 25, a newly discovered lump is unlikely to be cancer, whereas in a woman over the age of 70, it is likely to be cancer.

7. What initial diagnostic step can be taken to evaluate a newly discovered mass?

Needle aspiration of the palpable breast mass is easily and safely performed in an office or clinic setting. It distinguishes cystic from solid masses and provides cells for subsequent cytologic evaluation.

8. If a breast cyst is aspirated, should the fluid be sent for microscopic exam?

Only if it is bloody should the aspirant be sent for cytologic analysis.

9. What characteristics of an aspirated cyst require further workup?

As noted, aspiration of bloody fluid is suspicious. Also, if there is a residual mass after aspiration or if the cyst recurs, the likelihood of cystic cancer increases and further diagnostic studies should ensue.

10. If attempted aspiration of a palpable breast mass reveals a solid lesion, what further diagnostic studies can be performed?

The aspirated sample can be prepared on a slide and sent for cytologic analysis. The technique requires some experience and the availability of a cytopathologist.

11. What are the advantages of fine-needle aspiration of a solid breast mass over open biopsy?

Fine-needle aspiration is cheaper and more comfortable, has a better cosmetic result, and, in experienced hands, is very accurate.

12. What are the disadvantages of fine-needle aspiration of a solid breast mass over open biopsy?

A considerable amount of skill is required to obtain a satisfactory sample. An experienced cytopathologist is required to interpret the sample. There is a small but measurable number of false-negative and false-positive results compared with open biopsy.

13. What is the role of mammography in the evaluation of palpable breast masses?

The purpose of mammograms is to detect nonpalpable, suspicious areas in either breast.

14. Does a normal-appearing mammogram in a woman with a palpable mass exclude the possibility of cancer?

No. In general, the false-negative rate for mammograms is reported to be as high as 16%. Even in the presence of clinically evident cancer, mammograms can be interpreted as normal.

15. In what settings are mammograms particularly difficult to interpret?

Dense breasts are difficult for radiologists. Overall, this problem is found in 25% of women and is particularly common in younger women.

16. What role does ultrasound play in the evaluation of solid breast masses?

Ultrasound is useful for differentiating solid from cystic masses. The study can be used in women with large breasts who have deep, inaccessible lesions or who cannot undergo needle aspiration.

17. What is the approach to a woman whose mammogram shows a nonpalpable lesion that is read as "probably benign" by the radiologists?

There are two choices: biopsy or repeat mammography within 6 months. Recent studies indicate that the second approach is probably safe, but much depends on the comfort of the physician with the mammographic appearance and availability of the patient for follow-up.

18. If a lesion is regarded as suspicious on mammogram but is not palpable, how is it approached?

Mammographic localization techniques (including wires and dyes) are used to guide the surgeon for an open, excisional biopsy.

19. Are techniques other than open biopsy available to sample suspicious, nonpalpable breast lesions?

Recently, radiologists have developed techniques of stereotactic core biopsies of nonpalpable breast lesions. The technique is well tolerated and accurate, but its role in the approach to patients with suspicious, nonpalpable breast lesions is currently being defined.

20. What pathologic findings on breast biopsy put patients at a higher risk for subsequent development of breast cancer?

Most breast biopsies return as benign with some variation of fibrocystic disease. Of these lesions, approximately 30% show a proliferative pattern that is associated with an increased risk for the subsequent development of cancer. Of these lesions, atypical hyperplasia shows the highest relative risk.

BIBLIOGRAPHY

1. Donegan W: Evaluation of a palpable breast mass. N Engl J Med 327:937–942, 1992.
2. Dupont WD, Page DL: Risk factors for breast cancer in women with a proliferative breast disease. N Engl J Med 312:146–151, 1985.
3. Grant CS, Goellner JR, Welch JS, Martin JK: Fine needle aspiration of the breast. Mayo Clinical Proc 61:377–381, 1986.
4. Layfield LJ, Chrischilles EA, Cohen MB, Bottles K: The palpable breast nodule: A cost effective analysis of alternate diagnostic approaches. Cancer 72:1642–1651, 1993.
5. Parker SH, Lovin JD, Jobe WE, et al: Sterotactic breast biopsy with a biopsy gun. Radiology 176:741–747, 1990.
6. Sickles EA: Periodic mammographic follow-up of probably benign lesions: Results in 3,184 consecutive cases. Radiology 179:463–468, 1991.

22. LAPAROSCOPIC SURGERY IN GYNECOLOGY

Terry Johnson, D.O.

1. When the abdominal wall is viewed through the laparoscope, what are the important landmarks?

1. The **Urachus** (median umbilical ligament) is a fibrous strand that connects the apex of the bladder to the connective tissue of the umbilicus. It is a remnant of the original connection of bladder to allantois.

2. The **obliterated umbilical artery** (lateral umbilical ligament) begins just beyond the origin of the superior vesical artery. It is crossed by the round ligament.

3. The **inferior epigastric vessels**, a branch of the external iliac vessel, arise immediately above the inguinal ligament and just medial to the deep inguinal ring. The round ligament passes behind and lateral to these vessels to enter the inguinal canal. Internally, the vessels ascend obliquely toward the umbilicus in extraperitoneal connective tissue. Near the arcuate line they pierce the transversalis fascia and enter the rectus sheath between the muscle and posterior rectus sheath.

2. What is capacitive coupling? What are the implications in the use of electrosurgery in laparoscopy?

Capacitive coupling refers to an electrical charge radiating from one metal surface to another to place a charge on the outer metal surface. When unipolar electrosurgical current is delivered through the intact insulated probe passed through a channel of conductive material (e.g., a metal trocar sleeve or operating scope), the current may "couple" to the metal surface. In this situation, the sleeve or scope becomes a capacitor. The energy stored in the sleeve has no return pathway to ground; if a small piece of bowel, for example, touches the sleeve, the energy seeks ground through the tissue, and a burn may occur.

3. When electrosurgical energy is applied to tissue, three effects may occur: cutting, fulguration, and desiccation. What are the differences?

1. Cutting uses high-current, low-voltage (continuous–undamped) waveform energy that produces vaporization of tissue with minimal coagulation. The current passes through a steam bubble between the active electrode and tissue. Therefore, it is a noncontact form of desiccation.

2. Fulguration is application of high-voltage, low-current noncontinuous waveform energy, which achieves coagulation by spraying long electrical sparks to the surface of tissue. This is noncontact coagulation in which the electrode is held away from tissue. The peak voltage is high enough to arc or spark the tissue.

3. Desiccation is the application of electrosurgical current by means of direct contact of the electrode to tissue. As a result, all of the energy is converted to heat within the tissue, causing coagulation. Any waveform will desiccate when the electrode is in direct contact with tissue.

4. What are the different blends of current that can be delivered by electrosurgical units?

A pure cutting waveform is a simple sinusoidal, undamped, or unmodulated waveform and is generally produced by continuous energy. Modulation of the waveform is achieved by interrupting the current and increasing the voltage. As a result, the total energy remains the same, but the ratio of voltage to current is modified to increase hemostasis during dissection. The differences in blends (generally 1-2-3) represent increased modulation of waveforms, which results in less cutting (less necrosis) and more coagulation as the ratio changes.

5. What cardiovascular changes and potential complications are associated with laparoscopy?

1. A decrease in venous return and therefore an increase in CO_2 due to pneumoperitoneum and positive pressure ventilation.

2. Arrhythmia can result from hypercapnia induced by peritoneal absorption of CO_2 or hypoventilation.

3. A narrowing of pulse pressure due to cardiac compression caused by pneumoperitoneum.

4. Bradycardia may result from peritoneal stretching; in addition, electrical current passing through fallopian tubes or uterus can trigger a vagal response.

6. What is a "mill wheel" murmur?

Mill wheel murmur is a classic murmur associated with gas embolism. It is a rare but potentially lethal complication of laparoscopy with an estimated incidence of 15 per 113,253.

7. If one is concerned about subumbilical insertion of a Veress needle or trocar, what are the alternatives?

1. Open laparoscopy
   - Use of special cannulas (e.g., Hasson)
   - Cost-effective technique of using a pursestring fascial suture
2. Left upper quadrant
   - 3 cm below left costal margin, 3–5 cm left of midline near axillary line.
   - Place Veress needle in the 9th or 10th intercostal space, midway between midclavicular line and anterior axillary line. After insufflation, a 5-m scope is placed below last rib.
3. Place Veress needle through cul-de-sac of Douglas.
4. Place Veress needle through uterine fundus.

8. During the insertion of a laparoscope/Veress needle, the primary concern is the location of major vessels. What is the level of the bifurcation of the aorta and other major vessels?

The aortic bifurcation occurs at the level of L4 (75% of the time). L4 can be located at the level of the iliac crest; 85% will be within 1.25 cm above or below the crest. Be aware of the effect of Trendelenburg position and variation in patient habitus.

9. A thermal injury to bowel is devastating. How should it be repaired, given immediate recognition?

The involved area should be excised for at least 5 cm beyond the surrounding affected area.

10. A patient reports increasing abdominal pain after laparoscopy. What is the primary concern?

Any patient who has increasing abdominal pain after laparoscopy has bowel perforation until proved otherwise.

11. If a bowel injury occurs, how can one tell whether it is thermal or traumatic?

A classic study by Soderstrom et al. shows, via histology, that thermal injuries destroy full-thickness bowel wall and cause coagulation necrosis, whereas traumatic injury is more likely to cause hemorrhage and an acute inflammatory reaction.

12. The location of the ureter is of paramount importance. Are there any tricks to locating it?

1. The best rule of thumb is to look above the area of pathology. The ureter generally can be seen as it crosses the common iliac arteries before entering the pelvis.

2. The administration of metaclopramide (Reglan) stimulates peristalsis of the ureter and makes this action easier to identify.

13. Hemorrhage is always a concern. Laparoscopy is associated with a unique circumstance. The pressure of the pneumoperitoneum often exceeds venous pressure and small arterial vessel pressure. How can we compensate for this?

Very simple! After the procedure is completed, the pneumoperitoneum should be decompressed, then reinsufflated slowly under direct vision to detect bleeding. An alternative is to fill the abdomen with water (isotonic solutions will not lyse red cells) and look for streaming of lacerated vessels.

14. What is a laparoscopic-assisted vaginal hysterectomy (LAVH)?

A difficult question to answer. The procedure can vary from diagnostic laparoscopy to ensure that vaginal hysterectomy can be performed safely to a complete hysterectomy performed via the laparoscope. Recently, classification systems have been proposed. These efforts should be refined and a consensus reached by gynecologic pelviscopists.

15. What are the indications for LAVH?

In the most basic terms, any condition that generally would be performed by laparotomy. The use of the laparoscope can span the spectrum: simple diagnostic laparoscopy to determine feasibility of vaginal surgery, ancillary procedures to perform vaginal surgery (e.g., adhesiolysis), and portions of all operative maneuvers in vaginal hysterectomy.

16. Is LAVH cost-effective?

The major benefit of LAVH is avoidance of an abdominal incision, which has potential to reduce the length of hospital stay and recuperation. The comparative costs are difficult to quantitate as savings include not only hospital days saved but also earlier return to work. As the skills of laparoscopic surgeons increase, the cost benefit will increase as operative times decrease.

17. Does Veress needle insertion have an advantage over direct trocar insertion?

It depends on operator experience and/or performance. Operators who favor direct trocar insertion point to the fact that occult injury (vascular or visceral) may go unrecognized in Veress needle technique because of the tamponading effect of the pneumoperitoneum.

18. What is the hernia risk associated with trocar insertion?

Initially it was thought that incisional hernias would not occur in incisions < 1.0 cm. The risk of hernia development has not been calculated, but case reports of hernia development imply that all trocar sites > 7 mm require a deep fascial stitch. The umbilical incision is an exception to this rule.

19. Should all complications during endoscopic surgery be considered a laparoscopic complication?

Probably not. Only untoward events that result from the technique used to accomplish a particular operation should be considered a complication of laparoscopy. However, untoward events that result from the complexity of the surgical procedure are not considered to be complications of endoscopy; instead, they are considered complications of the pathologic condition. For example, opening the colon during resection of deep infiltrating endometriosis is a complication related to the disease process, but traumatic injury to the ilium by trocar insertion is a direct laparoscopic complication.

20. What is the role of patient position in primary insertion of Veress needle or trocar?

Most laparoscopists use the Trendelenburg position, which allows bowel contents to fall out of the pelvis. However, this position causes the sacral promontory and great vessels to rotate anteriorly. A more shallow angle of insertion is necessary to avoid retroperitoneal damage to large vessels (i.e., iliac artery).

21. How should bowel injuries associated with pelviscopy be managed?

1. In penetrating injury, as may occur with a trocar placed through the intestine, do not start by removing the trocar! A small laparotomy incision should be made, the damaged bowel exposed, and pursestring suture placed. The trocar can then be removed. A second layer of suture is then placed. Always inspect the opposite side of the bowel.

2. If a thermal injury occurs, the bowel should be resected for at least 5 cm around the area.

22. Is spillage of cyst contents at time of laparoscopy a problem?

A theoretical risk is always associated with spillage of fluid from a malignant tumor. It remains conjectural. Modern studies have shown that tumor grade, dense adhesions, and ascites affect relapse rates, whereas tumor rupture did not affect prognosis or rate of relapse. However, laparoscopic aspiration alone of cysts should not be condoned. It has been shown that 10–65% of aspirates are read as benign when, in fact, a malignancy is present.

23. What are absolute contraindications to laparoscopy?

1. **Multiple laparotomies**, especially for chronic conditions such as diverticulosis, peritonitis, or known adhesions.

2. Patients with **class IV cardiac disease** cannot tolerate the Trendelenburg position.

3. **Acute peritonitis with bowel distention** is a relative contraindication because of risk of bowel injury. If an open laparoscopy is done in a patient with bowel obstruction, it is possible to relieve the obstruction laparoscopically.

24. What is the role of laparoscopy in general gynecology?

1. **Ectopic pregnancy.** Randomized controlled studies have been done looking at the benefit of laparoscopy vs. laparotomy for management of ectopic pregnancies. Unfortunately the power in these studies was too low to detect important differences. There is evidence based on these studies that laparoscopy can be used to treat ectopic pregnancy. Laparoscopic treatment has not been shown to result in fewer adhesions or higher tubal patency rate than treatment by laparotomy.

2. **Ovarian biopsy.** When combined with diagnostic laparoscopy, ovarian biopsy increased complications. Risk of hemorrhage and ureteral injury and questionable risk of tumor spill need to be weighed.

3. **Treatment of polycystic ovarian syndrome.** This can be treated by electrocautery if patients have failed ovulation induction hormonally; it can be performed laparoscopically.

4. **Adnexal operations unrelated to ectopic pregnancy.** These procedures include salpingectomy, salpingostomy, oophorectomy and ovarian cystectomy.

5. **Ovarian cyst management.** Cyst management by laparoscopy is complicated by inadequacy of cytologic diagnosis of cyst fluid, recurrence of cysts, and potential for disseminating or delaying the diagnosis of ovarian cancer.

6. **Pelvic abscess.** Pelvic abscesses can be drained laparoscopically.

7. **Uterosacral nerve ablation for chronic pain.** This procedure has been done laparoscopically, but there is insufficient evidence to recommend this procedure because of complications and questionable benefit.

8. **Laparoscopic myomectomy.** Laparoscopic myomectomy can be performed and is indicated for infertility, but patients need to be selected carefully because the long term risks and benefits are not known.

25. What is the role of laparoscopy in gynecologic oncology?

1. **Cervical cancer.** Laparoscopic node dissection can diagnose metastatic disease in patients explored for radical hysterectomy, thus avoiding a laparotomy and allowing earlier treatment with radiation therapy if the radical hysterectomy is not indicated. In advanced-stage disease, high common and low paraaortic nodes can be sampled, thus extending the radiation field without an abdominal incision.

2. **Ovarian cancer.** Staging can be performed laparoscopically, especially in patients found to have grade I, unstaged ovarian cancer on final pathology, thus avoiding a second laparotomy. Use of laparoscopic second look is limited, but sometimes it may help limit abdominal incisions in second laparotomies for ovarian cancer.

3. **Endometrial cancer.** Laparoscopic staging with vaginal hysterectomy potentially decreases morbidity and allows earlier radiation therapy when indicated. The gynecologic oncology group presently is undertaking a carefully controlled randomized study of laparoscopic staging in endometrial cancer.

BIBLIOGRAPHY

1. Childers J, Brzechea R, Sorwill E: Laparoscopy using the left upper quadrant as the primary trocar site. Gynecol Oncol 50:221, 1993.
2. Dembo A, Davy M, Stenwig A, et al: Prognostic factors in patients with stage I epithelial ovarian cancer. Obstet Gynecol 75:263, 1990.
3. Grimes DA: Frontiers of operative laparoscopy: A review and critique of the evidence. Am J Obstet Gynecol 166:1062, 1992.
4. Hulka JF, Reich H: Textbook of Laparoscopy. Philadelphia, W.B. Saunders, 1994.
5. Jarrett JC: Laparoscopy: Direct trocar insertion without pneumoperitoneum. Obstet Gynecol 75:725, 1990.
6. Parker W: Management of ovarian cysts by operative laparoscopy. Contemp Obstet Gynecol 1991, p 47.
7. Parker WH, Berek JS: Laparoscopic management of the adnexal mass. Obstet Gynecol Clin North Am 21:79, 1994.
8. Reich H: Laparoscopic bowel injury. Surg Larprosc Endosc 2:74, 1992.
9. Sutton C: Power sources in endoscopic surgery. Curr Opin Obstet Gynecol 7:248, 1995.

II. Reproductive Endocrinology and Infertility

23. THE MENSTRUAL CYCLE

Kevin Bachus, M.D.

GENERAL QUESTIONS

1. What is the mean age of menarche and menopause?
The mean age of menarche is 12.7 years; the mean age of menopause is 51.4 years.

2. What is the mean duration and interval for menses?
Mean duration 5.2 days (3–8 day range); normal interval 28 days (range 21–35 days). Only 15% of women have a "typical" 28-day cycle.

3. In a woman's lifetime, when is the greatest variability in the menstrual cycle?
In the first 2 years after menarche and 3 years before menopause. Anovulatory cycles occur in up to 6 and 34% of these cycles, respectively.

4. What are the differences between the basal and functional layers of the endometrium with regard to hormonal responsiveness and presence throughout the menstrual cycle?
The basal layer is relatively unresponsive to hormonal stimulation and remains intact throughout the menstrual cycle. The functional layer is very responsive to hormonal stimulation, and most of this layer (subdivided into the compacta and spongiosa) is lost during menstruation.

5. How are prostaglandins involved in the process of menstruation?
Prostaglandins are maximal just prior to menses and appear to be important in initiating menstrual blood flow by causing constriction of the spiral arterioles and stimulating myometrial contractions.

6. How many germ cells are in the prenatal, neonatal, and pubertal ovary?
At 20 weeks' gestation, 6–7 million germ cells are present, which declines to 2 million by birth and 300,000 by puberty.

FOLLICULAR PHASE

7. What is a primordial follicle?
An oocyte arrested in the diplotene stage of the first meiotic prophase surrounded by a single layer of granulosa cells. Its growth is independent of gonadotropin stimulation.

8. What is the preantral follicle?
An oocyte surrounded by the zona pellucida with several layers of granulosa cells and a theca layer. Growth of the follicle in this stage becomes dependent on gonadotropins.

9. Which hormones are necessary for accumulation of granulosa cells and progressive follicular growth?
Follicle-stimulating hormone (FSH) is responsible for induction of luteinizing hormone (LH) receptors and aromatase enzyme, which are responsible for conversion of androgens to

estrogens within the developing follicle. Estrogen acts synergistically with FSH to increase the number of FSH receptors on the cells as well as to increase mitotic activity of the granulosa cell, which leads to proliferation of the granulosa cell layer.

10. Which hormone signals follicular recruitment and when in the menstrual cycle does it begin?

FSH, which is the signal of follicular recruitment, begins its increase in the late luteal phase of the preceding cycle.

11. What function does LH have in the follicular phase?

LH interacts with theca cells, which results in androgen production. These androgens serve as a substrate for aromatization to estrogen within the developing dominant follicle. These androgens, however, produce follicular atresia within nondominant follicles.

12. What is the two-cell, two-gonadotropin concept of ovarian steroidogenesis?

In response to LH, theca cells produce androgens (primarily androstenedione), which diffuse to the adjacent granulosa cells where they become aromatized to estrogen. This aromatization is facilitated in an estrogen microenvironment, which in turn is dependent on FSH stimulation of granulosa cells.

13. Which hormones are detrimental to progressive follicular maturation?

Androgens in high enough concentrations undergo 5α reduction to more potent androgens. Premature increases in LH also decrease mitogenic activity of granulosa cells. In both cases, degenerative changes occur.

ANTRAL FOLLICLE

14. What mechanisms promote the atresia of a nondominant follicle?

Selection of the dominant follicle occurs by days 5–7 of the menstrual cycle. As estrogen concentrations from the dominant follicle increase, FSH is inhibited centrally by negative feedback inhibition. This causes withdrawal of gonadotropin support of less developed follicles. The dominant follicle escapes the atretic consequences of falling FSH levels by having a greater number of FSH receptors via an increased mass of granulosa cells. Additionally, increased vascular development within the theca layer may offer preferential delivery of FSH to the dominant follicle. By altering the gonadotropin secretion by its own production of estrogen, the dominant follicle optimizes its own environment to the detriment of other follicles.

PERIOVULATORY FOLLICLE

15. What is the most reliable predictor of impending ovulation?

Ovulation occurs approximately 34–36 hours after the start of the LH surge or 10–12 hours after the peak of the LH surge.

16. What are the primary hormonal signals necessary for an adequate LH surge that will trigger ovulation?

Estradiol is necessary in threshold concentrations of > 200 pg/ml for approximately 50 hours and must be present until after the actual LH surge begins. This positive feedback response of estrogen upon the pituitary resulting in an LH surge is facilitated by low levels of progesterone.

17. What does an LH surge do?

It initiates resumption of meiosis in the oocyte, causes luteinization of granulosa cells, and synthesizes prostaglandins and progesterone essential for follicular rupture. Although antral fluid volume increases at the time of ovulation, the rupture of the follicle is not felt to be secondary to increased hydrostatic pressure. More likely, degenerative changes in the follicular wall result with destruction of collagen, which allows passive expansion and ultimate rupture of the follicle.

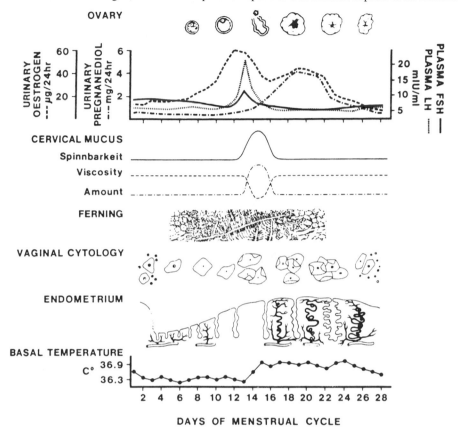

The cyclical biological consequences of the hypothalamic–pituitary–ovarian interactions. The physiologic and morphological events in the uterus, cervix and vagina are largely determined by the fluctuating levels of ovarian hormones. (From MacKay EV, et al (eds): Illustrated Textbook of Gynaecology. Artarmon, Australia, Holt-Saunders, 1983, with permission.)

OVULATION

18. When is the first polar body extruded from the oocyte?

Ovulation is accompanied by the completion of the first meiotic division with extrusion of the first polar body.

19. What causes the extrusion of the oocyte from the follicle?

The physical act of ovulation likely involves prostaglandins and lysosomal enzymes, which cause degenerative changes in the follicular wall. Contrary to what is believed by many, this process does not seem to involve a significant increase in hydrostatic pressure from within the follicle.

LUTEAL PHASE

20. Which hormone is necessary for normal corpus luteum function?

The lifespan and steroidogenic capacity of the corpus luteum are dependent on continued tonic LH secretion, which results in sustained progesterone output. Normal luteal function requires optimal preovulatory follicular development (i.e., adequate FSH stimulation) and continued tonic LH support. If human chorionic gonadotropin (hCG) is present in adequate concentrations, the corpus luteum of pregnancy can be maintained.

21. When in the luteal phase does progesterone peak?

Progesterone peaks approximately day 8 after the LH surge, mediates maturity of secretory endometrium, and suppresses new follicular growth. Light microscopic changes are so uniform that each of the luteal phase days can be identified by characteristic findings within the glands and stroma.

22. When is implantation likely to occur?

The most likely day of implantation is day 22–23, which coincides with peak intracellular apocrine secretory activity.

23. What is a luteal phase defect?

Corpus luteal insufficiency produces luteal phase defects. The role of luteal phase defect in causing infertility is unclear because of difficulty in diagnosis.

BIBLIOGRAPHY

1. Carpenter SE: Psychosocial menstrual disorders: Stress exercise and diet's effect on the menstrual cycle. Curr Opin Obstet Gynecol 6:121, 1994.
2. MacKay EV, et al (eds): Illustrated Textbook of Gynaecology. Artarmon, Australia, Holt-Saunders, 1983.
3. Mishell DR: Reproductive endocrinology. In Droegemueller W, et al (eds): Comprehensive Gynecology. St. Louis, Mosby, 1992, pp 79–140.
4. Seibel MM: Oocyte maturation and follicular genesis. In Seibel MM (ed): Infertility: A Comprehensive Text. Norwalk, CT, Appleton & Lange, 1990, pp 37–49.
5. Speroff L, Glass LRH, Kase NG: Regulation of the menstrual cycle. In Clinical Gynecologic Endocrinology and Infertility, 5th ed. Baltimore, Williams & Wilkins, 1994, pp 93–107.
6. Yen SSC: The human menstrual cycle. In Yen SSC, Jaffe RB (eds): Reproductive Endocrinology: Physiology, Pathophysiology, and Clinical Management, 3rd ed. Philadelphia, W.B. Saunders, 1991, pp 181–237.

24. PUBERTY

Catherine Stevens-Simon, M.D.

1. What is puberty?

Puberty encompasses the physiologic changes leading to the development of adult reproductive capacity; the process includes maturation of the hypothalamus, pituitary, and gonad.

2. What is adolescence?

Adolescence encompasses the psychologic, social, and cognitive changes leading to the development of an adult identity; the process includes individuation, the achievement of personal independence, and maturation of cognitive reasoning skills.

3. Are puberty and adolescence related?

Because puberty and adolescence proceed at the same time, they are often assumed to be identical. Although there is no evidence that young people who experience an early puberty also establish an independent adult identity and attain adult cognitive skills at an earlier age, some studies suggest that the events of puberty affect those of adolescence. Strict biologic determinism seems unlikely; rather, visible evidence of physical maturity probably alters adult expectations for behavior, and these expectations may, in turn, retard or accelerate adolescence. This may be problematic, particularly for early-maturing girls and late-maturing boys.

4. How does puberty start?

Puberty seems to be a gradual process. It starts long before we are aware of it in the teenager, perhaps as early as 7 to 8 years of age. The first event of puberty is thought to be the nocturnal release of luteinizing hormone releasing factor (LHRF) from the hypothalamus; this stimulates the release of luteinizing hormone (LH) and follicle-stimulating hormone (FSH) from the pituitary gland, and, in turn, the synthesis of estrogen and testosterone in the ovaries and testes of young girls and boys.

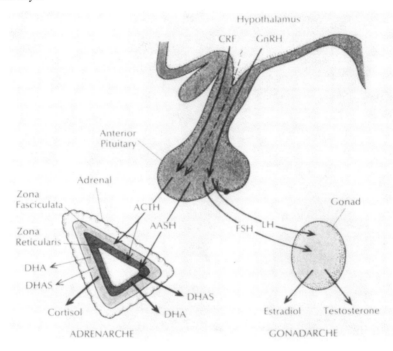

Pubertal development involves two temporally associated processes: adrenarche and gonadarche. The processes are controlled by different mechanisms, activation may be discordant, and either process may occur alone. (From Grumbach MM: The neuroendocrinology of pregnancy. Hospital Practice, March 1980, pp 51–60, with permission.)

5. What is Tanner staging?

Tanner staging is a rating system for pubertal development named after the man who proposed it, J. M. Tanner. Because young people mature at different rates, chronologic age is a poor index of physiologic maturity. The Tanner rating system is based on the orderly, progressive development of breasts and pubic hair in the female and genitalia and pubic hair in males. There are five developmental stages for girls and five for boys (see figures on pp 88–89).

6. What is sequencing?

Sequencing refers to the usual order in which the concurrent development of genitalia, breasts, pubic hair, and the soma occurs in girls and boys. Although the sequence is not exactly the same in all girls and boys, it is much less variable than the age at which the events occur.

Tanner Staging

Stages of Breast Development in Females

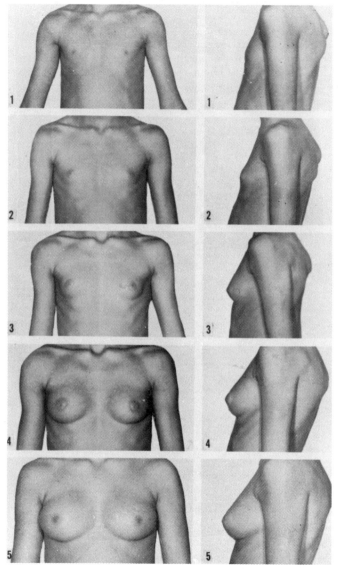

Stage 1: Prepubertal—no breast tissue
Stage 2: Appearance of a breast bud
Stage 3: Enlargement of breast and areola
Stage 4: Areola and nipple form a mound atop underlying breast tissue
Stage 5: Adult configuration, with areola and breast having smooth contour

(From Tanner JM: Growth at Adolescence, 2nd ed. Oxford, Blackwell, 1962, with permission.)

7. What is adrenarche?

Adrenarche is the maturational increase in the adrenal production of 17-ketosteroids, dehydroepiandrosterone (DHEA), and DHEA-sulfate (DHEAS); it accounts for the normal development of axillary and pubic hair, particularly in females.

8. What is the first visible sign of puberty in girls?

The breast bud; this usually appears first at about the age of 10–11 years, but may appear as early as 8 years of age or as late as 14 years of age.

Tanner Staging

Stages of Development of Pubic Hair in Females

Stage 1: Prepubertal—no pubic
hair
Stage 2: Sparse downy hair at
medial aspect of labia
majora
Stage 3: Darkening, coarsening,
curling of hair, which
extends upward and
laterally
Stage 4: Hair of adult consistency
limited to the mons
Stage 5: Hair spreads to medial
aspect of thighs

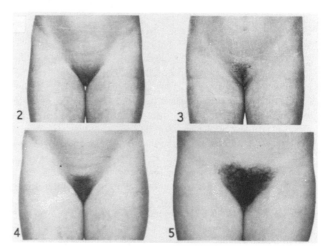

Development of Pubic Hair and Genitalia in Males

Pubic Hair
Stage 1: Prepubertal—no pubic
hair
Stage 2: Sparse downy hair at
base of phallus
Stage 3: Darkening, coarsening,
curling of hair, which
extends upward and
laterally
Stage 4: Hair of adult consistency
limited to the mons
Stage 5: Hair spreads to medial
aspect of thighs

Genitalia
Stage 1: Childhood size and configuration of genitalia
Stage 2: Enlargement of testes
and scrotum, the latter
reddening and thinning

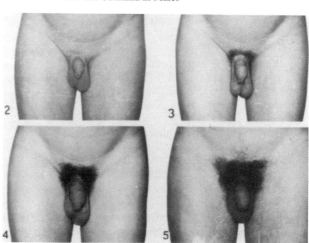

Stage 3: Lengthening of penis, associated with further enlargement of testes and scrotum
Stage 4: Widening as well as further lengthening of penis. Further enlargement of testes and scrotum, and
deepening pigmentation of scrotal skin
Stage 5: Adult configuration and size of genitalia

(From Tanner JM: Growth at Adolescence, 2nd ed. Oxford, Blackwell, 1962, with permission.)

9. What is the first visible sign of puberty in boys?

Darkening and thinning of the scrotum; this usually becomes evident at age 11–12 years, but
may appear as early as 9 years of age or as late as 14 years of age.

10. Do boys develop more slowly than girls?

Yes. Visible evidence of puberty usually becomes evident about 6–9 months earlier in girls
than boys (age 10½ compared with age 11 years). Additionally, once initiated, puberty usually is

completed within 3 years in girls and 5 years in boys. Differences in the rate of development are accentuated because the height spurt, one of the most obvious events of puberty, occurs earlier in the sequence of pubertal development in girls than boys.

11. Are there differences in physique between young people who mature early and those who mature late?

Yes, but these differences are usually evident prior to puberty. In general, mesomorphs begin to develop earlier and more rapidly than do ectomorphs. The result is that early-maturing girls and boys tend to have a rounder appearance and broader hips, whereas later maturing girls and boys tend to have broader shoulders and a more linear appearance. These differences are, however, only partly due to the timing and duration of the pubertal growth spurt. The prolonged growth spurt that allows for more leg and shoulder growth in the later maturers only adds finishing touches to a linear physique that is recognizable in childhood.

12. What is the theory of critical body fat?

The theory of critical body fat was proposed by Dr. Rose Frisch and colleagues; it suggests that girls must reach a certain level of body fat (17%) to menstruate, and a higher level (22%) to ovulate. The theory is teleologically appealing and helps to explain the association between body weight and menarche (fatter girls typically experience an earlier menarche than do thinner girls) and the loss of menstrual function associated with weight loss (e.g., anorexia, exercise, and starvation). However, current data do not support the concept that a certain level of body fat is a prerequisite for menarche (or menstruation); rather, it seems likely that the two events—increasing body fat and reproductive maturation—proceed together, undoubtedly stimulated by a third, common factor.

13. What is the secular trend?

The secular trend refers to the gradual decrease in the average age at menarche, which has been noted over the last three to four decades. The cause is unknown but has been attributed to better nutrition, improved sanitation, less physical work, and the electric light bulb.

14. Do girls stop growing after menarche?

No. Growth slows but does not cease at menarche. Although peak height velocity invariably precedes menarche, menarche is not a constant milestone and does not occur at the same point in the sequence of pubertal development in all girls. Growth continues at a decelerating rate for a number of years after menarche; this is particularly true for early-maturing girls.

15. Does menarche mark the attainment of reproductive maturity in girls?

No. Following menarche the female reproductive system continues to mature for approximately 3–5 years. During this time the number of ovulatory cycles increases from approximately 10% to 90%, and the duration of the menstrual cycle decreases. These postmenarcheal changes in the menstrual cycle are associated with a gradual rise in the follicular phase level of FSH and the luteal phase level of progesterone. These changes enable conception and also help to explain the frequent occurrence of dysfunctional uterine bleeding and subfecundity during early adolescence.

16. Do boys achieve reproductive maturity sooner than girls?

Yes; spermarche, unlike menarche, is usually an event of early puberty; in most males, sperm production begins prior to the development of significant pubic hair; thus a relatively physically immature appearing boy could father a child.

17. What is the pineal gland and does it affect pubertal development?

Descartes referred to the pineal gland as "the seat of the soul"; it has also been called "the third eye" by physiologists. The pineal gland produces a substance called melatonin, which suppresses gonadal development. Synthesis of melatonin is controlled by the day-night (circadian) cycle; light suppresses synthesis. The role of the pineal gland in controlling mammalian reproduction, especially among seasonal breeders, is well established, although prolonged and extreme diminution of the photo period reportedly reduces reproductive function in humans. Attempts to demonstrate a functional link between the pineal gland and human reproduction have yielded very equivocal results.

18. What is precocious puberty?

Precocious puberty is difficult to define because of the marked variation in the age at which puberty begins normally. Onset of puberty before age $8\frac{1}{2}$ years in girls and before 10 years in boys may be considered precocious; these are arbitrary guidelines. In about 80–90% of girls and about 50% of boys, no causative factor can be found. Presumably the normal hypothalamic mechanism that initiates puberty is just activated earlier; subtle cerebral abnormalities are detected in many children, suggesting a primary central nervous system dysfunction. New radiologic imaging techniques (magnetic resonance imaging) may reveal etiologies in these cases.

19. What is the difference between precocious puberty and precocious pseudopuberty?

Precocious pubertal development may be classified as true precocious puberty or precocious pseudopuberty. True precocious puberty is always isosexual (same sex) and involves the development of secondary sexual characteristics and an increase in the size and activity of the gonads. Precocious pseudopuberty involves the maturation of secondary sexual characteristics, but not the gonad, as there is no activation of the hypothalamic-pituitary-gonadal axis. Excessive exogenous synthesis of gonadal steroids (by the adrenal gland, tumors, or cysts) is the most common cause of precocious pseudopuberty; prolonged exposure to exogenous gonadal hormones may mature the central nervous system and cause true precocious puberty in some children.

20. What is McCune-Albright syndrome?

McCune-Albright syndrome is the association of fibrous dysplasia of the skeletal system with patchy cutaneous pigmentation and precocious pubertal development. The condition affects girls more often than boys. The endocrinologic manifestations of the disease appear to reflect the autonomous hyperfunctioning of the peripheral target glands. The average age at menarche in affected girls is about 3, but menarche may occur in infancy.

21. What is congenital adrenal hyperplasia?

Congenital adrenal hyperplasia is an autosomal recessive disorder caused by a defect in one of the adrenal enzymes necessary for the synthesis of cortisol. By far the most frequent form of the disorder is caused by a deficiency of the 21-hydroxylase enzyme. The defect not only causes a deficiency of cortisol, but also, in many cases, of aldosterone, which in turn leads to salt wasting. The adrenal gland produces excessive amounts of the precursors of cortisol and aldosterone, weak androgens. The syndrome is usually diagnosed in the newborn period; it is a common cause of virilization in females and isosexual precocious pseudopuberty in males.

22. What is premature thelarche? What causes it?

Premature thelarche is the early development of breast tissue only. It most often appears at birth or during the first year of life. Breast development may progress within the next 2–5 years in some girls. Premature thelarche is usually a benign condition and may be familial in some instances. Other aspects of pubertal development may not appear; plasma levels of gonadotropins, prolactin, and estrogen are within normal limits. The condition is thought to be caused by secretion of small amounts of estrogen by the ovaries. Although premature thelarche is a benign condition, enlargement of the breasts may be the first sign of precocious puberty or precocious pseudopuberty; a prolonged period of observation is therefore indicated.

23. What is delayed puberty?

Delayed puberty is difficult to define, again, because of the marked variation in age at which puberty normally begins. In girls and boys who show no signs of pubertal development by 14 years of age, puberty is usually considered to be delayed. Once initiated, pubertal development is usually completed in approximately 3 years in girls and 5 years in boys. Girls who require more than 4–5 years and boys who require more than 6 years to complete the pubertal process are usually considered to have delayed puberty. In over 90% of cases, no cause is found; a delay is presumed to exist in the initiation of the pubertal hypothalamic-pituitary, sleep-associated, LH secretory pattern. The latter condition is referred to as constitutionally delayed puberty and appears to be familial in many cases.

24. Is delayed puberty more of a problem for boys or girls? Why?

Boys. Boys who develop later and/or more slowly than their peers more often seek medical advice and many have significant psychosocial difficulties (behavioral problems, poor self-esteem, school phobia) related to their immature appearance and short stature. Slow-growing girls rarely exhibit these problems because they are less apt to be bullied and teased by peers. Both girls and boys may regress behaviorally, because adults tend to treat "late bloomers" like younger children.

25. Is precocious puberty more of a problem for boys or girls? Why?

Girls. Girls who develop earlier and/or more rapidly than their peers often exhibit psychosocial difficulties (behavioral problems, poor self-esteem, school phobia, precocious sexual activity), whereas boys who develop early often become the class president or the captain of the football team. The reasons appear to reflect the social norms and expectations of society rather than any physiologic differences between boys and girls.

BIBLIOGRAPHY

1. Apter D, Viinikka L, Vihko R: Hormonal pattern of adolescent menstrual cycles. J Clin Endocrinol Metab 47:944–954, 1978.
2. Cameron JL: Metabolic cues for the onset of puberty. Horm Res 36(3–4):97–103, 1991.
3. Carpenter SE: Psychosocial menstrual disorders: Stress, exercise and diet's effect on the menstrual cycle. Curr Opin Obstet Gynecol 6:536–539, 1994.
4. Denniston CR: Assessing normal and abnormal patterns of growth. Prim Care 21(4):637–654, 1994.
5. Litt IF: Evaluation of the Adolescent Patient. Philadelphia, Hanley & Belfus, 1990.
6. McCauley E: Disorders of sexual differentiation and development. Psychological aspects. Pediatr Clin North Am 37:1405–1420, 1990.
7. Morales AJ, Holden JP, Murphy AA: Pediatric and adolescent gynecologic endocrinology. Curr Opin Obstet Gynecol 4:860–866, 1992.
8. Reiter EO, Grumbach MM: Neuroendocrine control mechanisms and the onset of puberty. Annu Rev Physiol 44:595–613, 1982.
9. Remschmidt H: Psychosocial milestones in normal puberty and adolescence. Horm Res 41(Suppl 2): 19–29, 1994.
10. Roemmich JN, Rogol AD: Physiology of growth and development. Its relationship to performance in the young athlete. Clin Sports Med 14:483–502, 1995.
11. Rosenfield RL: Puberty and its disorders in girls. Endocrinol Metab Clin North Am 20:15–42, 1991.
12. Styne DM: Physiology of puberty. Horm Res 41(Suppl 2):306, 1994.
13. Tanner JM: Growth of Adolescence. Oxford, Blackwell, 1962.

25. AMENORRHEA

Nadine Burrington, M.D.

1. What is amenorrhea?

Complete absence of menstruation in a woman of reproductive age.

2. What is the most common cause of amenorrhea?

Pregnancy.

3. What is the difference between primary and secondary amenorrhea? What is the incidence of each?

Primary amenorrhea

- The absence of menses in a female who has not menstruated by the age of 16 years, regardless of normal growth and development of secondary sexual characteristics, *or*
- The absence of menses in a female who has not menstruated by the age of 14 years in the absence of normal growth or development of secondary sexual characteristics.
- The incidence of primary amenorrhea is less than 0.1%.

Secondary amenorrhea

- The absence of menses for longer than 6–12 months, *or*
- The absence of menses for a total of three previous cycle intervals.
- The incidence of secondary amenorrhea is approximately 0.7%.

4. What are the most common causes of primary amenorrhea?

Gonadal failure, such as Turner's syndrome. Gonadal agenesis accounts for one-third of all patients with primary amenorrhea. One-third of patients with gonadal failure have cardiovascular or renal abnormalities.

Müllerian anomalies, such as uterovaginal agenesis (Rokitansky-Kuster-Hauser syndrome), are the second most common cause, accounting for 20% of primary amenorrhea. They occur in 1 per 4000 female births.

5. A 14-year-old girl presents with complaints of monthly abdominal pain, but no menses. What is her diagnosis?

Imperforate hymen or transverse vaginal septum.

6. What is Kallmann's syndrome?

Primary amenorrhea secondary to inadequate release of gonadotropin-releasing hormone (GnRH) and anosmia. Patients have infantile sexual development. A pituitary tumor is rarely seen in patients with hypogonadotropic hypogonadism, but a craniopharyngioma may present with amenorrhea. Therefore, imaging of the hypothalamic-pituitary area is recommended.

7. Primary amenorrhea and breast development with absence of the uterus are found in which two syndromes?

1. Patients with androgen insensitivity or testicular feminization are XY genotype, but phenotypically are females because an androgen intracellular receptor is not functioning (a maternal X-linked recessive gene). Androgen induction of the Wolffian duct system does not occur despite normal male levels of testosterone. Because müllerian inhibiting factor (MIF) is still present, the müllerian system does not develop. Patients typically have large breasts with immature nipples but no axillary or pubic hair.

Incomplete testicular feminization with some pubic hair, axillary hair, and phallic development occurs in patients with Lubs, Reifensteins, Rosevaters, or Gilbert-Dreyfus syndrome.

Patients should be allowed to finish normal sexual maturity. After age 20, the gonads should be removed because 20% of patients develop gonadoblastoma or dysgerminoma.

2. Patients with müllerian agenesis have sexual hair and mature nipples. Because 40% have associated renal anomalies, intravenous pyelography or ultrasound should be performed.

8. What test can be used to distinguish between testicular feminization syndrome and congenital absence of the uterus?

Serum testosterone level is in the normal female range in congenital absence of the uterus and in the normal male range in testicular feminization syndrome. Only patients with testosterone levels in the normal male range need karyotype to confirm the diagnosis. Such patients need hormone replacement and removal of gonads.

9. What rare enzyme defects can cause amenorrhea?

1. Deficiency of 17-alpha-hydroxylase prevents the formation of sex hormones. In 46 XX patients, this leads to the absence of breast development, although the uterus is present. In 46 XY patients, there is also no breast development; the uterus is absent because of the presence of MIF. These patients also have hypernatremia, hypokalemia, and hypertension because of increased mineralocorticoid production. Sodium retention and potassium excretion are excessive. Cortisol production is decreased. Therefore, patients require cortisol as well as sex hormone replacement to attain breast development and to prevent osteoporosis.

2. Deficiency of 17-20-desmolase prevents the formation of estrogen and testosterone but not of aldosterone, cortisol, or progesterone. Patients do not have breast development (or uterus development in XY patients).

10. A 15-year-old girl complains of amenorrhea. She is in the 25th percentile for height and weight. She is not an athlete and has an appropriate diet. On physical examination, she has no evidence of breast growth or pubic hair, but vagina and uterus are present. What work-up will help to determine the cause of amenorrhea?

The patient has no evidence of estrogenization. Serum gonadotropin levels help to determine whether the patient has gonadal failure or unstimulated gonads.

An elevated serum gonadotropin level indicates gonadal failure. A karyotype usually shows an X-chromosome abnormality, causing gonadal dysgenesis. Patients should have a chest radiograph, electrocardiogram, intravenous pyelography, and thyroid function tests to evaluate the common problems associated with gonadal dysgenesis. If the patient has an XY-chromosome, the gonads must be removed after bone growth.

Hypogonadism indicates unstimulated gonads. Patients must be evaluated for intracranial tumors by checking thyroid function tests, growth hormone, prolactin, and cortisol. Pituitary stimulation tests also may be appropriate. Skull radiographs for calcifications and evaluation of the sella turcica region and CT of the pituitary region are also recommended.

11. Should athletic amenorrhea be treated?

The cause of amenorrhea in athletic women with no other etiology is not well understood, although many patients have eating disorders as well as high stress levels. Many patients are hypoestrogenic with significant loss of bone density that may lead to osteoporosis and stress fractures. Patients should be encouraged to improve their diet, to decrease stress levels, to decrease the amount of strenuous exercise, if possible, and to replace estrogen and progesterone, if other changes do not increase estrogen levels.

12. How do stress and exercise cause amenorrhea?

Stress and exercise cause an increase in levels of catecohol estrogens and beta endorphins; this influences the release of GnRH by acting on the neurotransmitters. Without appropriate GnRH release, follicle-stimulating hormone (FSH) and luteinizing hormone (LH) are not released appropriately; the result is anovulation, which may lead to amenorrhea.

13. How does weight loss cause amenorrhea?

At < 15% of ideal body weight, normal GnRH release does not occur. At < 25% of ideal body weight, not only is GnRH release abnormal, but pituitary release of LH and FSH is abnormal and the pituitary cannot be induced to secrete LH and FSH normally, even if GnRH is supplied in the normal pulsatile function.

14. Which drugs cause amenorrhea?

1. Any drug that stimulates prolactin secretion
2. Antipsychotics, such as phenothiazine derivatives, haloperidol, and droperidol (Inapsine)
3. Tricyclic antidepressants
4. Antihypertensives, such as reserpine and methyldopa
5. Antianxiety agents, such as benzodiazepines
6. Other drugs, such as metoclopramide (Reglan), opiates, barbiturates, and estrogens.

15. What psychiatric disorder in adolescents is a major cause of amenorrhea?

Anorexia nervosa is a major cause of amenorrhea. The incidence of anorexia nervosa is 1 per 1000 white female adolescents. Besides amenorrhea, patients have severe weight loss, often with bradycardia, hypotension, constipation, dry skin, hypothermia, and low levels of triiodothyronine (T_3) due to impaired peripheral conversion of thyroxine to T_3. The mortality rate is 5–15%.

16. What are the pituitary causes of amenorrhea?

1. Damaged cells—lack of LH and FSH secretion due to anorexia, thrombosis, or hemorrhage (as in Sheehan's syndrome; related to hypotension in pregnancy) or Simmonds syndrome (unrelated to pregnancy).
2. Neoplasms—most secrete prolactin but are not always associated with galactorrhea.
3. Amenorrhea—also associated with acromegaly and Cushing's syndrome.

17. What percentage of amenorrhea is due to hyperprolactinemia?

10–20%.

18. What initial blood tests should be performed on a patient with amenorrhea?

Thyroid function tests to rule out rare cases of asymptomatic hypothyroidism. Patients with hypothyroidism return to regular menses with thyroid replacement.

Prolactin levels to rule out hyperprolactinemia, which may occur even without galactorrhea. Patients with galactorrhea should also undergo a coned down view of the sella turcica or a CT scan to rule out a small pituitary adenoma.

19. What is "post-pill" amenorrhea?

Post-pill amenorrhea is due to suppression of the hypothalamic-pituitary axis, which can persist for several months after discontinuing oral contraceptive pills. The incidence of post-pill amenorrhea lasting > 6 months is equal to the incidence of secondary amenorrhea. It is no longer thought that oral contraceptive pills cause prolonged amenorrhea or infertility; thus other etiologies must be considered.

20. What is premature ovarian failure?

Ovarian failure and thus amenorrhea before age 40. Patients have symptoms of hypoestrogenism, increased FSH, and generalized sclerosis or only primordial follicles with no progression past the antrum stage on ovarian biopsy. Many patients have autoimmune diseases, such as Hashimoto's, Addison's, and hypoparathyroidism. If the patient is younger than 25, a karyotype should be performed to determine whether the patient is a 46XX/46XY mosaic. If so, the gonads must be removed to prevent malignancy after age 20.

Antithyroid antibodies, antinuclear antibody, and 24-hour cortisol levels also should be checked. Ovarian failure may result from irradiation or chemotherapy.

21. What is a progesterone challenge test?

A progesterone challenge test is an intramuscular injection of 100–200 mg of progesterone in oil or 10 mg of oral medroxyprogesterone acetate for 5 days. A positive test is any bleeding (even spotting) within 2 weeks of the test.

22. What does a positive progesterone challenge test indicate?

The patient has a serum estradiol level > 40 pg/ml; thus the anterior pituitary is producing LH and FSH and the endometrium and outflow tract are functioning. This indicates that, if the thyroid function tests and prolactin levels are normal, the patient is anovulatory.

23. What tests should be performed on a patient with amenorrhea after a progesterone challenge test reveals no bleeding?

A course of conjugated estrogen, 2.5 mg for 21 days prior to progesterone challenge, should be used to define a uterine defect as the cause of amenorrhea. This includes complete destruction of the endometrial lining by Asherman's disease or fibrosis after severe endometritis. This step need not be done if the patient has no history suggestive of any of these problems.

FSH level should next be assessed. If FSH is elevated, the patient has premature ovarian failure. If FSH is normal, a CT scan of the hypothalamus-pituitary area should be done to rule out a central nervous system tumor, such as craniopharyngiomas and granulomatous diseases (tuberculosis, sarcoid). Reserves of adrenocorticotropic hormone should be checked. If all of these tests are normal, the diagnosis of exclusion is hypothalamic-pituitary failure. All patients are hypoestrogenic and need hormone replacement.

BIBLIOGRAPHY

1. Frisch RE, McArthur JW: Menstrual cycles: Fatness as a determinant of minimum weight for height necessary for their maintenance or onset. Science 185:949, 1974.
2. Jacobs HS, Knuth UA, Hull MG, et al: Postpill amenorrhea: Cause or coincidence. BMJ 2:940, 1977.
3. Keltzky OA, Davajan V: Management of amenorrhea and associated disorders. Curr Opin Obstet Gynecol 2:386, 1990.
4. Kletzky OA, Davajan V, Makamura RM, Mishell DR: Classification of secondary amenorrhea based on distinct hormonal patterns. J Clin Endocrinol Metab 41:660, 1975.
5. Schacter M, Shoham Z: Amenorrhea during the reproductive years—is it safe? Fertil Steril 62:1, 1994.
6. Tulandi T, Kinch RA: Premature ovarian failure. Obstet Gynecol Surv 36:521, 1981.

26. ANOVULATION AND INDUCTION OF OVULATION

Sam E. Alexander, M.D.

1. How can lack of ovulation be clinically recognized?

The anovulatory woman may complain of lack of menses, irregular menses, or heavy menstrual flow. Molimina, the feeling of impending menstruation, and dysmenorrhea are typically absent in anovulatory cycles. In the absence of ovulation, there is no corpus luteum formation on the ovary. Without a functional corpus luteum, the ovary does not secrete enough progesterone to cause secretory transformation of the proliferative endometrium. Without withdrawal of progesterone support from the secretory endometrium, there is no organized endometrial shedding. This results in either amenorrhea or endometrial bleeding that is unpredictable in frequency and quantity.

2. What are the causes of anovulation?

Anovulation may originate from dysfunction at any level of the hypothalamic–pituitary–ovarian axis. Aberrations in the pulsatile release of gonadotropin-releasing hormone (GnRH) from the hypothalamus result in deficiency in the pituitary secretion of follicle-stimulating hormone (FSH) and luteinizing hormone (LH). Without appropriate gonadotropin stimulation, ovarian folliculogenesis and ovulation fail to occur. An interruption of this sequence of events at any step inhibits ovulation.

3. What are the causes of hypothalamic anovulation?

Hypothalamic anovulation may be caused by stress, strenuous exercise, weight loss, or eating disorders, any of which may result in decreased amplitude and frequency of the pulsatile secretion of GnRH from the hypothalamus. Isolated gonadotropin deficiency (Kallmann's syndrome) refers to a defect in GnRH secretion that is an autosomal dominant trait associated with anosmia.

4. How does hypothalamic anovulation differ from polycystic ovarian disease?

Polycystic ovarian disease (Stein-Leventhal syndrome) is characterized by the presence of multiple small follicles within the ovaries, none of which achieves the dominance necessary to develop into a preovulatory follicle. This condition results from tonically elevated LH levels and absence of the preovulatory surge that is necessary to achieve ovulation.

5. Can pituitary causes of anovulation be distinguished from hypothalamic causes?

Insufficient serum FSH and LH concentrations are usually due to poor stimulation of the pituitary by hypothalamic GnRH. If the gonadotropin deficiency is due to primary pituitary insufficiency, however, low serum concentrations of the other pituitary hormones also may be seen. Adrenal insufficiency may result from low levels of adrenocorticotropic hormone (ACTH), and hypothyroidism may arise from low levels of thyroid-stimulating hormone (TSH). This picture is seen with Sheehan syndrome, a type of hypopituitarism caused by pituitary ischemia at the time of postpartum hemorrhage. It also may be seen with neoplasms occupying the sella turcica and suprasellar area. Prolactin-secreting pituitary adenomas may result in galactorrhea and ovulatory disorders ranging from deficient luteal phase progesterone production to frank anovulation. The diagnosis is suspected by finding an elevated serum prolactin concentration and is confirmed by CT scan or MRI of the sella turcica.

6. Can the ovaries in a young woman fail to respond to stimulation by pituitary gonadotropins?

Yes. When the ovaries do not respond to gonadotropin stimulation by growth of follicles and production of estrogen and inhibin, secretion of FSH and LH increases because of absence of the normal negative feedback inhibition of estrogen and inhibin on the pituitary. Failure of ovarian response may result from gonadal dysgenesis, resistant ovary syndrome, or premature ovarian failure. In any case, poor ovarian estrogen production results in estrogen deprivation symptoms, including an increased risk of osteoporosis, unless estrogen replacement therapy is implemented.

7. What is the goal of therapy for the anovulatory woman with ovarian failure?

The choice of therapy for anovulation depends on the underlying cause of the anovulation and the patient's desire for fertility. In patients with ovarian failure, the main therapeutic aim is prevention of the consequences of estrogen deprivation, including vasomotor symptoms, urogenital atrophy, osteoporosis, and risk of cardiovascular disease. These conditions can be avoided with estrogen replacement therapy given in conjunction with a progestational agent to prevent endometrial hyperplasia and carcinoma. Likewise, estrogen replacement therapy should be considered in the hypoestrogenic woman with hypothalamic anovulation who is not desirous of pregnancy.

8. How should ovulation be induced in a woman found to have an elevation of serum prolactin?

After evaluating the sella turcica radiographically for the presence of a pituitary adenoma, ovulation usually can be induced by lowering the serum prolactin concentration with the dopamine agonist, bromocriptine. If the TSH level is elevated, indicating that the hyperprolactinemia is due to primary hypothyroidism, thyroid hormone replacement is appropriate.

9. What if the hyperprolactinemic woman has no evidence of an adenoma and is not interested in conception?

Some evidence suggests that hyperprolactinemia may place a woman at risk for osteoporosis even if she is not hypoestrogenic; thus normalization of the serum prolactin level with bromocriptine may be considered. No firm evidence, however, indicates that bromocriptine therapy is necessary in the ovulatory woman with mild hyperprolactinemia.

10. Does the well-estrogenized woman require treatment if she is not attempting pregnancy?

Yes, but it is not necessary to induce ovulation. If the woman has normal gonadotropin levels, copious cervical mucus, and withdrawal bleeding after progestin therapy, she is at risk for the development of endometrial hyperplasia because of constant endometrial stimulation unopposed by progesterone.

11. How can endometrial hyperplasia be avoided in this setting?

An oral progestin—such as medroxyprogesterone acetate, 10 mg—can be given for at least 10 days every 1–3 months. If the woman is sexually active and desires contraception, an oral contraceptive is ideal to provide contraception as well as cyclic progestational activity.

12. How is endometrial hyperplasia prevented if the woman wishes to attempt pregnancy?

After ovulation is induced, the ovarian production of progesterone effectively prevents the development of hyperplasia, as in a spontaneously ovulatory cycle. There is no indication, however, for induction of ovulation in a woman who is not actively attempting pregnancy.

13. If serum prolactin and gonadotropin levels are normal, how is ovulation induced?

Clomiphene citrate, a nonsteroidal antiestrogen, binds to pituitary and hypothalamic estrogen receptors to prevent the negative feedback effects of estrogen. This results in an elevation of FSH levels and subsequent follicular growth. Therapy is started with 50 mg daily on cycle days 5–9 and is increased in subsequent cycles by 50 mg/day to a maximum of 200–250 mg daily on cycle days 5–9 until ovulation occurs.

14. How is ovulation verified?

After ovulation, the basal body temperature rises by 0.4–0.6°F, the dominant follicle may be seen to collapse by ultrasound, serum progesterone rises to a level over 3 ng/ml, and the endometrium becomes secretory. Before ovulation, a surge of LH is released by the pituitary gland. Detection of this surge by home urinary LH testing and detection of a rise in basal body temperature are the two most common and cost-effective ways of detecting ovulation.

15. What other ancillary investigations should be performed before inducing ovulation?

Semen analysis and hysterosalpingography should be shown to be normal. In patients with a history of dysfunctional bleeding, an endometrial biopsy should be performed to rule out endometrial neoplasia.

16. What can be done if ovulation fails to occur with clomiphene?

After following follicular growth on clomiphene to a diameter of about 20 mm, an intramuscular injection of 10,000 IU of human chorionic gonadotropin (HCG) may be given to simulate the LH surge and trigger ovulation. In the hyperandrogenic woman, addition of low-dose dexamethasone (0.5 mg) nightly may enhance follicular development by diminishing the androgen milieu. If these methods fail to result in ovulation or pregnancy, therapy with gonadotropins (Pergonal, Metrodin, or Humagon) is indicated.

17. What is the role of wedge resection in the management of women with polycystic ovarian disease?

In the past, a wedge-shaped section of each ovary was removed by laparotomy to enhance ovulation by decreasing ovarian androgen production. This procedure often results in spontaneous ovulation for a few cycles, but the effect is short-lived and the surgery results in a high incidence of periovarian adhesions, which may adversely affect fertility. Laparoscopic cautery or laser destruction of ovarian stroma ("whiffle-balling") appears to have a similar effect on ovulation but is also associated with postoperative adhesion formation. Neither procedure should be considered as first-line therapy for polycystic ovarian disease; both should be reserved for the rare patient who does not respond to clomiphene citrate, cannot afford gonadotropin therapy, and has no other options.

18. How successful is clomiphene therapy?

Although 80% of women ovulate on clomiphene, only about 40% conceive. This discrepancy occurs primarily because other fertility factors are frequently found to be suboptimal in anovulatory women.

19. How is ovulation induced in the hypoestrogenic woman with hypothalamic amenorrhea?

Clomiphene is unlikely to be successful in such patients. The method of choice is to supply FSH directly by administering intramuscular gonadotropins such as Metrodin or Humagon. Administration is begun early in the follicular phase, with the dose titrated according to the individual's response as measured by follicular ultrasound and serum estradiol levels. HCG is given to trigger ovulation when the dominant follicle is 16–18 mm in diameter.

20. Are there other options for induction of ovulation?

GnRH may be given to stimulate the pituitary secretion of FSH and LH. It is administered either subcutaneously or intravenously in a pulsatile manner, with doses delivered every 60–120 minutes by a portable pump. The cost and effectiveness are similar to that of gonadotropin treatment, and the risk of multiple birth or ovarian hyperstimulation syndrome is lower. Because an indwelling catheter is required for about 2 weeks to deliver the medication, the method is unwieldy and not usually preferred by patients.

21. What are the risks of ovulation induction?

The risks include multiple gestation and ovarian hyperstimulation syndrome. Ovarian hyperstimulation syndrome is a potentially life-threatening condition characterized by ovarian enlargement, ascites, hemoconcentration, and hypercoagulability.

22. How are these risks minimized?

Because they occur more commonly with gonadotropin administration, it is important to monitor ovarian response to these medications by serial ultrasound measurement of follicular growth and serum estradiol levels.

BIBLIOGRAPHY

1. Adashi EY: Clomiphene citrate: Mechanism(s) and site(s) of action—a hypothesis revisited. Fertil Steril 42:331–334, 1984.
2. Adashi EY: Clomiphene citrate-initiated ovulation: A clinical update. Semin Reprod Endocrinol 4:255–276, 1986.
3. Berga SL, Mortola L, Girton L, et al: Neuroendocrine aberrations in women with functional hypothalamic amenorrhea. J Clin Endocrinol Metab 68:301–308, 1989.

 4. Coney PJ: Polycystic ovarian disease: Current concepts of pathophysiology and therapy. Fertil Steril 42:667–682, 1984.
 5. Fritz MA, Speroff L: The endocrinology of the menstrual cycle: The interaction of folliculogenesis and neuroendocrine mechanisms. Fertil Steril 38:509–529, 1982.
 6. Hammond MG, Halme JK, Talbert LM: Factors affecting pregnancy rate in clomiphene citrate induction of ovulation. Obstet Gynecol 62:196–202, 1983.
 7. Hanning RV, Strawn EY, Nolten WE: Pathophysiology of the ovarian hyperstimulation syndrome. Fertil Steril 66:220–224, 1985.
 8. Kerin JF, Liu JH, Pillipou G, Yen SSC: Evidence for a hypothalamic site of action of clomiphene citrate in women. J Clin Endocrinol Metab 61:265–268, 1985.
 9. Naether OGJ, Fischer R: Adhesion formation after laparoscopic electrocoagulation of the ovarian surface in polycystic ovary patients. Fertil Steril 60:95–98, 1993.
10. Navot D, Bergh PA, Laufer N: Ovarian hyperstimulation syndrome in novel reproductive technologies: Prevention and treatment. Fertil Steril 58:249–261, 1992.
11. Reid RL, Fretts R, Van Vugt DA: The theory and practice of ovulation induction with gonadotropin-releasing hormone. Am J Obstet Gynecol 158:176–185, 1988.

27. POLYCYSTIC OVARIAN SYNDROME

John Harrington, D.O., and George Betz, M.D., Ph.D.

1. List the common synonyms for polycystic ovarian syndrome (PCOS).

Stein-Leventhal syndrome
Chronic hyperandrogenism
Chronic oligo-ovulation

2. What are the criteria for diagnosing PCOS?

Perimenarcheal onset of menstrual irregularity
Increased body weight (in some women)
Physical and laboratory evidence of androgen excess
Chronic anovulation
Inappropriate gonadotropin secretions
Euprolactinemia

3. Which syndromes may be confused with PCOS?

Hyperprolactinemia
Late-onset adrenal hyperplasia
Ovarian and adrenal neoplasms
Cushing's syndrome
These conditions can be excluded by physical exam and the following tests:
  • Serum prolactin
  • 17-OH progesterone
  • Serum testosterone (elevated in both adrenal hyperplasia and neoplasms), dehydro-epiandosterone (DHEA-S)
  • 1-mg overnight dexamethasone suppression test

4. What are the most common clinical manifestations of PCOS?

Symptoms	Frequency (%)
Infertility	74
Hirsutism	69
Amenorrhea	51
Obesity	41

5. What laboratory values may be abnormal in patients with PCOS?
Elevated values may be found for:
- Testosterone
- Dehydroepiandrosterone (DHEA)
- Androstenedione
- Dehydroepiandrosterone sulfate (DHEA-S)
- Estrone
- Luteinizing hormone (LH)

Low values may be found for:
- Estradiol
- Follicle-stimulating hormone (FSH)

6. What is the LH/FSH ratio in PCOS?
The ratio is 3:1 (in contrast with the normal ratio of 1.5:1).

7. What is the basis for chronic anovulation in PCOS?
The secretion of excessive amounts of androgen and its subsequent conversion to estrogen or the secretion of abnormal levels of gonadotropin by the pituitary is the basis for chronic anovulation.

8. Where do the excessive androgens come from?
In about 50% of the cases the androgens come from both the ovary and the adrenal gland.

9. What percentage of patients with PCOS have elevated levels of DHEA-S?
50%.

10. Where is the DHEA-S produced?
Over 95% comes from the adrenal gland.

11. What causes the chronically elevated total estrogen levels found in PCOS?
Elevated androgens account for the elevated total estrogen levels through peripheral conversion of androstenedione to estrone.

12. What happens to sex hormone-binding globulin (SHBG) in patients with increased testosterone?
It decreases.

13. What increases SHBG?
Estrogen.

14. What is the relationship between obesity and free testosterone?
Increased weight causes a decrease in SHBG, which in turn releases more free testosterone.

15. What is the significance of an increase in free testosterone?
In contrast with protein-bound hormone, the free steroid readily enters target cells.

16. What three conditions may be found in women with elevated serum testosterone?
Hyperandrogenism
Insulin resistance
Acanthosis nigricans

17. Describe acanthosis nigricans.
A gray-brown, velvety area of hyperpigmented skin is found in skin folds and on the back of the neck and in the axillae.

18. What is the cause of the hyperplastic theca cells in the PCOS ovary?
Chronic stimulation of the ovary by elevated LH.

19. What are the "cysts" in PCOS?
Atretic follicles.

20. If PCOS is inherited, what is the pattern of the inheritance?
X-linked dominant.

21. What percentage of patients with PCOS who take clomiphene will ovulate? Achieve pregnancy?
90% and 50%, respectively.

22. If clomiphene is unsuccessful in stimulating ovulation, what is the next form of therapy?
Human menopausal gonadotropin.

23. What therapy is useful for hirsutism associated with PCOS?
Spironolactone
Analog of gonadotropin-releasing hormone (GnRH)
Low-dose birth control pills that do not use norgestril for the progestin (norgestril is the most androgenic progestin in use today)

BIBLIOGRAPHY

1. Barbieri RL: Hyperandrogenism, insulin resistance and acanthosis nigricans. J Reprod Med 39:327, 1994.
2. Bradehaw KD, Carr BR: Polycystic ovarian syndrome. In Schlaff W, Rock J, et al (eds): Decision Making in Reproductive Endocrinology. London, Blackwell Scientific, 1993.
3. Carr BR: Chronic anovulation with estrogen present. In Wilson JD, Foster DW (eds): Williams' Textbook of Endocrinology, 8th ed. Philadelphia, W.B. Saunders, 1992.
4. Cheung AP, Chang RJ: Polycystic ovaries and other ovarian causes of hyperandrogenism. Infertil Reprod Med Clin North Am 1991.
5. Dunaif A, Mandel J, Fuhr H, Dobjansky A: The impact of obesity and chronic hyperinsulinemia on gonadal steroid secretion in the polycystic ovarian syndrome. J Clin Endocrinol Metab 66:131, 1988.

28. INFERTILITY

Robert J. Wester, M.D.

1. In counseling a couple who have sought your opinion concerning infertility, what do you tell them when asked about the chances of becoming pregnant?
The normal fecundability rate—that is, the chance of conception per cycle attempted—is about 0.2 or 20% in normally fertile couples. This figure is particularly useful in trying to understand the success rates (or lack thereof) for treatment modalities offered to infertile couples.

2. Is fecundability in couples related to their age?
Most certainly in women, much less so in men. Studies of pregnancy rates in women (who have azospermic husbands and undergo artificial donor insemination) demonstrate that the success of pregnancy is related to the woman's age. For women under 30 years old, the pregnancy rates were in the range of 70–75% but fell to 60% in women between 30 and 35 years old and 50% in women over age 36. Other studies of couples having difficulty achieving pregnancy noted infertility rates of 10% in women under age 30, 15% in women between 30 and 35 years old, 30% in women between 35 and 40 years old, and 60% in women over age 40.

3. How is infertility defined? How common is it?
Failure to conceive after 1 year of unprotected intercourse is the general definition of infertility. This problem affects 10–15% of couples of reproductive age (i.e., 15–44 years old).

4. Describe three important goals that a generalist obstetrician-gynecologist may wish to achieve in working with an infertile couple.

1. **Patient education.** A couple needs to know the basics of human reproduction, the chances of becoming pregnant, when best to have intercourse, common causes of infertility, investigative tests, cost and discomfort associated with tests, and therapies available, with expected success rates.

2. **Basic patient evaluation.** Essential elements include documentation of ovulation and tubal patency, assessment of peritoneal factors (adhesions and endometriosis), and testing for male factor problems.

3. **Emotional support and guidance.** The clinician should counsel the couple in how far to go in the work-up, when referral for more elaborate testing and therapy is appropriate, and when to consider adoption.

5. What are the general causes of infertility? How common is each?

Ovulatory dysfunction (10–25%)
Pelvic factors (tubal disease or endometriosis; 30–50%)
Male factor (30–40%)
Cervical factors (5–10%)
Unknown (also called unexplained)

6. Couples with infertility can be categorized into two general groups: those with low fecundability (i.e., hypofertile) and those who are sterile. Give examples of each group.

Couples in the first group include couples with oligoovulation, unexplained infertility, mild endometriosis, or oligospermia. Couples in the second group include those with bilateral tubal occlusion, ovulatory failure, or azospermia.

7. What is the difference between primary and secondary infertility?

Primary infertility is a condition in which the woman has never been pregnant despite more than 1 year of unprotected intercourse. A woman with **secondary infertility** has a history of a proven pregnancy (liveborn, ectopic, or abortion), yet is currently unable to conceive after 1 year of unprotected intercourse.

8. What are the characteristics of a normal semen analysis?

Volume > 2 ml	Sperm motility ≥ 50% with active progression
pH of 7.2–7.8	Normal sperm morphology ≥ 50%
Sperm count ≥ 20 million/ml	

9. Define unexplained infertility and discuss the treatment options available.

Despite current tests and knowledge, about 10% of couples who have been thoroughly investigated have no demonstrable cause of childlessness. It is appropriate to offer such couples superovulation with gonadotropin therapy and intrauterine insemination after a careful discussion of the risks, costs, and success rates.

10. A couple has just stopped using birth control and asks for general information about trying to conceive. What information should you provide?

Explain the natural fecundability rate (20% chance per cycle of achieving pregnancy), importance of avoiding smoking and caffeine (both of which may decrease fertility), preconceptional use of folic acid (e.g., prenatal vitamins) to minimize neural tube defects, and information about the timing of intercourse and when to return if not pregnant.

11. Ovulation dysfunction accounts for 10–15% of infertility. How is the adequacy of ovulation tested?

Presumptive evidence of ovulation can be determined by a biphasic basal body chart or noted by an elevated progesterone (> 5 ng/ml) in the luteal part of the menstrual cycle.

12. Of the causes of infertility, which is most consistently treated with success?

Treatment of ovulation disorders is successful in as many as 80–90% of cases, whereas the rate of successful treatment for other causes of infertility is closer to 30%.

13. What evidence from a patient's history is suggestive of ovulation?

Menses at regular monthly intervals
Mittelschmerz (localized lower quadrant discomfort during ovulation)
Moliminal symptoms (breast tenderness and pelvic discomfort)
Mild dysmenorrhea

14. Describe the most commonly used ovulation-inducing drug.

Clomiphene citrate is the most commonly used ovulation-inducing drug. It is a weak anti-estrogen that works at the hypothalamic level to initiate the changes needed to produce an ovulatory cycle. Complications and side effects include hot flashes, mood swings, multiple pregnancy (5–10% twins), ovarian cysts, and, rarely, visual disturbances.

15. Documentation of tubal patency is an important aspect of the infertility work-up. How is this initially done?

A hysterosalpingogram (HSG) is a radiographic procedure performed on an outpatient basis several days after the onset of menses. A radiopaque dye is injected transcervically into the uterine cavity. This allows assessment of the endometrial cavity structure, tubal patency, and tubal architecture.

16. What are the contraindications to an HSG? The possible complications?

Acute pelvic infection is an absolute contraindication. Women with adnexal tenderness demonstrated on pelvic exam or with a history of pelvic infection may benefit from a course of antibiotics (e.g., doxycycline) before the procedure. Possible complications include pain (which can be minimized by premedication with a nonsteroidal agent) and development of acute salpingitis (1–3% of procedures).

17. An HSG can demonstrate various uterine lesions. What are the more common ones?

Intrauterine adhesions
Submucous fibroids
Polyps

18. In choosing a dye for the performance of an HSG, why do most clinicians prefer a water-soluble contrast agent over an oil-based agent?

A water-soluble agent allows ideal visualization of the tubal mucosa, whereas an oil-based media obscures this detail of tubal anatomy.

19. When is it appropriate to offer laparoscopy to an infertile woman?

Laparoscopy allows endoscopic visualization of the internal female anatomy, thereby assessing the pelvis for peritubal or periovarian adhesions, endometriosis, and external structure of the uterus. Generally this test is offered to a woman after male factor and ovulatory functions have been noted to be normal or corrected. If distal tubal occlusion is found, it may be treated laparoscopically. Implants of endometriosis can be diagnosed and treated at the time of laparoscopy.

20. Does endometriosis cause infertility?

Although endometriosis is a relatively common gynecologic condition affecting 5–10% of women and a documented cause of pelvic pain and dysmenorrhea, the exact relationship between endometriosis and infertility is unclear. Treatment of mild endometriosis does not enhance infertility, but severe endometriosis can structurally damage the anatomic relationship between tubes and ovaries, leading to decreased fertility.

21. What is the postcoital test?

Within 12 hours of intercourse and at midcycle, a woman's cervical mucus is assessed for quality, quantity, and number of motile sperm. A normal postcoital test demonstrates abundant, clear, watery, relatively acellular cervical mucus with > 5 motile sperm present per high-powered field.

22. What is the most common cause of an abnormal postcoital test? How helpful is this test in the work-up of an infertile couple?

The most common cause of an abnormal postcoital test is mistiming. The value of the test has been called into question because many normally fertile couples have abnormal tests. Furthermore, the increasing use of intrauterine insemination with ovulation induction makes results of the test of less diagnostic benefit for many couples undergoing investigation of infertility.

23. How does the treatment of proximal and distal tubal disease differ?

Distal tubal disease is best treated surgically with distal salpingostomy. Proximal tubal disease may be treated with hysteroscopic tubal canalization. The presence of both proximal and distal disease is best treated with referral to reproductive endocrinology for in vitro fertilization.

24. What clues in the patient's history should alert the physician to the possibility of tubal factor?

A history of previous ectopic pregnancy, previous tubal surgery, ruptured appendix, tuberculosis, use of an intrauterine device, septic abortion, and sexually transmitted diseases, such as chlamydial infection and gonorrhea. Fifty percent of women with tubal damage and/or pelvic adhesions have no history of these factors.

25. What does the term ART mean?

ART—assisted reproductive technology—refers to retrieval of an ovum (usually after superovulation with gonadotropins), fertilization in vitro with sperm, then return of the fertilized ovum into the uterus. It is important to inform patients of the cost, overall success rates (defined as infants delivered), and complications.

26. The evaluation of the infertile couple can be divided into four basic or primary tests (for which therapy is available and of proven benefit) and a series of secondary tests, the results of which do not consistently provide evidence of a causal relationship. What are these tests?

In the first group are the tests that should be offered to all couples who fit the definition of infertility: semen analysis to assess male factor, documentation of ovulation, assessment of tubal patency (HSG), and assessment of peritoneal factors (laparoscopy). Depending on the specific abnormality, treatment of these problems may lead to an enhanced pregnancy rate. In the second level of testing are assessment of cervical factor, immunologic factors, luteal phase defects, hamster egg penetration assay, and cultures of the cervix and semen. Treatment of abnormal results of these tests has not proved conclusively to enhance fertility.

BIBLIOGRAPHY

1. Agarwal SKk, Haney AF: Does recommending timed intercourse really help the infertile couple? Obstet Gynecol 84:307, 1994.
2. Jones HW Jr, Toner JP: The infertile couple. N Engl J Med 329:1710, 1993.
3. Seibel MM: Workup of the infertile couple. In Seibel MM (ed): Infertility: A Comprehensive Text. Norwalk, CT, Appleton & Lange, 1990, pp 1–21.
4. Swerdloff RS, Wang C, Kandee FR, Evaluation of the infertile couple. Endocrinol Metab Clin North Am 17:301, 1988.

29. INFERTILITY SURGERY

Sam E. Alexander, M.D.

1. When should diagnostic laparoscopy be performed in the course of an infertility evaluation?

After failing to conceive after at least 1 year of unprotected intercourse, a couple should be investigated for possible causes of infertility. If reproductive age is advanced or if there is a history of an obvious abnormality such as amenorrhea or previous pelvic surgery, the evaluation should begin even sooner. Areas of investigation should include the male factor, anatomy of the fallopian tubes and uterus, ovulatory adequacy, and cervical mucus-sperm interaction. This evaluation includes one or more semen analyses, hysterosalpingogram, and evaluation of ovulation with a late luteal phase endometrial biopsy, early follicular phase levels of follicle-stimulating hormone (FSH) and estradiol, and possibly luteal phase serum progesterone levels or serial ultrasounds to assess follicular development. The diagnostic benefit of the postcoital test has recently been called into question. If no abnormality is found, pelvic endometriosis and pelvic adhesions should be excluded by diagnostic laparoscopy. If there is a history of progressively worsening dysmenorrhea, dyspareunia, premenstrual spotting, pelvic inflammatory disease, or previous ectopic pregnancy, diagnostic laparoscopy should be considered earlier in the course of evaluation.

2. Who should perform diagnostic laparoscopy?

Diagnostic laparoscopy should be performed by a gynecologist trained and experienced in diagnostic laparoscopy and capable of treating the abnormalities that may be found. Preferably this is the physician who is managing the rest of the infertility evaluation and treatment.

3. Which surgical method is most effective for treatment of endometriosis?

Pelvic endometriosis may be treated by sharp scissor excision, laser ablation, or electrocautery. No data suggest that one method of treatment is superior to others for the relief of pelvic pain or infertility. The surgeon's choice is a matter of training and experience, although it is beneficial to master more than one technique in case the need arises.

4. How successful is the surgical treatment of endometriosis in infertile women?

The surgical treatment of minimal or mild endometriosis does not appear to improve the chance of pregnancy in infertile women. Correction of anatomic abnormalities associated with more severe endometriosis may enhance fecundity, however. With the advent of more sophisticated laparoscopic technology, endometriosis is usually treated laparoscopically rather than by laparotomy.

5. Can endometriomas be treated laparoscopically?

Laparoscopic treatment of endometriomas involves opening the endometrioma with cautery, scissors, or laser. After drainage of the cyst contents, the cyst wall may be stripped from the underlying ovarian stroma. Alternatively, the cyst wall may be ablated with the laser or cauterized. Simple drainage of an endometrioma is not successful; the endometrioma will refill and grow after surgery.

6. What is the role of laparotomy in the treatment of infertility?

Endometriosis and pelvic adhesions are not commonly treated by laparotomy to enhance fertility. If the disease is so severe that it cannot be treated successfully by laparoscopy, in vitro fertilization-embryo transfer is the procedure of choice for the infertile couple. Laparotomy is required for tubal ligation reversal and is usually the best approach for myomectomy in the woman who desires fertility.

7. What is the role of laparoscopy in the evaluation of recurrent pregnancy loss?

None.

8. What surgical technique is used to correct a bicornuate uterus?

The classic Strassman metroplasty is the procedure used to unify a bicornuate uterus. At the time of laparotomy, an incision is made through the myometrium from the tip of one uterine horn to the other. The myometrium is then closed in layers from front to back. This results in a single uterine cavity.

9. What surgical technique is used to correct a septate uterus?

A uterine septum may be incised hysteroscopically using either scissors, laser, or cautery. After the septum is incised, it retracts, so that no tissue is actually removed. This hysteroscopic dissection is carried out under laparoscopic guidance to decrease the risk of uterine perforation. Some surgeons may use postoperative adjuncts such as an intrauterine Foley catheter balloon or estrogen supplementation to decrease the risk of intrauterine adhesion formation. No firm evidence indicates that either is necessary.

10. What is the indication for metroplasty?

Neither septate nor bicornuate uteri have been shown to be a cause of infertility. Either may be found in women with recurrent pregnancy loss, however, and metroplasty may increase the chance of live birth.

11. How is proximal tubal occlusion corrected?

Approximately 80% of women with proximal tubal occlusion can be treated successfully by fallopian tube catheterization. The catheter can be guided either fluoroscopically or by direct vision through the operative hysteroscope. About 25% of tubes that are successfully catheterized reocclude within 6 months. If the occlusion is bilateral and neither tube can be successfully catheterized, in vitro fertilization-embryo transfer is the alternative treatment.

12. How is distal tubal occlusion managed surgically?

Ascending inflammation secondary to sexually transmitted disease may result in complete distal fallopian tube occlusion. Because of damage to the mucosa of the fallopian tube, simply opening the tube surgically may not result in normal tubal function. Hysterosalpingogram fails to show the striated appearance of normally rugated tubal mucosa if the mucosa has been significantly damaged by previous infection. The success of surgical tubal repair is related to the radiographic appearance of the tubal mucosa and the amount of dilatation seen on hysterosalpingogram.

Distal salpingostomy is performed laparoscopically by piercing the distal occluded end of the fallopian tube with cautery, laser, or laparoscopic scissors. Radial incisions are carried proximally from that point, and the resulting flaps are folded back to the more proximal tubal serosa. The flaps may be held in place by laparoscopic sutures, or the serosa may be heated slightly with the laser or cautery to create a curling effect known as the **Bruhat technique.**

Although 90% of fallopian tubes remain open after this procedure, only about 25–30% of patients can be expected to conceive, depending on the amount of mucosal damage. Approximately 5–10% of those who do conceive have ectopic pregnancies.

13. What is the preferred method for removal of uterine fibroids?

Myomectomy may be performed either by laparoscopy or laparotomy. Because myomectomy subjects the woman to a significant risk of postoperative adhesion formation, it should be performed in the manner that results in the least trauma to the uterus, the neatest closure, and the best hemostasis. Unless the fibroids are small and immediately subserosal, laparoscopic myomectomy is not likely to be the procedure of choice in an infertile woman. Submucosal myomas may be removed hysteroscopically. Pretreatment for 12 weeks with an agonist of gonadotropin-releasing hormone (GnRH) may result in shrinkage of the myomas by 40–50% of their pretreatment size as well as decreased operative time and blood loss.

14. How can postoperative adhesions be prevented?

Gentle tissue handling, irrigation rather than sponging or rubbing serosal surfaces, meticulous hemostasis, limited suturing and cautery, and keeping serosal surfaces moist are surgical principles that minimize postoperative adhesion formation. Adjuncts at the time of surgery include instillation of crystalloid solutions or 32% dextran 70 (Hyskon) or placing barriers such as oxidized regenerated cellulose (Interceed) or expanded polytetrafluoroethylene (Goretex surgical membrane) over serosal surfaces that have been damaged or sutured. None of these adjuncts replaces the need for meticulous surgical technique, because none has been shown to totally prevent adhesions. Although barriers have been shown to decrease the extent of postoperative adhesion formation, their effect on subsequent fertility has yet to be proved.

BIBLIOGRAPHY

1. Flood JT, Grow DR: Transcervical tubal cannulation: A review. Obstet Gynecol Surv 48:768–776, 1993.
2. Friedman AJ, Rein MS, Harrison-Atlas D, et al: A randomized, placebo-controlled, double-blind study evaluating leuprolide depot treatment before myomectomy. Fertil Steril 52:728–733, 1989.
3. Khalifa E, Toner JP, Jones HW: The role of abdominal metroplasty in the era of operative hysteroscopy. Surg Obstet Gynecol 176:208–212, 1993.
4. Nezhat C, Nezhat F, Silfen SL, et al: Laparoscopic myomectomy. Int J Fertil 36:275–280, 1991.
5. Operative Laparoscopy Study Group: Postoperative adhesion development after operative laparoscopy: Evaluation of early second-look procedures. Fertil Steril 55:700–704, 1991.
6. Pagidas K, Tulandi T: Effects of Ringer's lactate, Interceed (TC7) and Gore-Tex surgical membrane on postsurgical adhesion formation. Fertil Steril 57:199, 1992.
7. Richard-Davis G, Leach RE: Surgical principles that reduce postoperative adhesion formation. Infertil Reprod Clin North Am 5:427–436, 1994.
8. Schlaff WD, Hassiakos DK, Damewood MD, Rock JA: Neosalpingostomy for distal tubal obstruction: Prognostic factors and impact of surgical technique. Fertil Steril 54:984–990, 1990.
9. Vercellini P, Vendola N, Colombo A, et al: Hysteroscopic metroplasty with resectoscope or microscissors for the correction of septate uterus. Surg Gynecol Obstet 176:439–442, 1993.

30. IN VITRO FERTILIZATION

William Schoolcraft, M.D., and Craig Stark, M.D.

1. What is in vitro fertilization and embryo transfer (IVF-ET)?

IVF-ET is a process in which oocytes from preovulatory follicles are exposed to sperm in a laboratory setting, with fertilization and subsequent cleavage of the embryo. The embryo is then returned to the endometrial cavity.

2. What are the major steps of an IVF-ET cycle?

1. Controlled ovarian hyperstimulation
2. Transvaginal oocyte retrieval
3. Fertilization of the oocyte
4. Embryo culture until cleavage (4–8 cell)
5. Transcervical transfer of the embryos into the uterine cavity

3. What are the essential requirements for a couple considering IVF-ET?

1. Normal day-3 levels of follicle-stimulating hormone (FSH), luteinizing hormone (LH), and adequacy of egg quality.

2. Semen analysis, including strict morphology, and antisperm antibodies assessment.

3. Assessment of the uterine cavity: both structural assessment by hysterosalpingography or hysteroscopy and functional assessment by visualization of an 8-mm or greater "triple pattern" of the endometrium on ultrasound during the late proliferative phase of the menstrual cycle.

4. How often does IVF-ET result in the delivery of a viable infant?

The delivery rate per oocyte retrieval averages 15–20% nationally. In several programs, however, the rate exceeds 30%. Delivery of a viable infant occurs in 12% nationally.

5. What are the major indications for the use of IVF-ET in the infertile couple?
- Tubal disease
- Endometriosis unresponsive to standard medical and/or surgical therapy
- Male factor infertility
- Cervical factor
- Immunologic factor
- Idiopathic infertility
- Ovulatory dysfunction
- Genetic disorders

6. In infertile women undergoing tubal surgery, which preoperative findings are associated with lower rates of subsequent successful pregnancy?
- Presence of a large hydrosalpinx (> 3 cm)
- Absence of discernible fimbria
- Severe pelvic adhesive disease
- Salpingostomy after distal tubal obstruction
- Infertility after tuboplasty (A second procedure generally is not beneficial to these patients.)
- < 4 cm of total tube remaining after tubal ligation
- Tubal ligation performed using monopolar cautery
- Repeated ectopic pregnancies
- Endometriosis with tubal or ovarian involvement

If the preoperative estimate of a successful outcome of tubal surgery in terms of delivery of a viable infant is believed to be < 20%, IVF-ET appears to be a reasonable substitute for surgery.

7. What is the effect of maternal age on success rates for IVF-ET?

Success declines with age, particularly after age 35. Indeed, the delivery rate nationally in women 40 years of age and older is 4%. Assisted hatching has been shown to improve significantly the pregnancy rates in older women by creating an artificial gap in the zona pellucida of an 8-cell embryo before transfer, thereby promoting hatching and implantation.

8. What role does IVF-ET play in infertile couples in whom ovarian disorders appear to be of major importance?

Women with hypogonadotropic anovulation, oligoovulation, and luteal phase defects may benefit from IVF-ET, although it is rarely indicated when any of these appears to be the only factor associated with infertility. IVF-ET or gamete intrafallopian transfer (GIFT) is the procedure of choice in patients with unruptured luteinized follicle syndrome who are unresponsive to gonadotropin therapy. Women with menopause secondary to premature ovarian failure, gonadal dysgenesis, and resistant ovary syndrome also benefit from IVF with donated oocytes.

9. How can the woman who either has or is a carrier of a genetic disorder benefit from IVF-ET?

By the use of donated oocytes the woman who carries a defective gene lowers her chances of delivering a genetically affected child to the same rate as that of the general population.

10. Why is ovulation induction used almost exclusively to obtain oocytes in IVF-ET programs?

Although the initial IVF-ET successes used oocytes recovered from natural unstimulated cycles, presently stimulation of multiple preovulatory follicles with recovery of 3 or 4 oocytes and implantation of the same number of embryos is the rule. Successful pregnancy rates after embryo transfer are directly related to the number of embryos transferred (up to a maximum of 4 embryos). The recovery of multiple oocytes allows cryopreservation of excessive embryos. This decreases the risks and expenses when more than one IVF-ET cycle is required. Finally, successful

IVF-ET procedures require the precise coordination of several different specialists and technologies for oocyte retrieval, fertilization, and embryo transfer to be as successful as possible. This task is made even more difficult when the timing of ovulation cannot be controlled.

11. What are the major agents used in ovulation induction in the patient undergoing IVF-ET?
1. Clomiphene citrate
2. Human menopausal gonadotropins (HMG)
3. Gonadotropin-releasing hormone analogs (GnRH)
4. Combinations of the above agents
5. Human chorionic gonadotropins (HCG)

12. What is the most common protocol for controlled ovarian hyperstimulation during IVF-ET?
Downregulation with GnRH analog, followed by gonadotropin stimulation, is the most common protocol used today. Its advantages include (1) greater number of synchronous oocytes, (2) avoidance of premature surges of luteinizing hormone (LH), and (3) lower incidence of premature luteinization.

13. How and why are human menopausal gonadotropins (HMGs) used to induce ovulation in patients undergoing IVF-ET?
HMG contains both LH and follicle-stimulating hormone (FSH) in equal amounts. It has three advantages over clomiphene citrate: (1) more reliable ovarian response, (2) no associated antiestrogen effects, and (3) production of multiple preovulatory follicles. The major disadvantages are the expense and the need for closer monitoring of the status of the ovaries. HMG must be started early in the cycle (before selection of the dominate follicle) for maximal effect of dosages. Dosage schedules vary with the patient but generally involve injection of 2–4 ampules/day. Completion of oocyte maturation, initiation of ovulation, and luteinization require appropriately timed administration of HCG in a dose of 5,000–10,000 IU.

14. Which criteria are used to monitor administration of HMG and to determine the appropriate timing for administration of HCG?
Established criteria include evaluation of (1) the number and sizes of the lead follicles, (2) serum estrogen concentration and rate of increase, (3) length of ovarian stimulation, (4) status of vaginal cytology and cervical mucus characteristics, and (5) evidence of an increase in LH or progesterone levels.

15. How is ultrasound used to monitor the patient treated with HMG?
Ultrasound is used early in the follicular phase before the start of therapy to assess the structural state of the ovary. If the initial evaluation suggests dominant follicle selection and development, ovulation induction therapy is delayed until the next cycle. Ultrasound is used once the patient begins to manifest a biologic response to therapy (based on either physical exam or serum estrogen levels) on a daily basis until oocyte retrieval to assess follicular response. Follicles are assessed in terms of either diameter or volume. Follicular growth is linear for approximately 1 week before ovulation, and slower than expected growth may reflect inadequate HMG dosage. The majority of normal pregnancies arise from follicles with diameters of 1.7–2.3 cm. Small follicles generally contain immature ova and are not associated with high embryo transfer rates. Large follicles are associated with high spontaneous abortion rates. Ultrasound may be helpful in detecting an earlier than expected ovulation and prevent further unnecessary treatment in the current cycle.

16. How is monitoring of serum estradiol used to guide HMG therapy?
A baseline estradiol level ≥ 100 pg/ml suggests active follicular development. In this setting, HMG or clomiphene citrate therapy is often associated with rapid enlargement of the single dominant follicle. Ovulation induction therapy is therefore postponed until the next treatment cycle.

Rapid follicular development is associated with an exponential rise in serum estradiol levels. Low estradiol levels on 2 or more days suggest that the HMG dosage may be inadequate and needs to be increased. A peak estradiol level < 500 pg/nl is associated with the poorest outcomes. Cancellation of HCG administration and attempted retrieval are strongly considered in patients who fail to demonstrate a significant rise in estradiol concentrations after 5 days of HMG therapy or in patients whose estradiol levels fall in the final stages of ovarian stimulation.

The serum estrogen pattern associated with the highest pregnancy rate includes (1) a progressive rise in estrogen levels throughout HMG administration, (2) a continued rise between the last day of HMG dose and the administration of HCG, and (3) further elevation in estrogen levels on the day after HCG administration.

Serum estradiol levels > 3000 pg/ml are associated with a high risk of severe ovarian hyperstimulation syndrome. Further hormonal therapy is generally stopped until resolution.

17. What is the role of embryo cryopreservation in IVF-ET?

With controlled ovarian hyperstimulation, approximately 40% of patients have a surplus of embryos beyond the number needed for a fresh embryo transfer. Surplus embryos can be stored in liquid nitrogen indefinitely and transferred later, giving the infertile couple a second chance at pregnancy (approximately 20% per frozen embryo transfer).

18. What is intracytoplasmic sperm injection (ICSI)?

A single sperm is injected with a micropipette into the center (cytoplasm) of the oocyte. Approximately 60% of injected eggs fertilize normally. The rate of implantation and development of the embryo is equal to that of conventionally fertilized embryos.

19. What is the limit to which IVF can treat male factor infertility?

Now that ICSI is available, any man with any motile sperm can induce pregnancy. Even in men with azoospermia due to obstruction, sperm can be aspirated from the vas deferens, epididymis, or testicle and then used for the injection of the oocyte.

20. What is ovarian age?

Ovarian age is the assessment by FSH, LH, and estradiol, measured on day 2 or 3 of the menstrual cycle, of the number and quality of oocytes in the ovary. These levels also predict the number of eggs that a woman will produce on a given amount of ovarian hyperstimulation.

21. Which techniques are used for oocyte retrieval?

In most centers ultrasonic guidance is used for oocyte retrieval. Transabdominal, transvaginal, and transvesical routes are available. Success rates in oocyte retrieval with these methods vary from 75–85%. Ultrasound-guided oocyte retrieval avoids the risks of general anesthesia and the costs associated with the use of an operating room. Oocytes often can be recovered from the patient with a "frozen pelvis." Oocyte retrieval is often impossible in these patients if laparoscopy is used. Oocyte retrieval via laparoscopy is generally reserved for situations that require concurrent treatment of pelvic disease. Successful retrievals range from 85–95%.

22. How is the embryo transfer accomplished?

Embryo transfer usually takes place approximately 43–48 hours after insemination. The embryos are generally at the four-cell stage. Although the number of embryos transferred varies, often no more than four are transferred at one time. Surplus normal-appearing embryos are cryopreserved for use in a later cycle. The embryos are loaded into an open-ended Teflon catheter with media and air. The catheter is placed through the cervix into the uterine cavity and the embryos are gently deposited in the area of the fundus.

23. Why has four been chosen as the number of embryos to be transferred at one time?

Transfer of < 4 embryos has been associated with lower pregnancy rates. Increases in the number of transferred embryos have been associated with an increase in the number of multiple gestations as well as the number of fetuses per pregnancy. Below is a description of the relationship between the number of embryo transfers and subsequent pregnancy rates.

Number of embryos transferred	Pregnancy rate (5)
1	9–10
2	12–15
3	15–20
4	20–25

24. What problems are associated with the luteal phase in patients after IVF-ET?

A shortened luteal phase and a decrease in progesterone production often complicate gonadotropin-stimulated cycles. This may be due to the effect of high luteal phase estrogen production on pituitary gonadotropin secretion. Patients are often treated with progesterone in oil, 25 mg intramuscularly every 12 hours, started the day before embryo transfer to combat this problem.

25. What are the major risks of IVF-ET?

1. Ovarian hyperstimulation syndrome (OHSS), resulting from the production of an excessive number of oocytes, may lead to ovarian enlargement and ascites as well as respiratory compromise and may be life threatening.

2. Hemorrhage, infection, and, rarely, bowel injury from the transvaginal oocyte procedure.

3. 3–4% of patients undergoing embryo transfer will develop multiple gestations (triplet or greater) from an IVF-ET cycle.

26. When should a couple be referred for IVF-ET?

1. When a complete infertility evaluation has been completed.

2. When all abnormalities have been treated for 6–12 months by conventional means (i.e., intrauterine insemination for male factor and cervical factor disorders, surgical treatment of uterine and tubal disease, and ovulation induction for ovulatory disorders).

3. In cases of unexplained infertility, at least 3 cycles of HMG/intrauterine insemination have been attempted.

BIBLIOGRAPHY

1. Damewood M (ed): The Johns Hopkins Handbook of In Vitro Fertilization and Assisted Reproductive Technologies. Boston, Little, Brown, 1990.
2. Kohen J, et al: Implantation enhancement by selective assisted hatching using zona drilling of human embryos with poor prognosis. Hum Reprod 5:685–691, 1992.
3. Meldrum D (ed): Assisted reproductive technologies. Infertil Reprod Med Clin North Am 4(4):1993.
4. Schoolcraft W: Efficacy of assisted hatching in the treatment of poor prognosis IVF candidates. Fertil Steril 1962:551–554, 1994.

31. MENOPAUSE

Robert E. Wall, M.D., and Donna E. Okuda, M.D.

1. How does menopause differ from the climacteric?

Strictly speaking, menopause is defined as cessation of menses for a minimum of 6 months because of inadequate ovarian follicular development and waning estrogen production. The climacteric is an extended period of gradually declining ovarian function often beginning years before and lasting years after menopause itself.

2. At what age does menopause usually occur?

The average age of menopause in the United States is 51 years, with a large majority of women experiencing menopause between the ages of 45 and 55. Natural menopause prior to the age of 40 is termed **premature ovarian failure**. Surgical castration prior to natural menopause produces dramatic symptoms of estrogen deficiency that usually require hormonal supplementation.

3. How many women in the U.S. are postmenopausal?

With the average life expectancy of women in the United States exceeding 81 years, a woman will spend more than a third of her life without endogenous estrogen production. It is estimated that in the United States alone, the number of postmenopausal women presently approaches 40 million.

4. Which changes in uterine bleeding patterns are considered normal during the perimenopausal period?

For some women, menopause occurs abruptly without any premenopausal change in menstrual bleeding. In many women the normal climacteric is accompanied by menstrual periods that are lighter, shorter, and less frequent. Perimenopausal women with complaints of heavier, longer menstruation or periods more frequent than every 21 days require endometrial sampling to exclude hyperplasia and adenocarcinoma of the endometrium.

5. Which symptoms are frequently associated with menopause?

Eighty to ninety percent of menopausal women experience hot flashes, an overwhelming uncomfortable sensation of heat and perspiration over the face, neck, and chest. For some women, hot flashes are uncommon and may last only a few months. Others experience multiple flashes each day and night that become truly disabling. Although the cause is not well understood, hot flashes appear to be a manifestation of unstable hypothalamic control of the heat regulatory mechanisms brought about by estrogen withdrawal. Increases in circulating levels of luteinizing hormone (LH), adrenocorticotropic hormone (ACTH), cortisol, and norepinephrine are associated with, but are not the cause of, the hot flash.

Anxiety, irritability, fatigue, depression, headaches, and insomnia are typical menopausal complaints. After prolonged estrogen deficiency, dyspareunia, vulvar pruritus, urinary frequency, and dysuria are commonly experienced.

6. Which laboratory studies are helpful in confirming the diagnosis of menopause?

Although in most women the clinical diagnosis of menopause is readily apparent and highly accurate, laboratory confirmation may be necessary or desirable. The physiologic mid-cycle LH surge may occasionally be confused with the elevated gonadotropins associated with menopause. However, follicle-stimulating hormone (FSH) levels persistently above 40 mIU/ml are indicative of endogenous estrogen deficiency and menopause. Measurement of circulating estradiol levels is usually not helpful. If warranted by clinical findings, laboratory studies to rule out pregnancy, thyroid dysfunction, and prolactin disorders must always be considered in the evaluation of peri-menopausal women with amenorrhea.

7. What is osteoporosis? How common is it?

Osteoporosis is a reduction in the quantity of structural bone; specifically, loss of protein fibers and calcium, which provide strength and resistance to fracture. By age 60, 25% of white and Asian women develop spinal compression fractures. By age 80, 20% of all white women develop hip fractures. In the United States, it has been estimated that there are 1.2 million osteoporosis-related fractures annually. Femoral neck fractures are the twelfth leading cause of death in women in the United States; 50% of these fractures cause permanent disability.

8. Who is at risk for osteoporosis?

Factors known to increase the risk of osteoporosis are race (white or Asian), reduced weight for height, early menopause, family history, smoking, sedentary lifestyle, long-term heparin or steroid therapy, endocrine disorders (diabetes, hyperthyroidism, Cushing's disease), and diet (low calcium or vitamin D intake; high caffeine, protein, or alcohol intake).

9. What steps should be taken to prevent osteoporosis in postmenopausal women?

The single most important way to minimize the rate of osteoporosis in postmenopausal women is supplemental estrogen. Ideally, estrogen replacement therapy (ERT) should be instituted soon after the onset of menopause, especially in women who are at increased risk for osteoporosis. Regular weight-bearing exercise, daily calcium supplementation (1500 mg/day in hypoestrogenic women), elimination of cigarette smoking, and moderation of caffeine and alcohol intake help to retard osteoporosis. In women with osteoporosis, safety precautions should be taken to prevent falls. Calcitonin augments bone mass and is recommended in women who cannot take estrogen. Alendronate sodium (Fosamax) has recently been approved for treatment of osteoporosis in postmenopausal women. Alendronate sodium interferes with osteoclast activity, allowing normal bone to be formed.

10. Which conditions are contraindications to ERT?

Active thromboembolism, chronic liver impairment, and abnormal uterine bleeding without tissue diagnosis are contraindications to the initiation of estrogen therapy. For some women with active migraines or active seizure disorders, ERT may aggravate their problems. For women with a history of estrogen-dependent tumors (breast or endometrial), the use of estrogen is controversial; the benefits of its use should be weighed against the risks on an individual basis. Use of estrogen replacement in women with previous endometrial cancer is widespread, despite the lack of randomized controlled studies. No adverse effects of estrogen replacement in these patients have been reported. No data document the effect of ERT in women with previously treated breast cancer.

11. When do perimenopausal women require endometrial sampling? Is it safe to assume that irregular bleeding during climacteric years is normal?

Any trend toward more bleeding requires endometrial sampling. If an episode of bleeding occurs more often than every 21 days, lasts longer than 8 days, is heavy, or occurs after a 6-month interval of amenorrhea, sampling must be done. It is never safe to assume that irregular bleeding is "normal." Endometrial cancer must be ruled out with sampling.

12. Do women on ERT require endometrial sampling?

Women with abnormal premenopausal bleeding require endometrial sampling. Endometrial biopsy by aspiration curettage performed in the office is diagnostically reliable and cost-effective and usually preferred to dilatation and curettage (D&C). Most authorities do not recommend routine pretreatment biopsy or routine endometrial sampling while patients are taking estrogen and progesterone. Women who bleed irregularly should undergo endometrial sampling. Women on unopposed estrogen should be sampled before initiation of therapy and yearly thereafter.

13. In what other forms can estrogen replacement be given?

Transdermal administration of estradiol (Estraderm) is effective. Some authorities contend, however, that eliminating the first-pass effect on the liver that occurs with oral estrogens reduces the beneficial rise in levels of high-density lipoproteins (HDLs). Vaginal administration of estrogen is erratic and unpredictable and should be restricted to short-term supplemental treatment in women with severe vaginal dryness and dyspareunia. The use of parenteral depot forms of estrogen for hormonal replacement during menopause is to be condemned. Newer sustained-release subcutaneous estrogen pellets may soon be available in the United States after studies are completed. Regardless of the route of administration, patients with a uterus receiving long-term estrogen treatment also need progestin withdrawal to prevent the development of endometrial hyperplasia or adenocarcinoma.

14. What is the role of estrogen and testosterone replacement?

A preparation combining an esterified estrogen with methyltestosterone is used most commonly in younger women who have undergone surgical menopause or premature ovarian failure as well as in postmenopausal women complaining of decreased libido. Methyltestosterone is not a substitute for progesterone and has not been proved to change libido.

15. What are the possible side effects of low-dose ERT?

About 5–10% of women given low-dose estrogen/progestin report breast tenderness, bloating, edema, weight gain, increased appetite, or dysmenorrhea. Most symptoms decrease after several months of therapy. If patients continue to have side effects, changing the prescribed dose or altering the specific estrogen or progestin usually improves tolerance. With cyclic administration of estrogen and progesterone, about 90% of patients have period-like withdrawal bleeding. If patients are well educated about the benefits of ERT, most will tolerate mild side effects and the scheduled breakthrough bleeding that they usually experience. No documented evidence indicates that estrogen replacement causes weight gain.

16. Which patients should be offered ERT?

All women who develop estrogen deficiency should be considered for ERT. After careful evaluation and counseling, most patients are willing to accept the occasional side effects and minimal health risks of ERT in exchange for the symptomatic relief and long-term health benefits.

17. Are any health risks associated with low-dose ERT?

Yes. Continuous estrogen administration in postmenopausal women is associated with a 4–8-fold risk of endometrial adenocarcinoma. Most estrogen-induced endometrial cancers are well differentiated and detected at an early stage of disease. Monthly addition for 10–14 days of a progestational agent for women with a uterus decreases the risk of uterine malignancy or premalignant atypical adenomatous hyperplasia.

Epidemiologic evidence indicates the possible association of a slightly increased risk of breast cancer with long durations of postmenopausal estrogen use. Meta-analysis of estrogen use and breast cancer yields no definitive answer regarding breast cancer risk, but if the risk is increased it is increased only slightly. Women on estrogen at the time of breast cancer diagnosis have improved survival rates. Women who have taken estrogen replacement have a longer life expectancy than women who have never taken estrogen.

18. What cardiovascular effects are observed with postmenopausal oral estrogen replacement?

In recent years, repeated studies have demonstrated an increase in HDL levels and concomitant decrease in low-density lipoprotein (LDL) levels associated with the postmenopausal administration of oral estrogens. This alteration in lipoprotein fractions has a beneficial effect on coronary artery disease and stroke. In women receiving postmenopausal low-dose estrogen supplementation, the incidence of myocardial infarction, stroke, and death resulting from these complications is reduced at least 50%. Estrogen may retard atherosclerotic processes indirectly by

affecting lipid metabolism and/or directly by inhibiting intimal hyperplasia and other components of vessel pathology.

**19. Does ERT have any known benefit for mood or cognitive function in postmenopausal
women?**

Yes. Estrogen influences the biochemistry of the brain by altering the concentrations and
availability of neurotransmitter amines, including serotonin. This evidence suggests that estrogen
enhances mood in women and maintains verbal memory.

BIBLIOGRAPHY

1. American College of Obstetricians and Gynecologists: Hormone replacement therapy. Tech Bull 166, 1992.
2. American College of Obstetricians and Gynecologists: Osteoporosis. Tech Bull 167, 1992.
3. Creasman WT: Estrogen replacement therapy: Is previously treated cancer a contraindication? Obstet
    Gynecol 77:308–312, 1991.
4. Droegemueller W, Herbst AL, Mishell DR, Stenchever MA, et al (eds): Comprehensive Gynecology, 2nd
    ed. St. Louis, Mosby, 1992.
5. Ettinger B: Optimal use of postmenopausal hormone replacement. Obstet Gynecol 72:31s–36s, 1989.
6. Hazzard WR: Estrogen replacement and cardiovascular disease: Serum lipids and blood pressure effects.
    Am J Obstet Gynecol 161:1847–1853, 1989.
7. Menopause and hormone replacement. Obstet Gynecol 87(5):1, 1996.
8. Sarrel PM: Sexuality and menopause. Obstet Gynecol 75:26s–35s, 1990.
9. Speroff L, et al (eds): Clinical Gynecologic Endocrinology and Infertility, 5th ed. Baltimore, Williams &
    Wilkins, 1994.

III. Gynecologic Oncology

32. PREMALIGNANT DISEASE OF THE CERVIX, VAGINA, AND VULVA

David M. Terry, M.D.

CERVIX

1. What is meant by premalignant cervical disease?

In 1967 the term *cervical intraepithelial neoplasia* (CIN) was introduced to define a continuum of abnormalities seen within the epithelium of the cervix. Normally, an orderly progression of maturation extends from the basement membrane to the epithelial surface layer. A pathologic diagnosis of CIN is made when the polarity of cellular differentiation is lost and the cells are characterized by enlarged, pleomorphic nuclei and scant cytoplasm. A crowding of cells is observed with increases in the mitotic number and nuclear-to-cytoplasmic (N:C) ratio. Carcinoma in situ is defined as cytologic atypia similar to that seen in invasive carcinoma without evidence of invasion beneath the basement membrane. Lesions composed of similar atypical cells but maintaining some degree of surface maturation are termed dysplasia and are graded as mild, moderate, or severe. Such changes, no matter how severe, are limited to the epithelial layer and may include the endocervical glandular epithelium.

2. How much is known about the cause of preinvasive disease of the cervix?

Cervical carcinoma certainly appears to be a sexually transmitted disease. Most women who develop the disease seem to be in the same grouping as women at high risk for other sexually transmitted diseases. The most statistically pertinent risk factors seem to be (1) early age at first coitus, (2) multiple sexual partners, (3) frequent coitus with multiple partners, (4) smoking, and (5) lower socioeconomic status. Independent covariables, at present, are limited to multiple male sexual partners and smoking.

Viral causes have been postulated. Herpes simplex was formerly thought to be the causative organism, but this has not been proved. Currently, much research is focused on the role of human papillomavirus (HPV) as a cofactor, because HPV DNA has been isolated in many women with preinvasive and invasive cervical lesions.

3. Does infection with HPV result in progression to cancer?

No. All HPV serotypes that have an affinity for the cervical epithelium may manifest themselves as condylomata or dysplasia, but not all serotypes progress to carcinoma. Clinicians screen for cervical dysplasia and infer a viral etiology. They detect varying degrees of dysplasia, i.e., mild, moderate, or severe. Depending on the degree of dysplasia, the progression to invasive cancer is very different. Mild dysplasia has been found to regress spontaneously in 60–80% of cases. In contrast, severe dysplasia progresses to cervical cancer in up to 12% of cases. Moderate dysplasia falls somewhere between the two. This concept has an important bearing on patient counseling and treatment.

4. How much time is usually required for CIN to progress to invasive cancer?

Although there are certainly exceptions, cervical neoplasia is a slowly progressive disease, with invasion generally occurring at the end of the progression. Estimates range from 1–20 years, but some neoplasia never become invasive.

5. How is cervical dysplasia diagnosed?

Cervical dysplasia is a pathologic diagnosis made from biopsy of the cervix. Colposcopic exam consists of painting the cervix with an acetic acid solution (generally 3%) and visualizing the cervix under magnification (5–40 ×). Acetic acid has a dehydrating effect on the epithelial cells, allowing cells with increased N:C ratio to become white in contrast with normal cervical epithelium. This phenomenon is given the term *acetowhite epithelium* (AWE). In addition to AWE, vascular changes associated with dysplasia may also be observed. These changes are called punctations and mosaicism. Clinicians with expertise in colposcopic exams may be able to characterize the lesion by the severity of vascular patterns seen during colposcopic exam. Colposcopy provides a guided approach to cervical biopsy.

6. What constitutes an adequate colposcopic exam?

Several features must be addressed during the colposcopic exam. First, the clinician must state whether the full transformation zone has been visualized. The transformation zone comprises all tissue between the original and current squamocolumnar junction. If the full transformation zone has been visualized, the exam is considered satisfactory. If not, the exam is considered unsatisfactory. Second, the full ectocervix needs to be evaluated. A diagram of the cervix and its abnormalities may be drawn, describing the clinician's impression of the lesion. A biopsy of the lesions may be performed at this time. Third, evaluation of the endocervix must be made by endocervical curettage. A repeat Papanicolaou (Pap) smear is generally performed before the biopsy is made. The three features of the colposcopic exam which must be evaluated are the endocervix, ectocervix, and transformation zone.

7. What is the significance of the transformation zone?

The transformation zone is the region of the cervix in which squamous epithelium develops from glandular epithelium. It is a region of high cellular activity and is susceptible to HPV and subsequent development of cervical dysplasia. Classically, this is the region where all cervical dysplasia develops.

8. What are the treatment options for cervical dysplasia?

In general, there are two treatment patterns, excisional and ablative. Excisional techniques include cold knife cone biopsy (CKC), loop electrosurgical procedures (LEEP), and laser cone biopsy. Ablative techniques include cryosurgery and laser ablation of the cervix. The most appropriate method of treatment depends on the size of the lesion, presence of dysplastic cells within the endocervical canal, whether the colposcopic exam was satisfactory, and degree of difference between the Pap smear and cervical biopsies. Laser cone, CKC, and Leep allow the clinician to evaluate tissue to determine whether disease extends to the margins of treatment. Ablative therapies eliminate the epithelium of the entire transformation zone. Relapse rates after cryotherapy vary between 7–16%. Laser ablation has an overall success rate of 87–99%. Ablative therapy must destroy the epithelium to a depth of 5 mm to destroy the epithelium in cervical gland crypts.

9. Once a patient is treated, what then?

Follow-up is of utmost importance in patients treated for cervical dysplasia. Pap smears should be repeated every 3–4 months for 1 year. If after this time cytology has remained negative, cure may be presumed, and patients can resume yearly screenings.

10. What are the indications for cone biopsy of the cervix?

The indications for cone biopsy are (1) findings of dysplastic cells in the endocervix (a positive endocervical curette); (2) features suggestive of invasive disease (evaluation of microinvasive cervical carcinoma); (3) an unsatisfactory colposcopy; and (4) a two-degree difference of abnormality between the pap smear and cervical biopsies. Cone biopsy must be done to confirm the diagnosis of microinvasion and ultimately to rule out more invasive disease.

11. What are the contraindications to cone biopsy of the cervix?

A cervical lesion suggestive of or biopsy-proven carcinoma is a contraindication to cone biopsy of the cervix. Conization of the cervix would add expense and delay definitive treatment. By definition, gross lesion of the cervix is most certainly not microinvasive disease. Conization of the cervix is a means of evaluating microinvasive carcinoma of the cervix. To direct treatment adequately, either surgically or with radiation therapy, cone biopsy must be obtained to evaluate depth and size of the lesion in patients with microinvasion on biopsy.

12. What are koilocytes? What is their significance?

Koilocytes, cells found in the epithelial layer, have at least one and probably two of the following three characteristics: (1) pyknotic raisinoid nucleus,(2) perinuclear cytoplasmic halo, and (3) multinucleation. These cells indicate probable infection with HPV. Therefore, they may indicate the presence of a possible cofactor in the development of invasive cervical carcinoma.

13. What is the incidence of positive condyloma in male partners of females with cervical condyloma?

50–75% via colposcopic examination.

14. Are there different types of HPV?

Yes. At least 50 types have been identified, and there is increasing evidence that many more types exist. When one considers lower reproductive tract problems in women, several HPV types come to the forefront:

1. Types 6 and 11 are generally associated with typical raised genital condylomata (warts); they are mostly benign.

2. Types 16 and 18, seen more commonly with flat warts, may be rapidly progressive and are often found in association with invasive cervical lesions.

3. Types 30, 31, 33 and 35 seem to have a less rapidly progressive potential but are not necessarily benign.

15. Should koilocytotic atypia be considered a preinvasive lesion?

No.

VAGINA

16. Name two conditions associated with neoplasia of the vagina.

Vaginal intraepithelial neoplasia (VAIN) and adenosis.

17. What is vaginal adenosis? With what is it associated?

Vaginal adenosis is the presence of glandular columnar epithelium and its mucinous secretory products in the vagina. Vaginal adenosis is associated with prenatal exposure to diethylstilbestrol (DES), which apparently interferes with the normal development of the vagina.

18. Can vaginal adenosis progress to cancer?

No. It is generally accepted that vaginal adenosis does not progress to cancer, but it is found in association with clear cell adenocarcinoma. The risk of developing clear cell adenocarcinoma of the vagina is approximately 1:1000. Adenosis of the vagina is found in over 90% of women exposed to DES. Because of this association, adenosis should be followed closely with cytologic and clinical examination but requires treatment only when symptomatic. Epidemiologic studies also have found that CIN and VAIN occur in higher rates in women exposed to DES.

19. What is a field response? How does this concept apply to VAIN?

Fifty percent of women with VAIN have a neoplasia at other sites in the lower female genital tract. Most of these lesions involve the vulva and cervix, which therefore must be closely evaluated for the presence of disease. This finding follows a field response in that tissues originating from a common embryologic origin are susceptible to common carcinogens, namely HPV.

20. How is VAIN diagnosed?

VAIN is screened with the Pap smear and diagnosed with colposcopically directed biopsies. Lugol's solution, an iodine formula, may occasionally be used to help delineate areas of VAIN. Normal cells of the vagina have high glycogen content and thus take up the solution and stain brown, whereas dysplastic cells have a low glycogen content and remain a lighter color. VAIN is generally found in the upper third of the vagina. Careful full evaluation of the upper vagina and fornices is mandatory if VAIN is suspected.

21. What is the most common clinical and historical presentation of VAIN?

1. Patients are usually asymptomatic; less often, postcoital bleeding occurs.
2. VAIN usually occurs in women with current or previous history of CIN or cervical cancer.
3. HPV, radiation, and immunosuppressive therapy are thought to increase the risk for development of VAIN.
4. VAIN is most commonly found by Pap smear.

22. What treatment regimens are available for VAIN?

Surgical excision has been the mainstay of therapy with an 80% success rate. Other methods of treatment include laser ablation to a depth of 2–4 mm with a success rate of 70–80% or topical 5-fluorouracil (5-FU) with a success rate of 85%.

VULVA

23. What are the most common symptoms of vulvar intraepithelial neoplasia (VIN)?

Vulvar itching is the most common symptom associated with VIN. Grossly lesions may be white, red, pigmented, flat, or raised. For this reason, abnormal-appearing areas of the vulva should be liberally biopsied. Colposcopic examination with acetic acid highlights areas of dysplasia. It is also important to evaluate the anal canal for VIN, because up to 57% of women with VIN have anal involvement.

24. What other terms have been used to describe VIN?

Bowen's disease, Bowenoid papulosis.

25. What is the relationship between HPV and VIN?

Approximately 20–30% of patients who develop vulvar cancer have a history of condylomata; 90% of VIN lesions have evidence of HPV DNA. In a recent study, 7.4% of patients with vulvar HPV infections had VIN lesions; the authors suggest that HPV may play a similar role in VIN as in CIN.

26. How common is the progression to invasive disease?

The pathogenesis of VIN is poorly understood. It is generally believed that progression to invasive disease occurs infrequently. The frequency of progression to cancer is unknown but may be in the 6% range. Warty and basaloid types of vulvar intraepithelial neoplasia are associated with HPV infection. These changes are more often seen in younger women who smoke than in older nonsmoking women whose lesions do not appear to be HPV-related.

27. What are the treatment options for VIN?

Wide local excision has been the traditional therapy for unifocal disease. Laser ablation also may be used after adequate tissue biopsies have been taken to rule out invasive cancer. For patients with recurrent disease, 5% 5-FU cream has been used topically. Skinning vulvectomy with skin graft has been used for extensive lesions, but recurrences are common in the grafted skin.

28. What type of follow-up is appropriate for women treated for VIN?

Examination with biopsies as indicated every 4–6 months because recurrences of this disease are very common.

BIBLIOGRAPHY

1. Dickinson LE: Control of cancer of the uterine cervix by cytologic screening. Gynecol Oncol 3:1, 1975.
2. Durst M: The human papillomaviruses. Classification and molecular biology. Clin Pract Gynecol 9892:29, 1989.
3. Felix JC, Muderspach LI, Duggan BD, et al: The significance of positive margins in loop electrosurgical cone biopsies. Obstet Gynecol 84:996, 1994.
4. Gunasekera P: Large loop excision of the transformation zone (LLETZ) compared to carbon dioxide laser in the treatment of CIN: A superior mode of treatment. Am J Obstet Gynecol 97:995, 1990.
5. Kaufman RH: Intraepithelial neoplasia of the vulva. Gynecol Oncol 56:8, 1995.
6. Krebs H: Treatment of vaginal intraepithelial neoplasia with laser and topical 5-flourouracil. Obstet Gynecol 73:657, 1989.
7. Lenehan P: Vaginal intraepithelial neoplasia: Biological aspects and management. Obstet Gynecol 68:143, 1986.
8. National Cancer Institute Workshop: The 1988 Bethesda system for reporting cervical/vaginal cytologic diagnosis. JAMA 262:931, 1989.
9. Richart RM: Natural history of cervical intraepithelial neoplasia. Clin Obstet Gynecol 10:748, 1967.
10. Sillman F: A review of lower genital intraepithelial neoplasia and the use of topical 5-flourouracil. Obstet Gynecol Surv 40:190, 1985.
11. Stillman R: In utero exposure to diethylstilbestrol: Adverse effects on the reproductive tract and reproductive performance in male and female offspring. Am J Obstet Gynecol 42:905, 1982.
12. Wright TC, Richart RM: Role of human papillomavirus in the pathogenesis of genital tract warts and cancer. Gynecol Oncol 37:151, 1990.

33. CARCINOMA OF THE UTERINE CERVIX

Helen Frederickson, M.D.

1. What are the presenting signs of cervical carcinoma?

The most frequent symptom is a bloody discharge presenting as postcoital bleeding, intermenstrual bleeding, or menorrhagia. Symptoms of more advanced disease include backache, leg pain, leg edema, or hematuria.

2. What are the risk factors for cervical carcinoma?

First coitus at a young age
Multiple sexual partners
Lower socioeconomic status
Human papillomavirus (HPV) probably acts as a cofactor in cervical carcinogenesis.

3. How is the diagnosis of cervical cancer made?

All cervical lesions should be biopsied, regardless of the Pap smear. Pap smear and colposcopically directed biopsies are used for microscopic (or occult) lesions. Cervical biopsy consistent with microinvasion requires cone biopsy to rule out frankly invasive carcinoma.

4. What is the definition of microinvasion? How does it determine necessary treatment?

Microinvasion is defined by the International Federation of Gynecology and Obstetrics (FIGO) as measurable microscopic lesions not exceeding 5 mm from the base of the epithelium or 7 mm of horizontal spread. The 1995 FIGO staging system further defines cervix cancer stage IA-1 as measured invasion of stroma no greater than 3 mm in depth and no wider than 7 mm.

Patients may be treated with conservative surgery, i.e., simple hysterectomy or, in selected cases, cone biopsy with free margins to preserve childbearing ability.

5. What is the 1995 FIGO staging system for carcinoma of the cervix?

Stage I: The carcinoma is strictly confined to the cervix (extension to the corpus should be disregarded).

Stage IA: Invasive cancer identified only microscopically. All gross lesions, even with superficial invasion, are stage IB cancers. Invasion is limited to measured stromal invasion with maximal depth of 5.0 mm and maximal width of 7.0 mm.

Stage IA1: Measured invasion of stroma no deeper than 3.0 mm and no wider than 7.0 mm.

Stage IA2: Measured invasion of stroma deeper than 3.0 mm but no deeper than 5.0 mm and no wider than 7.0 mm.

Stage IB: Clinical lesions confined to the cervix or preclinical lesions larger than stage IA.

Stage IB1: Clinical lesions no larger than 4.0 cm.

Stage IB2: Clinical lesions larger than 4.0 cm.

Stage II: The carcinoma extends beyond the cervix but has not extended to the pelvic wall. The carcinoma involves the vagina but not as far as the lower third.

Stage IIA: No obvious parametrial involvement.

Stage IIB: Obvious parametrial involvement.

Stage III: The carcinoma has extended to the pelvic wall. Rectal examination reveals no cancer-free space between the tumor and pelvic wall. The tumor involves the lower third of the vagina. All cases with hydronephrosis or nonfunctioning kidney are included unless kidney disease is known to be due to other causes.

Stage IIIA: No extension to the pelvic wall.

Stage IIIB: Extension to the pelvic wall and/or hydronephrosis or nonfunctioning kidney.

Stage IV: The carcinoma has extended beyond the true pelvis or has clinically involved the mucosa of the bladder or rectum. Bullous edema does not assign a case to stage IV.

Stage IVA: Spread of carcinoma to adjacent organs.

Stage IVB: Spread to distant organs.

6. What is the prognosis for 5-year survival based on stage of disease?

Stage I	80–85%	Stage III	25–35%
Stage II	50–65%	Stage IV	8–14%

7. Which patients are candidates for primary surgical management? What if paraaortic nodes are positive on frozen section?

Patients with stage I and stage IIA cervical carcinoma are candidates for primary surgical treatment. Positive paraaortic nodes prevent cure with radical hysterectomy; therefore, the procedure should be abandoned and the patient treated with pelvic radiation therapy with an extended paraaortic field. Although no definitive data document improved survival, some gynecologic oncologists treat these patients with adjuvant chemotherapy as a radiation sensitizer.

8. How does radical hysterectomy differ from simple hysterectomy? Are the ovaries always removed at the time of radical hysterectomy?

In radical hysterectomy, the uterine artery is ligated at its origin from the internal iliac artery, uterosacral ligaments are resected back toward the sacrum, cardinal ligaments are resected at the pelvic sidewall, and the upper one-third of the vagina is removed. Pelvic lymphadenectomy is routinely performed. Ovaries may be preserved with this procedure; this is one of the major advantages of surgery over radiation therapy in young patients.

9. What are the common complications of a radical hysterectomy?

The most common complication is bladder dysfunction. Lymphocyst formation may occur. Risk of pulmonary embolus, hemorrhage, and infection is increased. Ureteral fistula is also a complication of radical hysterectomy but has become less frequent as surgical techniques improve.

10. What is the alternative to surgical therapy for early-stage disease? Is there a difference in cure rates?

Primary radiation therapy can be used to treat early-stage carcinoma of the cervix with the same survival rates as surgery.

11. What is the theory on which radiation therapy for cervical cancer is based?

The cervix is accessible to application of radiation techniques and is surrounded by normal tissue (cervix and vagina) that is highly radioresistant. Because of the anatomy of the cervix, intracavitary doses of 10,000 rads may be delivered to the tumor. The dose of radiation falls off by the inverse square of the distance from the source; the bowel and bladder are protected by packing.

12. Does postoperative radiation therapy in patients with positive pelvic nodes at the time of radical hysterectomy improve survival?

No. Postoperative radiation therapy increases pelvic control but does not improve long-term survival.

13. What are the advantages and disadvantages of high dose-rate (HDR) brachytherapy vs. low dose-rate (LDR) brachytherapy?

The advantages of HDR brachytherapy include outpatient treatment, less anesthesia, less potential for displacement, and decreased personnel exposure. HDR brachytherapy delivers therapy with shorter exposure than the repair half-time of sublethal damage, which may increase the risk of complications. More insertions are required for HDR therapy because of the loss of the dose-rate effect. Preliminary studies of HDR vs. LDR brachytherapy suggest nearly equal 5-year efficacy without increased late tissue response. Initial expense for HDR equipment may prove to be a major limitation to this therapy.

14. What is the most common location of recurrence after radical hysterectomy? After radiation therapy?

After radical hysterectomy, approximately one-third of recurrences are in the pelvic sidewall and approximately one-fourth in the central pelvis. Recurrence after radiation therapy is in the parametrial area in 43% of cases; 27% of recurrences are in the cervix, uterus, or upper vagina.

15. What is the prognosis for a patient with persistent or recurrent cervical carcinoma?

The 1-year survival rate is 10–15%.

16. What treatment options are available for patients with recurrent tumor?

Patients with pelvic recurrence after radical hysterectomy may be treated with radiation therapy. Patients with central recurrence after radiation therapy are candidates for pelvic exenteration.

17. Which patients are candidates for pelvic exenteration?

Pelvic exenteration for recurrent carcinoma of the cervix is indicated only when pelvic recurrence is centrally located. The triad of unilateral leg edema, sciatic pain, and ureteral obstruction indicates unresectable disease.

18. What are the absolute contraindications for pelvic exenteration?

Extrapelvic disease
Triad of unilateral leg edema, sciatica, and ureteral obstruction
Tumor-related pelvic sidewall fixation
Bilateral ureteral obstruction

19. Does chemotherapy have a role in treatment of recurrent cervical cancer?

Chemotherapy has traditionally had low response rates and short duration. The prognosis for patients with unresectable recurrent disease is so poor that new combinations of chemotherapeutic agents are being evaluated. Cisplatin had been shown to be the best single agent against squamous cell carcinoma. The use of chemotherapeutic agents (cisplatin, 5-fluorouracil, and hyroxyurea) as radiosensitizers is being evaluated for prolonged survival or increased cure rates in patients with poor prognosis. The combination of bleomycin, ifosfamide, and cisplatin has shown initially encouraging results in recurrent disease. The use of chemotherapy as neoadjuvant therapy has been considered but to date has shown no significant improvement over standard therapies.

20. Is the prognosis of adenocarcinoma of the cervix worse than the prognosis of squamous carcinoma? If so, should the two lesions be treated differently?

Stage for stage there is no significant difference in survival of patients with adenocarcinoma vs. squamous cell carcinoma, but lesions tend to be initially bulky and more poorly differentiated. Local recurrence is more common in adenocarcinomas; as a result, many oncologists consider combined radiotherapy and surgery for these lesions.

21. Should the treatment of adenocarcinoma in situ and microinvasive adenocarcinoma differ from the standard treatment of the squamous counterparts?

Adenocarcinoma in situ of the cervix can be a difficult pathologic diagnosis to make. Present data suggest that cone biopsy with negative margins or simple hysterectomy is adequate therapy. The patient with adenocarcinoma in situ who elects to preserve her uterus should be followed closely, because the disease may be multifocal, with lesions above the negative margin. Pap smears tend to be less reliable in adenocarcinoma. Microinvasive adenocarcinoma of the endocervix is not well defined. There are essentially no data to support less than radical treatment of invasive adenocarcinoma.

BIBLIOGRAPHY

1. Buxton EJ, Meanwell CA, Hilton C, et al: Combination bleomycin, ifosfamide and cisplatin chemotherapy in cervical cancer. J Natl Cancer Inst 81:359–361, 1989.
2. Curtin JP, Hoskins WF, et al: Adjuvant chemotherapy versus chemotherapy plus pelvic irradiation for high-risk cervical cancer patients after radical hysterectomy and pelvic lymphadenectomy (RH-PLND): A randomized phase III trial. Gynecol Oncol 61:3, 1996.
3. Delgado G, Bundy B, Zairo R, et al: A prospective surgical pathological study of Stage I squamous carcinoma of the cervix: A Gynecologic Oncology Group study. Gynecol Oncol 35:314, 1989.
4. Keys H, Bundy B, Stehman FB, et al: Adjuvants to radiation therapy in the treatment of locally advanced carcinoma of the cervix: The Gynecologic Oncology Group (GOG) experience. In Salmon SE (ed): Adjuvant Therapy of Cancer VI. Philadelphia, W.B. Saunders, 1990, pp 544–555.
5. Marrow CP [panel report]: Is pelvic radiation beneficial in the postoperative management of stage IB squamous cell carcinoma of the cervix with pelvic lymph node metastasis treated by radical hysterectomy and pelvic lymphadenectomy? Gynecol Oncol 37:74, 1990.
6. Perez CA, Camel HM, Kuske RR, et al: Radiation therapy alone in the treatment of carcinoma of the uterine cervix: A 20-year experience. Gynecol Oncol 23:127–140, 1986.
7. Potter MD, Alvarez R, Shingleton HM, et al: Early invasive cervical cancer with pelvic lymph node involvement: To complete or not to complete radical hysterectomy? Gynecol Oncol 37:78, 1990.
8. Rotman M, Pajak TF, Choi K, et al: Prophylactic extended-field irradiation of para-aortic lymph nodes in stages IIB and bulky IB and IIA cervical carcinomas. Ten-year treatment results of RTOG 79-20. JAMA 274:387, 1995.
9. Shingleton HM, Orr JW: Cancer of the Cervix. Philadelphia, J.B. Lippincott, 1995.
10. Yazigi R, Sandstad J, Munoz AK, et al: Adenosquamous carcinoma of the cervix: Prognosis in Stage IB. Obstet Gynecol 75:1012, 1990.

34. ENDOMETRIAL CARCINOMA

Susan A. Davidson, M.D.

1. What is the incidence of endometrial carcinoma? How does the incidence compare with other gynecologic and nongynecologic malignancies in women?

The incidence of endometrial carcinoma is about 72 per 100,000 women per year. It is estimated that in 1995 there will be 32,800 new cases and 5,900 deaths. This makes endometrial cancer the most common gynecologic malignancy and the fourth most common cancer in women after breast, lung, and colon carcinomas. It occurs primarily in postmenopausal women, with an average age at diagnosis of 61.

2. Describe the hypothesis for development of endometrial carcinoma. .

It is hypothesized that unopposed estrogen leads to the development of endometrial cancer. Women on unopposed exogenous estrogen replacement therapy have a greater risk than women in whom exogenous estrogen is opposed by progesterone therapy. Excessive endogenous estrogen, which occurs with obesity, also increases the risk of endometrial cancer. The risk is 10-fold or higher in these two groups of women. The risk is increased 2–3-fold in women with other risk factors, which include nulliparity, history of infertility (especially if due to anovulation and amenorrhea), early menarche or late menopause, and diabetes mellitus.

3. Why are obese women at greater risk of developing endometrial cancer?

Adipose tissue is a primary site of conversion of adrenal androstenedione to estrone, a weak estrogen. Obese women also have lower levels of sex-hormone-binding globulin, which lead to greater bioavailability of estrogens. Obese premenopausal women may have a greater risk of anovulatory cycles, therefore losing the protective effect of progesterone.

4. What is the most common presenting symptom of endometrial carcinoma? How often does it occur?

Ninety percent of patients with endometrial cancer present with abnormal uterine bleeding. Any bleeding in a postmenopausal woman is suspect. Premenopausal women may give a history of oligomenorrhea, amenorrhea, intermenstrual bleeding, or bleeding patterns that suggest anovulatory cycles. Perimenopausal women may present with bloody menopause.

5. How is the diagnosis of endometrial carcinoma made?

Office endometrial biopsy, using any of the many available biopsy devices, is the diagnostic procedure of choice. Endocervical curettage also should be performed. Occasionally dilatation and curettage (D&C) must be performed in the office or operating room if the endometrial biopsy is unsatisfactory or the patient cannot tolerate the office procedure.

6. Is the Pap smear useful in diagnosing endometrial carcinoma?

The Pap smear is not a useful screening test for endometrial cancer. Only 30–50% of patients with endometrial cancer have an abnormal Pap smear. Also, if the Pap smear is abnormal, the cancer is more likely to be in an advanced stage. If normal endometrial cells are seen on Pap smear from a postmenopausal woman, endometrial biopsy should be performed; about 6% of these women have endometrial cancer.

7. Is there a precursor state of the endometrium before the onset of endometrial carcinoma?

Yes. Atypical endometrial adenomatous hyperplasia is thought to be a precursor lesion. The risk factors for development of this condition are the same as those for endometrial carcinoma.

The treatment of choice is hysterectomy; up to 43% of patients with a preoperative diagnosis of atypical hyperplasia have endometrial carcinoma in the hysterectomy specimen.

8. **How is endometrial carcinoma staged? What is the FIGO staging system?**
   Endometrial carcinoma is staged surgically.
   FIGO Stage and Grade Description

IA	G 1, 2, 3	Tumor limited to endometrium
IB	G 1, 2, 3	Invasion of < ½ myometrium
IC	G 1, 2, 3	Invasion of > ½ myometrium
IIA	G 1, 2, 3	Endocervical glandular involvement only
IIB	G 1, 2, 3	Cervical stromal invasion
IIIA	G 1, 2, 3	Tumor invades serosa and/or adnexa and/or positive peritoneal cytology
IIIB	G 1, 2, 3	Vaginal metastases
IIIC	G 1, 2, 3	Metastases to pelvic and/or paraaortic lymph nodes
IVA	G 1, 2, 3	Tumor invasion of bladder and/or bowel mucosa
IVB	G 1, 2, 3	Distant metastases, including intraabdominal and/or inguinal lymph nodes

9. **What percentage of endometrial carcinomas are stage I at diagnosis?**
   Approximately 75%.

10. **What are the significant prognostic factors in endometrial adenocarcinoma?**
    The most important prognostic factors are histologic differentiation (tumor grade), histologic type, depth of myometrial invasion, and cervical stromal involvement. High-grade tumors and tumors that deeply invade the myometrium or involve the cervix are more likely to have spread to the adnexa or lymph nodes, therefore placing the patient in a more advanced stage.

11. **How does endometrial carcinoma spread?**
    Endometrial carcinoma arises from the glands of the endometrium and initially grows slowly. Eventually it invades the underlying myometrium. Extrauterine spread occurs by lymphatics and blood. Lymphatic invasion results in metastasis to the parametrial, pelvic, aortic, or inguinal nodes. Hematogenous spread usually results in pulmonary metastasis but may involve bone and liver. Peritoneal implants may be caused by lymphatic spread or transtubal or transmural penetration.

12. **How is endometrial carcinoma treated?**
    The initial treatment is surgical staging with abdominopelvic washings for cytology, total abdominal hysterectomy, and bilateral salpingo-oophorectomy. Pelvic and paraaortic lymph node sampling is also performed except in patients with grade 1 tumors invading < 50% of the myometrium (gross inspection and frozen section evaluation are used to assess myometrial invasion and cervical/adnexal spread). After surgery, adjuvant radiation, chemotherapy, and/or hormonal therapy may be used, based on the surgical findings.

13. **What is the incidence of pelvic and paraaortic lymph node metastases in patients with tumors confined to the uterus (presumed stage I)?**
    The risk depends on many factors, the most important of which are grade and depth of myometrial invasion. The risk of deep invasion by tumor grade is 10% for G1, 20% for G2, and 42% for G3. If the tumor is deeply invasive, the risk of pelvic node metastases is 11% for G1, 19% for G2, and 34% for G3. If the tumor is deeply invasive, the risk of paraaortic node metastases is 6% for G1, 14% for G2, and 23% for G3.

14. **Can radiation alone be used to treat endometrial carcinoma?**
    Yes, but the cure rate drops from about 80% for all stage I patients to about 50%. It is therefore used only in patients too debilitated to undergo surgery.

15. What are the most common sites of recurrence in patients treated with surgery and adjuvant radiation therapy? In patients treated with surgery alone?

After surgery plus radiation: lung, abdomen, liver, or bone. After surgery alone: vaginal apex, pelvic side wall, and parametrium.

16. What is the most active chemotherapy agent against endometrial carcinoma?

The response rate to doxorubicin is as high as 38%. Unfortunately, the duration of response is short.

17. What is the role of hormonal therapy in the treatment of endometrial carcinoma?

Many endometrial carcinomas, especially low-grade tumors, have estrogen and progesterone receptors and respond to progestational therapy. The overall response rate is < 30%, but side effects of treatment are minimal. Thus it is often the first treatment used for metastatic disease. Responses to progestins can be prolonged; therefore, treatment is continued as long as the disease remains stable.

18. What is uterine papillary serous adenocarcinoma? How does it commonly spread?

Uterine papillary serous adenocarcinoma is a variant of endometrial carcinoma characterized by histology that resembles ovarian serous carcinomas. This variant tends to spread intraperitoneally, like ovarian carcinoma, and has a higher incidence of nodal spread and distant metastases.

19. Is hormone replacement therapy appropriate after treatment of endometrial carcinoma?

Yes, in select patients. Women with early-stage disease have an excellent long-term prognosis. It is therefore important to protect them from the deleterious effects of estrogen deprivation, namely osteoporosis and cardiovascular disease.

20. How is tamoxifen related to endometrial cancer?

Tamoxifen (a nonsteroidal antiestrogen) therapy can induce or promote the development of endometrial adenocarcinoma. The increased risk seems to be dose- and time-dependent. The risk is 2–3 times that of the general population.

BIBLIOGRAPHY

1. Barakat RR, Wong G, Curtin JP, et al: Tamoxifen use in breast cancer is not associated with a higher incidence of adverse histologic features. Gynecol Oncol 55:164, 1994.
2. Behbakht K, Hordan EL, et al: Prognostic indicators of survival in advanced endometrial cancer. Gynecol Oncol 55:363, 1994.
3. Brinton LA, Berman ML, Mortel R, et al: Reproductive, menstrual, and medical risk factors for endometrial cancer: Results from a case-control study. Am J Obstet Gynecol 167:1317, 1992.
4. Burke TW, Heller PB, Woodward JE, et al: Treatment failure in endometrial carcinoma. Obstet Gynecol 75:96, 1990.
5. Creasman WT, Morrow CP, Buncy BN, et al: Surgical pathologic spread patterns of endometrial cancer. A Gynecologic Oncology Group study. Cancer 60:2035–2041, 1987.
6. Grady D, Gebretsadik T, Kerlikowske K, et al: Hormone replacement therapy and endometrial cancer risk: A meta-analysis. Obstet Gynecol 85:304, 1995.
7. Janicek MF, Rosenshein NB: Invasive endometrial cancer in uteri resected for atypical endometrial hyperplasia. Gynecol Oncol 52:373, 1994.
8. Kadar N, Malfetano JH, Homesley HD: Determinants of survival of surgically staged patients with endometrial carcinoma histologically confined to the uterus: Implications for therapy. Obstet Gynecol 80:655, 1992.
9. Lee RB, Burke TW, Park RC: Estrogen replacement therapy following treatment for Stage I endometrial carcinoma. Gynecol Oncol 36:189, 1990.
10. Moore TD, Phillips PH, Nerenstone SR, Cheson BD: Systemic treatment of advanced and recurrent endometrial carcinoma: Current status and future directions. J Clin Oncol 9:1071, 1991.
11. Wingo PA, Tong T, Bolden S. Cancer statistics, 1995. Cancer J Clin 45:8, 1995.

35. OVARIAN CANCER

Helen Frederickson, M.D.

1. What is the incidence of ovarian cancer? Which women are at increased risk for developing the disease?

The incidence of ovarian cancer increases with age. Lifetime incidence is 1 of 70 women (1.4%). The median age at diagnosis is 61. Nulliparous women have an increased risk, whereas use of oral contraceptives confers a protective effect. Thus, the probability of developing ovarian cancer is related to the total number of ovulatory cycles.

Patients with breast cancer have a twofold increase in risk of developing ovarian cancer. A small percentage of ovarian cancer is familial (< 5%); patients in families with true familial ovarian cancer have a 50% risk (autosomal dominant) of developing the disease.

Environmental factors play an unknown role in development of ovarian cancer. Ovarian cancer has its highest incidence in industrialized countries, possibly because of high animal fat diets.

2. How does the typical patient with ovarian cancer present?

Most patients have vague abdominal complaints. Early satiety and abdominal bloating signal ascites and often omental spread of disease. Usually, a pelvic mass is present. Serum CA125 levels are elevated in 80% of patients with epithelial cancers; 75% of patients present with stage III disease.

3. Is there a screening test for ovarian cancer?

No. Pelvic examination may detect an ovarian cancer before it becomes disseminated, but there are no data on the frequency with which ovarian cancer is detected in asymptomatic women by pelvic exam. Ultrasonography is not sufficiently specific to be useful as a screening procedure in asymptomatic women. The specificity of ultrasound diagnosis may be improved by transvaginal sonography and color-flow Doppler studies, but to date no data imply a decrease in mortality in screened populations.

CA125 is not a good screening test because the incidence of the disease in the general population is so low that the majority of positive tests are false positives.

Even in women with two first-degree relatives with ovarian cancer (i.e., true familial ovarian cancer syndrome with a risk of 50%), the ability of screening tests to detect earlier-stage ovarian cancer has not been established.

4. How is ovarian cancer staged?

Surgical staging in the absence of obvious stage III disease includes (1) peritoneal washings; (2) multiple peritoneal biopsies (in the upper abdomen, bilateral colic gutters and diaphragm assessment [may be by Pap smear]; in the pelvis, bilateral pelvic sidewall, cul-de-sac, and bladder peritoneum); (3) pelvic and paraaortic node sampling; and (4) infracolic omentectomy.

5. Describe the stages of ovarian cancer.

Stages	Description
I	Confined to the ovaries
IA	Confined to single ovary
IB	Both ovaries involved
IC	No gross spread beyond ovaries
	Malignant cells in cytologic washings or ascites
	Spread to ovarian surface
	Tumor ruptured at surgery

II	Spread in pelvis beyond ovaries
IIA	Spread to uterus or fallopian tube
IIB	Spread to other pelvic structures
IIC	Malignant cells in cytologic washings or ascites
	Tumor ruptured at surgery
III	Extrapelvic spread confined to abdominal cavity or inguinal nodes
IIIA	No gross spread beyond pelvis, with microscopic implants to upper abdomen
IIIB	Gross intraabdominal extrapelvic implants < 2 cm
IIIC	Gross intraabdominal extrapelvic implants > 2 cm
	Retroperitoneal spread to pelvic or aortic lymph nodes or inguinal nodes
IV	Distant spread

6. Why is aggressive cytoreductive surgery pursued in the initial treatment of advanced-stage ovarian cancer?

Survival rates are better in patients with smaller residual disease than in patients with larger residual disease, despite identical chemotherapeutic regimens postoperatively. This difference relates to the Goldie-Coldman hypothesis, which predicts that smaller tumor nodules are more likely to be chemosensitive than larger nodules because of a higher percentage of spontaneous mutations to a resistant phenotype in larger nodules. Most gynecologic oncologists consider maximal nodule diameter of < 2 cm as optimal debulking.

7. Which chemotherapy regimens are used postoperatively?

Presently, platinum-based regimens are the first-line chemotherapy for ovarian cancer. Studies comparing single-agent chemotherapy with combination therapy suggest that combination therapy prolongs survival and progression-free interval. Until recently, the standard chemotherapeutic regimen has been the combination of cisplatin plus cyclophosphamide (Cytoxan). The doses of cisplatin ranged from 50–100 mg/m^2. The major dose-limiting toxicity of cisplatin is neurotoxicity. Carboplatin is an analog of cisplatin with less neurotoxicity; thus it is more suitable for dose intensity studies. The activity of the new drug, paclitaxel (Taxol), in previously treated patients has led to studies using combinations of platinum and paclitaxel as first-line therapy. Data suggest that this combination is better than cisplatin and cyclophosphamide in suboptimally debulked patients. The optimal length of therapy has not been established. A prospective randomized trial compared 5 cycles with 10 cycles of platinum-based therapy and showed no statistical difference.

8. Is there a role for a second-look laparotomy?

Yes, when a patient is part of a research protocol for either first- or second-line therapy. In about one-half of patients with a complete clinical response (including a negative CA125), malignancy is found at second-look. In 50% of patients with a negative second-look laparotomy, treated with platinum-based regimens, tumor will recur. Surgical assessment of residual disease remains the only way to determine treatment effectiveness and thus the only way to determine the benefit of new treatment regimens. The survival benefit of second-look laparotomy has not been proved.

Second-look laparotomy should be performed by a gynecologic oncologist who has a complete understanding of ovarian cancer and has defined the goals of second-look laparotomy for the individual patient. Plans for further therapy should be made before the procedure; some protocols treat patients with negative second-look laparotomy. Secondary debulking has shown survival benefits in a small subset of patients.

9. What is the prognosis of patients with ovarian cancer?

The 5-year survival rate for patients with stage III or IV disease is only 25–30%. The most common cause of death is related to ascites, bowel obstruction, and essentially slow starvation. Distant metastases, including bone, lung, liver, and brain, are unusual.

The 5-year survival of patients with stage I disease is 80%. Grade 1 stage I tumors have a 95% 5-year survival rate.

10. Is there any benefit to secondary debulking at second-look laparotomy or in patients with recurrent disease after first-line therapy?

The benefit of secondary debulking has not been proved. Patients who progress on platinum therapy are unlikely to survive, regardless of further therapy. Patients with bulky residual disease at second surgery are also unlikely to survive, but some studies suggest that if bulky disease can be converted to microscopic residual disease, patients may have a survival advantage with second-line treatments.

11. What second-line therapies are available?

Patients with minimal residual disease after second surgery are candidates for intraperitoneal chemotherapy. The most common agent used for intraperitoneal therapy is cisplatin. About 50–75% of patients survive 2–4 years after intraperitoneal salvage. More recently taxol has become available for second-line therapy; 30% of platinum-resistant patients respond to taxol with an average response duration of 7 months. Other second-line drugs include hexamethylmelamine, VP-16, and 5-fluorouracil. Topotecan has recently been approved for second-line therapy in ovarian cancer. Whole abdominal radiation therapy has had significant response rates in patients with small-volume disease, but the rate of bowel obstruction after this therapy is about 20–30%.

12. Does autologous bone marrow transplant have a role in patients with ovarian cancer?

Patients with minimal residual disease who are chemoresponsive may be good candidates for treatment with high-dose chemotherapy with bone marrow transplant. Presently, no data suggest that this therapy is superior to intensive traditional chemotherapy. The Gynecologic Oncology Group plans to look at the role of bone marrow transplant in a randomized study of chemotherapy-sensitive patients at completion of first-line therapy.

13. What is the significance of an ovarian tumor of low malignant potential?

Tumors of low malignant potential or borderline malignancy are epithelial tumors of the ovary with an excellent prognosis but histologic features of cancer. Even if the tumor has spread to the abdomen, the 5-year survival rate is 80%. Patients may die of disease, however, as long as 20 years later. These tumors do not benefit from adjuvant chemotherapy in early or advanced stages. The indolent clinical course of these tumors suggests a low growth fraction and thus accounts for their lack of responsiveness to chemotherapy.

BIBLIOGRAPHY

1. Bast RC, Klug TL, St. John E, et al: A radioimmunoassay using a monoclonal antibody to monitor the course of epithelial ovarian cancer. N Engl J Med 309:883, 1983.
2. Benjamin I, Rubin SC: Management of early stage epithelial ovarian cancer. Obstet Gynecol Clin North Am 21:107, 1994.
3. Cancer and Steroid Hormone Study of the Centers for Disease Control and the National Institute of Child Health and Human Development: The reduction in risk of ovarian cancer associated with oral contraceptive use. N Engl J Med 316:650, 1987.
4. Goldie JH, Coldman AJ: A mathematic model for relating the drug sensitivity of tumors to their spontaneous mutation rate. Cancer Treat Rep 63:1727, 1979.
5. Granai CO: Ovarian cancer—unrealistic expectations. N Engl J Med 327:197, 1992.
6. Griffiths CT, Parker LM, Fuller AF: Role of cytoreductive surgical treatment in the management of advanced ovarian cancer. Cancer Treat Rep 63:235, 1979.
7. McGuire WP, Hoskins WJ, Brady MF, et al: Cyclophosphamide and cisplatin compared with pacitaxil and cisplatin in patients with Stage III and Stage IV ovarian cancer. N Engl J Med 334:1, 1996.
8. NIH Consensus Development Conference on Ovarian Cancer: Screening, treatment, and follow-up. Gynecol Oncol 55:S173, 1994.
9. Nguyuen HN, Averette HE, Janicek MF: Ovarian carcinoma: A review of the significance of familial risk factors and the role of prophylactic oophorectomy in cancer prevention. Cancer 74:545, 1994.
10. Potter ME, Soong SJ, et al: Second-look laparotomy and salvage therapy: A research modality only? Gynecol Oncol 44:3, 1992.
11. Potter ME, Partridge EE, Hatch KD, et al: Primary surgical therapy of ovarian cancer: How much and when. Gynecol Oncol 40:195, 1991.

36. GERM CELL, STROMAL, AND OTHER OVARIAN TUMORS

Thomas W. Montag, M.D.

GERM CELL TUMORS

1. What is the incidence of ovarian germ cell tumors? How often are they malignant?
Germ cell tumors constitute approximately 20% of all benign and malignant ovarian neoplasms. Only 3–5% of ovarian germ cell tumors are malignant. Germ cell tumors are more frequent in children and adolescents, comprising 60–70% of ovarian neoplasms in females under the age of 20. One-third of germ cell tumors in patients in this age range are malignant.

2. What are the histologic types of germ cell tumors?
The World Health Organization (WHO) Classification is presented in decreasing order of frequency below. Mixtures of these histologic types occur in 10–15% of cases.

WHO Histologic Classification of Ovarian Germ Cell Tumors

I. Teratomas	II. Dysgerminoma
A. Immature (solid, cystic, or both)	III. Endodermal sinus tumor
B. Mature	IV. Embryonal carcinoma
1. Solid	V. Choriocarcinoma
2. Cystic	VI. Polyembryoma
a. Dermoid cyst (mature cystic teratoma)	VII. Mixed forms
b. Dermoid cyst with malignant transformation	
C. Monodermal or highly specialized	
1. Struma ovarii 3. Struma ovarii and carcinoid	
2. Carcinoid 4. Others	

3. What is the most common germ cell tumor?
Cystic teratomas (dermoids) account for over 95% of teratomas and 10–12% of all ovarian neoplasms. Dysgerminoma is the most common *malignant* ovarian germ cell neoplasm, accounting for about 1% of all ovarian neoplasms.

4. What is the histogenesis of germ cell tumors?
The most commonly accepted proposed derivation of germ cell tumors is depicted below.

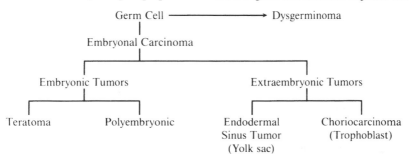

The histogenesis of germ cell neoplasms. (From Teilum G: Special Tumors of Ovary and Testis and Related Extragonadal Lesions: Comparative Pathology and Histological Identification, 2nd ed. Philadelphia, J.B. Lippincott, 1977, with permission.)

5. What are the presenting symptoms of ovarian germ cell tumors?

Most frequently, young patients report pelvic fullness or urinary symptoms such as frequency or dysuria. Diffuse, nonspecific abdominal pain, rectal pressure, menstrual irregularities, or a palpable mass may be present. Torsion or rupture may result in acute symptoms.

6. What diagnostic studies should be performed when germ cell tumors are suspected?

A thorough history and physical examination should be performed, searching for evidence of metastases. Ultrasonographic evaluation will determine the size and consistency of pelvic/abdominal masses. Lesions that are solid or solid and cystic are likely to be neoplastic and require exploratory laparotomy. Adnexal masses that are 2 cm or larger in premenarcheal females or 8 cm or larger in postmenarcheal women require surgical exploration. If menstruating patients have predominantly cystic lesions up to 8 cm in diameter, hormonal suppression with oral contraceptives may be attempted. Persistent masses after two cycles require surgical exploration.

A chest x-ray may demonstrate pulmonary or mediastinal metastases. A karyotype should be obtained for all premenarcheal patients, because these tumors have a propensity to arise in dysgenetic gonads. Routine blood studies and serum for tumor markers should be drawn preoperatively. (A preoperative CT scan may disclose retroperitoneal lymphadenopathy or liver metastases, but would not change management, as these patients need exploration.)

7. Which tumor markers are associated with ovarian germ cell tumors?

Lactic dehydrogenase (LDH), alpha-fetoprotein (AFP), human chorionic gonadotropin (HCG), and CA-125 have been found to be elevated in germ cell tumors. All patients with germ cell malignancies should be monitored during and after treatment with serial LDH, AFP, HCG, and CA-125 determinations, because these markers are not specific, and pure and mixed tumors may be difficult to determine histologically.

Tumor Markers in Ovarian Germ Cell Tumors

TUMOR	HCG	AFP	LDH	CA-125
Mixed germ cell tumor	+	+	+	+
Embryonal carcinoma	+	+	±	+
Endodermal sinus tumor	–	+	±	?
Dysgerminoma	±	–	+	+
Immature teratoma	–	±	±	+
Choriocarcinoma	+	–	±	?

Modified from Morrow CP, Curtin JP, Townsend DE (eds): Synopsis of Gynecologic Oncology. New York, Churchill Livingstone, 1993.

8. What is the staging system employed for germ cell tumors?

The International Federation of Gynecology and Obstetrics (FIGO) staging system for epithelial ovarian carcinoma is also used for germ cell tumors. The main route of dissemination for germ cell tumors is by regional lymphatics, most commonly to the paraaortic and iliac nodes. This is especially true for dysgerminomas. Nondysgerminomatous germ cell tumors also commonly spread to peritoneal surfaces. Peritoneal spread with dysgerminomas may also occur. Hematogenous spread of all germ cell tumors occurs late in the disease process.

9. Describe the clinical management of germ cell tumors.

1. **Benign cystic teratomas** (dermoids) should be removed intact. Cystectomy, oophorectomy, or salpingo-oophorectomy may be performed, depending on the contralateral adnexa and the salvageability of the involved ovary. If bilateral involvement is present overtly, bilateral cystectomy should be performed when it is desirous to preserve ovarian function. Previous recommendations to bivalve an apparently normal contralateral ovary are outdated, because the incidence of covert bilateral disease is low and the risk of infertility from adhesions or ovarian failure is high.

2. **Dysgerminomas** are overtly bilateral in 10–15% of cases and covertly bilateral in an additional 15% of cases. Thus, if the diagnosis of dysgerminoma is known intraoperatively, bilateral salpingo-oophorectomy should be performed if both ovaries clearly contain tumor. Surgery for dysgerminoma apparently confined to one ovary should involve obtaining peritoneal fluid/washings for cytology, unilateral salpingo-oophorectomy, wedge biopsy of the contralateral ovary, infracolic omentectomy, and ipsilateral pelvic and paraaortic node dissection. Total abdominal hysterectomy and bilateral salpingo-oophorectomy (TAH/BSO) may be performed if the patient does not desire future fertility. Tumor reductive surgery should be attempted for disseminated disease.

Pelvic or paraaortic nodal metastases may be treated with radiation therapy, as dysgerminomas are highly radiosensitive tumors. Techniques to preserve fertility with shielding of the uninvolved ovary or oophoropexy of the remaining ovary can be done in these women. Disseminated disease requires chemotherapy with vincristine, actinomycin D, and cyclophosphamide (VAC) or bleomycin, etoposide, and cisplatin (BEP). There may be a role for primary chemotherapy rather than radiation therapy to preserve ovarian function.

3. The majority of **nondysgerminomatous malignant germ cell tumors** are confined to the ovary at the time of diagnosis. Unilateral salpingo-oophorectomy, subtotal omentectomy, peritoneal cytology, and ipsilateral pelvic and paraaortic node biopsies should be performed when preservation of fertility is desired. TAH/BSO may be performed in older patients who do not desire fertility. Careful evaluation of the entire peritoneal cavity is essential. Tumor reductive surgery should be performed for disseminated disease. The addition of hysterectomy and contralateral salpingo-oophorectomy does not alter the outcome when the uterus and contralateral ovary appear grossly normal. When fertility is an issue, the uterus and contralateral ovary should not be removed.

Combination chemotherapy with VAC or BEP should be given to all patients with germ cell tumors, except those with stage IA, grade 1 immature teratomas. BEP or VBP (vinblastine, bleomycin, and cisplatin) appear to be more effective than VAC.

10. Is the clinical management different when a germ cell tumor is diagnosed during pregnancy?

Dysgerminoma accounts for 25–35% of all ovarian cancers coexisting with pregnancy. The nondysgerminomatous germ cell tumors occur predominantly in the second and third decades, and thus will also be associated with pregnancy. When an ovarian mass is discovered in the first trimester and does not resolve, laparotomy with resection should be performed in the early second trimester. If the mass is noted in the second or third trimesters, laparotomy with resection is indicated. In the third trimester, some delay is usually acceptable until fetal maturity is documented, at which time surgical resection and cesarean section may be performed. In any trimester, staging procedures should be performed for disease confined to the ovary. Tumor reductive surgery should be performed for disseminated disease. Pregnancy termination for disseminated disease is controversial and depends largely on gestational age. Because of the rapid growth of germ cell tumors, chemotherapy should be initiated within 2 weeks of surgery. When conservative surgery is performed in the first half of pregnancy, the potential risks to the developing fetus must be considered and pregnancy termination offered. Risk of congenital abnormalities is highest in the first trimester, especially with antimetabolites and alkylating agents. During the second half of pregnancy, chemotherapy can be given in the same dosages as for nonpregnant patients and is generally not associated with an increase in fetal abnormalities, although the number of patients reported is relatively small.

11. What is the duration of chemotherapy?

The optimal number of treatment cycles has yet to be established. In the past, VAC was given for 2 years, then shortened to 12 months without reduction in survival rates. Based on the efficacy of 3 or 4 courses of multi-agent chemotherapy in testicular germ cell malignancies, there is a trend toward employing 4–6 courses of VAC or BEP for ovarian germ cell tumors. Recent data support the use of 4 cycles of BEP and the use of VAC for BEP failures or those patients unable to take BEP.

12. What are the effects of chemotherapy on subsequent menstrual function and reproductive capacity?

The incidence of menstrual dysfunction or ovarian failure in young women treated with chemotherapy is variable, with the risk increasing with patient age and duration of therapy. When short-term invasive chemotherapy is employed, reproductive injury is uncommon. Oral contraceptives taken during chemotherapy may reduce the risk of ovarian failure. Many reports of normal pregnancy following completion of combination chemotherapy have appeared in the literature. With short-term multi-agent therapy, there does not appear to be increased risk of pregnancy complications or fetal abnormalities.

13. Is there a role for second-look laparotomies in ovarian germ cell tumors?

Second-look laparotomy has been recommended in the past for patients with Stage I endodermal sinus tumor, embryonal cell carcinoma, mixed germ cell tumors, and incompletely staged, immature teratomas following completion of chemotherapy. Recently the value of the operation has been questioned. On the GOG protocol for germ cell tumors, the requirement for second look was made optional. In addition, second-look exploratory laparotomy may be appropriate in patients at high risk for failure, such as those with advanced stage and especially those with large amounts of residual disease after the initial surgery. If these patients have positive tumor markers, there would be no role for a second-look laparotomy.

14. What is the association between gonadal dysgenesis and ovarian germ cell tumors?

Approximately 5% of dysgerminomas are discovered in phenotypic females with abnormal gonads, i.e., pure dysgenesis (46XY, bilateral streak gonads), mixed gonadal dysgenesis (45X/46XY, unilateral streak gonad, contralateral testes), and androgen insensitivity syndrome (46XY). A karyotype should be obtained in premenarcheal patients with a pelvic mass. Dysgerminomas in patients with gonadal dysgenesis arise in gonadoblastomas, which are benign tumors characterized by germ cells mixed with sex cord elements. If gonadoblastomas are left in situ, approximately 50% will develop into ovarian malignancies. Choriocarcinoma, embryonal carcinoma, and mixed germ cell tumors have all been reported to arise in gonadoblastomas. Prophylactic bilateral gonadectomy before puberty is recommended in all intersex patients with a Y chromosome, except in those with testicular feminization, in whom delay to age 30 can be considered.

SEX CORD–STROMAL TUMORS

15. How common are the sex cord–stromal tumors of the ovary?

Ovarian sex cord–stromal tumors account for about 5–8% of all ovarian malignancies.

16. What are the histologic types of sex cord–stromal tumors?

This group of tumors is derived from the sex cords and ovarian stroma. A classification is presented below:

Classification of Sex Cord–Stromal Tumors

I. Granulosa–stromal cell tumors	II. Sertoli-Leydig cell tumors (androblastomas)	III. Gynandroblastoma
A. Granulosa cell tumors	A. Well-differentiated	IV. Unclassified
B. Tumors in the thecoma–fibroma group	1. Sertoli cell tumors	A. Sex cord tumor with annular tubules
1. Thecoma	2. Sertoli-Leydig cell tumor	B. Lipid cell tumors
2. Fibroma–fibrosarcoma	3. Leydig cell tumor; hilus cell tumor	
3. Sclerosing stromal tumor	B. Moderately differentiated	
4. Unclassified	C. Poorly differentiated (sarcomatoid)	
	D. With heterologous elements	

17. How are sex cord–stromal tumors of the ovary staged?

The FIGO staging system for epithelial ovarian carcinomas is employed.

18. How can an ovarian tumor be composed of cells commonly found in the testes, i.e., Sertoli and Leydig cells?

The embryonic gonad can develop into either an ovary or testes. The parenchyma of the ovary and the testicle are derived from the same primitive parenchymal stroma. Granulosa and Sertoli cells are homologous, as are theca and Leydig cells.

19. Why are sex cord–stromal tumors called "functioning" tumors?

Many of these tumors synthesize estrogen, progesterone, testosterone, other androgens, and occasionally corticosteroids. Hormone production is not consistent and cannot be used to classify these tumors, because occasionally a tumor composed of "female" cells (granulosa or theca) produces androgens and vice versa. About 15% of stromal tumors do not produce hormones.

20. How do sex cord–stromal tumors present?

Approximately 50% of granulosa cell tumors occur in postmenopausal women and less than 5% develop in premenarcheal girls, most of whom develop isosexual precocity associated with estrogen production. Granulosa cell tumors have a high frequency of rupture, especially in pregnancy, causing pain and bleeding. Fibromas and thecomas are rare in children and adolescents. They can cause amenorrhea, menometrorrhagia, or postmenopausal bleeding. Occasional patients will present with signs of androgen production. Sertoli-Leydig cell tumors are most often virilizing, resulting in oligomenorrhea, breast and genital atrophy, clitoromegaly, hirsutism, acne, deepened voice, and increased libido.

21. What is Meigs' syndrome?

The combination of clinically detectable ascites, hydrothorax, and a benign ovarian tumor, commonly an ovarian fibroma, is popularly known as Meigs' syndrome. The benign nature of this syndrome is important, because some women have not undergone surgery owing to the mistaken impression of far advanced malignancy.

22. Are there known associations with any of the sex cord–stromal tumors of the ovary and other disorders?

Adenocarcinoma of the endometrium is associated with 10–15% of granulosa (and theca) cell tumors. Up to 50% have endometrial hyperplasia or polyps. Juvenile granulosa cell tumors are associated with Ollier's disease (multiple endochondromatosis). Ovarian fibromas occur commonly in young women with Gorlin syndrome, an autosomal dominant syndrome characterized by basal cell nevi, carcinomas, skeletal abnormalities, and dental cysts. One-third of patients with sex cord tumors with annular tubules have been reported to have Peutz-Jeghers syndrome: gastrointestinal polyposis with oral and cutaneous melanin pigmentation. Adenoma malignum of the cervix is also associated with sex cord tumors with annular tubules.

23. How are sex cord–stromal tumors managed surgically?

If abnormal uterine bleeding is present, a fractional curettage should be performed preoperatively to rule out cervical or endometrial cancer. Because the majority of these tumors are unilateral, conservation of the contralateral ovary and uterus may be considered after proper surgical staging in those patients desirous of preserving fertility. Wedge biopsy of the contralateral normal appearing ovary is not recommended. In perimenopausal and postmenopausal women, a hysterectomy and bilateral oophorectomy should be performed. Although insufficient data exist regarding tumor reductive surgery (debulking) for disseminated disease, if feasible, it should be performed. Hormone receptors on the fresh specimen may be helpful for subsequent management.

24. Which patients are candidates for adjuvant postoperative chemotherapy?

It is difficult to determine the role of adjuvant chemotherapy in stromal tumors of the ovary because of the rarity and indolent behavior of these tumors. Adjuvant therapy should be considered for patients with ruptured granulosa cell tumors, granulosa cell tumors with > 2 mitoses/10 HPF, positive cytology, or size greater than 10–12 cm in diameter, Sertoli-Leydig cell tumors with poor differentiation or heterologous elements, lipid cell tumors with large size, high mitotic counts, or pleomorphism, or in any patient with disease beyond Stage I.

25. Which chemotherapeutic regimens are active in sex cord–stromal tumors?

VAC: vincristine, actinomycin D, and cyclophosphamide
AcFuCy: actinomycin D, 5-fluorouracil, and cyclophosphamide
VBP: vinblastine, bleomycin, and cisplatin (Platinol)
CAP: cyclophosphamide, adriamycin, and cisplatin have been used with responses in patients with measurable disease.

26. What about radiation therapy or hormonal therapy?

There is no evidence to support the use of adjuvant radiation therapy, although radiation may be employed to palliate focal recurrent disease. The use of progestins or antiestrogens has theoretical value, but no data are available to suggest efficacy.

27. Are there tumor markers for sex cord–stromal ovarian tumors?

Serum CA-125 has been found to be elevated in some of these tumors, especially granulosa cell tumors. Follicle regulatory protein (FRP) may be useful for granulosa cell tumors when it becomes commercially available. When a stromal tumor produces measurable hormone levels, serial values may be useful in long-term surveillance for recurrence.

OTHER OVARIAN MALIGNANCIES

28. What other primary tumors may originate in the ovaries?

Mesenchymal tumors not specific to gonadal stroma may arise in the ovaries but are extremely rare. Examples include myxoma (connective tissue origin), endometrioid stromal sarcomas, malignant mixed mesodermal sarcomas (endometrioid stromal origin), leiomyomas, leiomyosarcomas, rhabdomyosarcomas (muscle origin), hemangioma, lymphangioma, hemangiopericytomas, angiosarcoma (vascular origin), neurofibroma, neurilemmoma, neurofibrosarcoma, ganglioneuroma, pheochromocytoma (neural origin), osteoma, osteogenic sarcoma, and chondrosarcoma (skeletal origin).

29. Which tumors commonly metastasize to the ovaries?

About 5% of ovarian tumors are metastatic from other organs, most frequently from the female genital tract, the breast, or the gastrointestinal tract. Lymphoma and leukemia can involve the ovaries, usually in advanced stage disease. In about 75% of ovarian secondaries, both ovaries are grossly involved, and usually metastatic disease is found in other parts of the body.

30. What is Krukenberg tumor?

This term should be restricted to ovarian neoplasms characterized by mucin-containing signet-ring cells with a sarcoma-like stromal hyperplasia. The primary tumor is most frequently from the stomach, and less commonly from the colon, breast, or biliary tract. Rarely the cervix or bladder may be the primary site.

BIBLIOGRAPHY

1. Berek JS, Hacker NF (eds): Practical Gynecologic Oncology. Baltimore, Williams & Wilkins, 1994.
2. Gershenson DM, Morris M, Burke T, et al: Treatment of poor-prognosis sex cord–stromal tumors of the ovary with the combination of bleomycin, etoposide, and cisplatin. Obstet Gynecol 87:527, 1996.

3. Malmstrom H, Hogberg T, Risberg B, Simonsen B: Granulosa cell tumors of the ovary: Prognostic factors and outcome. Gynecol Oncol 52:50, 1994.
4. Morrow CP, Curtin JP, Townsend DE (eds): Synopsis of Gynecologic Oncology. New York, Churchill Livingstone, 1993.
5. Stenwig JT, Hazekamp JT, Beecham JB: Granulosa cell tumors of the ovary: A clinicopathological study of 118 cases with long-term follow-up. Gynecol Oncol 136:52, 1979.
6. Zambetti M, Escobedo A, Pilotti S, De Palo G: Cisplatinum/vinblastine/bleomycin combination chemotherapy in advanced or recurrent granulosa cell tumors of the ovary. Gynecol Oncol 36:317, 1990.

37. VULVAR CARCINOMA

Kevin Davis, M.D.

1. How common is vulvar carcinoma?

Vulvar carcinoma accounts for 1% of all carcinomas in women and approximately 5% of all female genital malignancies.

2. What are the significant risk factors for vulvar carcinoma?

Vulvar carcinomas are more common in elderly (average age at diagnosis = 65), obese, hypertensive, and diabetic women. Vulvar dysplasia, low socioeconomic class, and history of vulvar dystrophies are associated with an increased incidence of vulvar carcinoma. Cigarette smoking has recently been implicated.

3. Do venereal warts increase the risk of vulvar carcinoma?

Unknown. Human papillomavirus (HPV) has been found in up to 60% of squamous cell carcinomas. There appears to be a similar association of HPV DNA with vulvar malignancy and squamous cell cervical carcinoma, but a direct causative mechanism has not been found.

4. What are the common presenting symptoms of patients with vulvar carcinoma?

Patients presenting without symptoms are rare. Most women with vulvar carcinoma complain of pain or itching (pruritus) associated with a raised area or ulcer.

5. How is the diagnosis made?

A high degree of suspicion, together with a required biopsy of the lesion.

6. List the different histologic subtypes and their incidence.

Squamous cell	86%	Basal cell carcinoma	2%
Melanoma	6%	Sarcoma	2%
Adenocarcinoma (Bartholin gland)	3.5%	Paget's disease	0.5%

7. What is the most important prognostic indicator for vulvar carcinoma?

Inguinal node involvement.

8. What increases the risk of node involvement?

Depth of invasion, tumor diameter, and decreasing degree of differentiation.

Depth of invasion (mm)	Groin node metastasis (%)
< 1	0
1–2	8
2–3	11
3–4	26

9. Describe the current staging system.

Since 1988, surgical staging has been used in vulvar carcinoma. The rules for staging are similar to those for carcinomas of the cervix.

Staging for Carcinoma of the Vulva

Stage 0		
Tis	Carcinoma in situ; intraepithelial carcinoma	
Stage I		
T1N0 M0	Tumor confined to the vulva and/or perineum; ≤ 2 cm in greatest dimension; nodes not palpable	
Stage II		
T2N0 M0	Tumor confined to vulva and/or perineum—> 2 cm in greatest dimension; nodes are not palpable	
Stage III		
T3N0 M0	Tumor of any size with	
T3N1 M0	(1) adjacent spread to lower urethra and/or vagina or anus and/or	
T1N1 M0	(2) unilateral regional lymph node metastasis	
T2N1 M0		
Stage IVA		
T1N2 M0	Tumor invades any of the following:	
T2N2 M0	Upper urethra, bladder mucosa, rectal mucosa, pelvic bone, and/or	
T3N2 M0	bilateral regional node metastasis	
T4 any N M0		
Stage IVB		
Any T	Any distant metastasis, including pelvic lymph nodes	
Any N, M1		

TNM Classification of Carcinoma of the Vulva

T	**Primary tumor**	**N**	**Regional lymph nodes**
Tis	Preinvasive carcinoma (carcinoma in situ)	N0	No lymph node metastasis
T1	Tumor confined to vulva and/or perineum; ≤ 2 cm in greatest dimension	N1	Unilateral regional lymph node metastasis
T2	Tumor confined to vulva and/or perineum; > 2 cm in greatest dimension	N2	Bilateral regional lymph node metastasis
T3	Tumor of any size with adjacent spread to urethra and/or vagina and/or to anus	**M**	**Distant metastasis**
		M0	No clinical metastasis
T4	Tumor of any size infiltrating bladder mucosa and/or rectal mucosa, including upper part of urethral mucosa and/or fixed to bone	M1	Distant metastasis (including pelvic lymph node metastasis)

From International Federation of Gynecology and Obstetrics: Annual report on the results of treatment in gynecological cancer. Int J Gynecol Obstet 28:189–190, 1989.

10. What is the therapy for vulvar carcinoma?

The trend over the past 10–15 years appears to be a less radical approach. For large lesions, radical vulvectomy, together with inguinal node dissection, has traditionally been the method of treatment. Smaller lesions (< 2 cm) that are not located in the clitoral region or midline (lateral only) can be less radically treated (e.g., radical hemivulvectomy with ipsilateral inguinal node dissection).

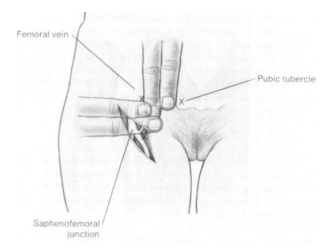

Femoral vein

Pubic tubercle

Saphenofemoral
junction

Incision can be made as noted so that superficial inguinal nodes can be removed easily. (From DiSaia PJ, Creasman WT: Clinical Gynecologic Oncology, 3rd ed. St. Louis, Mosby, 1989, p 256, with permission.)

11. When is a groin node dissection necessary?
Suspicious nodes should be pathologically assessed, along with nodes in patients with squamous cell carcinomas that are more deeply invasive than 1 m. Ipsilateral node dissections can be done for lateral lesions, because lymphatic flow is anterior and lateral, rarely crossing the midline to involve contralateral nodes.

12. Describe the lymphatic drainage of the vulva.
Superficial vulvar lymphatics extend over the perineal body, labia minora, forchette, and prepuce of the clitoris and drain toward the anterior portion of the labia minora. From there the lymphatics form several trunks extending toward the mons, turning laterally, and ending in the superficial nodes in the groins. The superficial inguinal and femoral nodes drain into the deep femoral nodes below the fascia lata and cribriform fascia. Drainage from the deep femoral nodes then proceeds to the deep pelvic nodes. The lymphatics of the clitoris may drain to either groin and have been found to drain directly to the deep pelvic nodes. Clinical experience has shown that the deep pelvic nodes are not involved without involvement of inguinal nodes.

13. What are some key anatomic landmarks of the femoral canal?
Superiorly—inguinal ligament
Medially—adductor longus muscle
Laterally—sartorius muscle
Floor (medial to lateral)—pectineus, iliopsoas muscles

14. What is Cloquet's node?
Cloquet's node (also called Rosenmuller's node, sentinal node) is the deepest node of the femoral group. It is located in the femoral canal, just medial and deep to the terminal branch of the femoral vein.

15. What are the most common complications of surgery in vulvar carcinoma?
Wound breakdown and lymphedema of the lower extremities.

16. Is radiation therapy used in vulvar carcinoma?
Radiation therapy is rarely used for stage I and II lesions. Its usefulness has been for locally advanced carcinomas in combination with surgery. Patients with metastasis to groin nodes benefit from adjuvant inguinal and pelvic radiation therapy.

17. How effective is chemotherapy for vulvar carcinoma?

Chemotherapy is relatively ineffective except when combined with radiation therapy. Chemotherapy has been used as salvage therapy, but recent studies suggest that it may have a role in management of advanced squamous carcinomas, combined with radiation therapy and surgery.

18. How common is Bartholin's gland carcinoma?

Bartholin's gland carcinomas account for approximately 3–5% of all vulvar carcinomas and are predominantly adenocarcinomas.

19. Discuss malignant melanoma of the vulva. What is the best staging system?

Malignant melanoma is the second most common malignancy of the vulva. Survival is based on depth of invasion and metastatic spread at diagnosis (e.g., nodes, urethra, vagina). Treatment is primarily surgical, because radiation and chemotherapy have not been proved beneficial. Estrogen receptors have been demonstrated in human melanoma, and responses to tamoxifen have been reported. Interferon is now used in high-risk patients with a 10% increased survival rate.

The Breslow microsurgical staging (millimeter measure of vertical thickness) appears to be the best system for predicting prognosis in malignant melanoma.

20. Discuss Paget's disease of the vulva.

Extramammary Paget's disease is a rare intraepithelial adenocarcinoma that often appears as a velvety red lesion with areas of superficial white coating ("cake-icing" effect). An underlying adenocarcinoma has been reported in 15–20% of patients. Noninvasive lesions are usually treated with wide excisions, having 1-cm margins by frozen section. Because of the propensity for node involvement, invasive lesions are more radically treated with bilateral inguinal lymphadenectomy and radical vulvectomy.

BIBLIOGRAPHY

1. Binder SW, Huang I, Yao S, et al: Risk factors for the development of lymph node metastasis vulvar squamous cell carcinoma. Gynecol Oncol 37:9, 1990.
2. DiSaia PJ, Creasman WT: Clinical Gynecologic Oncology, 4th ed. St. Louis, Mosby-Year Book, 1993.
3. Homesley HD, Bundy BN, Sedlis A, et al: Assessment of current International Federation of Gynecology and Obstetrics staging of vulvar carcinoma relative to prognostic factors for survival: A Gynecologic Oncology Group study. Am J Obstet Gynecol 164:997, 1991.
4. Homesley HD, Bundy BN, Sedlis A, et al: Prognostic factors for groin node metastasis in squamous cell carcinoma of the vulva: A Gynecologic Group study. Gynecol Oncol 49:279, 1993.
5. Morrow CP, Curtin JP, Townsend DE: Synopsis of Gynecologic Oncology, 4th ed. Edinburgh: Churchill Livingstone, 1993.
6. Podratz KC, Symmonda RE, Taylor WF, et al: Carcinoma of the vulva: Analysis of treatment and survival. Obstet Gynecol 61:63, 1983.
7. Thomas G, Dembo A, DePetrillo A, et al: Concurrent radiation and chemotherapy in vulvar carcinoma. Gynecol Oncol 34:263, 1989.

38. GESTATIONAL TROPHOBLASTIC DISEASE

Judith McCarthy, M.D.

1. What are the two types of molar pregnancy?

The two types of molar pregnancy are complete and partial. A **complete hydatidiform mole** arises from the fertilization of an empty ovum; i.e., the nucleus is absent or nonfunctional. The sperm duplicates its own chromosomes. The most common chromosomal pattern is 46XX, all paternally derived. No embryonic tissue is present. A **partial mole** is much rarer. Fetal and/or embryonic structures are identifiable. The chromosomal pattern is usually triploid, again paternally derived. The fetus usually survives only to 8–9 weeks—rarely to term—and often has multiple anomalies.

2. How often do malignant sequelae occur in patients with a partial mole? A complete mole?

Malignant sequelae occur in 5–10% of patients with a partial mole and 20% with a complete mole.

3. What is the histologic appearance of a hydatidiform mole?

The tissue of a hydatidiform mole consists of diffusely hydropic chorionic villi and hyperplastic trophoblasts. Grossly, the cystic villi give the appearance of clusters of grapes.

4. What is the most common presenting symptom of complete moles?

Vaginal bleeding is the most common symptom and occurs in approximately 97% of patients. Other symptoms, in descending order of frequency, include uterine size greater than dates, hyperemesis gravidarum, preeclampsia, hyperthyroidism, and trophoblastic pulmonary emboli.

5. What are the medical complications of molar pregnancy?

Medical complications include pregnancy-induced hypertension, hyperthyroidism, anemia, and hyperemesis. About 15–25% of patients have theca lutein cysts of the ovaries with enlargement > 6 cm. The cysts regress as the levels of human chorionic gonadotropin (HCG) fall and do not need surgical intervention.

6. What causes the hyperthyroidism?

The answer is not fully known. The presence of a thyrotropin in chorionic membranes has been investigated but not isolated. Some think that high levels of HCG can stimulate the thyroid, but this has not been proved in animal studies. It is important, nonetheless, to treat patients who are hyperthyroid before evacuation of a molar pregnancy, because thyroid storm may develop in some patients. A beta-adrenergic blocking agent is used.

7. How is molar pregnancy diagnosed?

Ultrasound has replaced all other means of diagnosing molar pregnancy. It typically reveals the absence of a fetus and multiple echogenic areas of villi and clots. This has been described as the classic "snowstorm" pattern on ultrasound.

8. What laboratory tests should be obtained before evacuation of a molar pregnancy?

Complete blood count with platelets	Antibody screen
Renal and liver function studies	Quantitative HCG level
Blood type	Chest radiograph

9. Describe the treatment of a patient with molar pregnancy.

Dilatation and suction evacuation of the uterus should be carried out as soon as the diagnosis is made. Sharp curettage of the uterus should be performed after suction to remove all tissue. If the patient does not wish to preserve fertility, hysterectomy may be undertaken to remove the mole, but it is not necessary. Dilatation should be done at the time of the procedure, not beforehand with laminaria, because of the markedly increased risk of hemorrhage. Oxytocin should be started at the beginning of the procedure to decrease bleeding.

10. What are the potential causes of adult respiratory distress syndrome in patients at the time of evacuation?

Trophoblastic embolization may be an underlying cause of respiratory distress. Respiratory distress also may result from high-output congestive failure caused by anemia, hyperthyroidism, preeclampsia, or iatrogenic fluid overload.

11. What is the appropriate follow-up after evacuation?

The beta subunit of the HCG molecule is followed weekly until three consecutive values are normal. Then values are tested monthly until normal for 6–12 consecutive months.

12. What about birth control during the follow-up period?

Prevention of pregnancy is essential to track HCG levels adequately. Barrier methods or oral contraceptives are used. A Gynecologic Oncology Group (GOG) prospective, randomized study of 216 patients concluded that there is no increase in postmolar gestational trophoblastic disease.

13. What is the rationale for monitoring HCG levels for 6–12 months before attempting pregnancy?

This time frame allows identification of the rare patient who develops postmolar malignancy after achieving a normal HCG. Almost all malignant sequelae occur within 6 months of molar evacuation. Patients with a prior partial or complete mole have a 10-fold increased risk (1–2%) of a second mole in subsequent pregnancies.

14. Should prophylactic chemotherapy be given to prevent persistent disease?

This is an area of definite controversy. Between 15–25% of patients with complete moles develop persistent tumor. Not everyone feels that a potentially toxic drug should be given to all patients with molar pregnancies. The commonly used agents are methotrexate or actinomycin D. One possible solution is to treat only patients who are at high risk for persistent disease or unreliable for long-term follow-up. Because only about 20% of molar pregnancies require chemotherapy and the cure rate is almost 100% with adequate follow-up treatment, prophylactic chemotherapy is hard to justify.

15. What should be done if β-HCG titers plateau or rise over more than 2 weeks?

A plateau or rise in β-HCG titers is an indication for immediate work-up for malignant postmolar gestational trophoblastic disease. Repeat curettage does not induce remission and frequently results in uterine perforation.

16. Do only patients with moles get gestational trophoblastic tumors (GTTs)?

No. GTTs may develop after any gestation, including term and ectopic pregnancy or spontaneous abortion. A majority, however, occur after molar pregnancy. Women with gestational trophoblastic disease (GTD) after nonmolar pregnancies may present with subtle signs and symptoms of disease, making diagnosis difficult. Abnormal bleeding after any pregnancy should be evaluated promptly with β-HCG testing and endometrial sampling to determine the presence of GTD.

17. What is the clinical classification system for identification of patients with risk factors?
Malignant GTD is divided into nonmetastatic GTD and metastatic GTD. Metastatic GTD is further divided into good-prognosis, low-risk disease and poor-prognosis, high-risk disease. Poor-prognosis disease is associated with one or more of the following factors: (1) duration > 4 months; (2) pretherapy level of β-HCG in serum > 40,000 mU/ml; (3) brain or liver metastases; (4) GTD after term pregnancy; or (5) prior failed therapy.

18. Describe the three types of GTD.
   1. **Invasive mole.** Molar villi and trophoblasts invade local myometrium. Invasive moles account for 5–15% of molar pregnancies
   2. **Choriocarcinoma.** Malignant tumor arises from the trophoblasts of any gestational event (most commonly molar pregnancy). Choriocarcinoma consists of proliferation of cytotrophoblast and syncytiotrophoblast, but no villi are present.
   3. **Placental site tumor.** This type, which is extremely rare, occurs only after nonmolar gestations. Tumor growth is indolent over a long period, but when metastases occur, they are usually fatal. The causes are poorly understood, because few cases exist.

19. What is the staging of GTD?

Stage I	Confined to the uterine corpus	Stage III	Metastases to the lung
Stage II	Metastases to the pelvis or vagina	Stage IV	Distant metastases

Metastatic sites, in order of frequency, are lung, vagina, pelvis, brain, and liver.

20. What are the treatment options?
Chemotherapy is the mainstay of treatment and is determined by risk stratification. Nonmetastatic GTD is usually treated with single-agent therapy. A regimen of either methotrexate, 40–50 mg/m^2/week, or dactinomycin, 1.25 mg/m^2 intravenously every 2 weeks, is efficacious, minimally toxic, and cost-effective. Treatment should be continued until β-HCG values have achieved normal levels and two further cycles of chemotherapy have been given.

Low-risk metastatic disease can be treated successfully with single-agent regimens. The traditional choice is a 5-day cycle of methotrexate or dactinomycin. Forty percent of patients require alternative therapy to achieve remission.

Patients with one or more high-risk factors require combination chemotherapy. A high success rate has been achieved by alternating etoposide, methotrexate, and dactinomycin with cyclophosphamide and vincristine (EMA/CO).

Management of cerebral and hepatic metastases is controversial. Whether radiation therapy to the liver or brain is necessary in patients treated with newer combinations of chemotherapy is debatable. Disease recurs in up to 13% of high-risk patients despite aggressive chemotherapy for three cycles after a negative HCG test.

21. Does surgery have a role in therapy? What about radiation?
Surgery is limited mostly to removing a focus of disease that is resistant to chemotherapy, such as the uterus or a pulmonary nodule. Hysterectomy shortens the duration of chemotherapy needed in nonmetastatic disease. If childbearing is complete, hysterectomy should be considered. Radiation is rarely used but occasionally may be needed to control hemorrhage from brain or liver lesions.

22. Do all patients survive GTD?
Based on data from the New England Trophoblastic Disease Center, the overall survival rate since 1975 for stages I, II, and III is virtually 100%. For stage IV disease, the survival rate is approximately 70–73%.

23. Can patients who are cured have a normal pregnancy?
Yes. Rates of pregnancy loss and complications of pregnancy are not increased after treatment. In addition, even after chemotherapy, no increase in congenital malformations has been reported.

BIBLIOGRAPHY

1. Berkowitz RS, Bernstein NR, Laborde O, et al: Subsequent pregnancy experience in patients with gestational trophoblastic disease—New England Trophoblastic Disease Center, 1965–1992. J Reprod Med 39:228, 1994.
2. Berkowitz RS, Goldstein DP: Gestational trophoblastic disease. In Ryan K, Berkowitz R, Barbieri R (eds): Kistner's Gynecology—Principles and Practice. St. Louis, Mosby, 1995, p 377.
3. Homesley HD, et al: Weekly intramuscular methotrexate for nonmetastatic gestational trophoblastic disease. Obstet Gynecol 72:413, 1988.
4. Miller DS, Lurain JR: Classification and staging of gestational trophoblastic tumors. Obstet Gynecol Clin North Am 15:477, 1988.
5. Newlands ES, Bagshawe KD, Begent RHJ, et al: Results with the EMA/CO (etoposide, methotrexate, actinomycin D, Cyclophosphamide, vincristine) regimen in high risk gestational trophoblastic tumours, 1979–1989. Br J Obstet Gynaecol 98:550, 1991.
6. Palmer JR: Advances in the epidemiology of gestational trophoblastic disease. J Reprod Med 39:155, 1994.
7. Parazzini F, Mangili G, LaVecchia C, et al: Risk factors for gestational trophoblastic disease: A separate analysis of complete and partial hydatidiform moles. Obstet Gynecol 78:1039, 1991.
8. Watson EJ, Hernandez E, Miyazawa K: Partial hydatidiform moles: A review. Obstet Gynecol Surv 42:540, 1987.

39. CANCER IN PREGNANCY

Helen Frederickson, M.D.

1. Is the natural history of malignancy affected by pregnancy?

Usually not. Melanoma may be one exception.

2. Is the fetus affected by the cancer?

The fetus is not affected by the neoplasm but may be affected by the therapy. Less than 100 cases of metastasis to the fetus or placenta have been reported. The most common malignancies to metastasize to the placenta or fetus (even more rare) are melanoma, leukemia or lymphoma, and breast cancer.

3. Does termination offer any therapeutic value?

No. The pregnancy may need to be terminated to carry out standard therapies (i.e., radiation or chemotherapy in the first trimester). No data suggest that termination of the pregnancy affects the clinical course of the malignancy, including breast cancer and melanoma.

4. How is the fetus affected by treatment?

Radiation therapy is known to cause abortion, growth retardation, or major physical abnormalities. Injuries are less harmful later in gestation than in early stages (during organogenesis). The central nervous system, eye, and mesenchymal tissues appear more sensitive to radiation.

All chemotherapeutic agents are theoretically teratogenic and mutagenic. Thus, they are contraindicated in the first trimester but relatively safe later in pregnancy. The risk of obstetric complications, but not of congenital abnormalities, increases if chemotherapeutic agents are used in the second or third trimesters.

5. May patients treated with chemotherapy have future pregnancies?

Yes. Studies to date have shown no adverse outcomes in patients with histories of previous malignancies who become pregnant after treatment. This includes patients with breast cancer and melanoma, both of which are estrogen-stimulated. The estrogen levels of pregnancy do not appear to stimulate potentially malignant cells.

Ovarian function after treatment varies with the drugs used. At least 50% of women treated with single-agent alkylating agents develop ovarian failure. Adjuvant chemotherapy in patients with breast cancer may result in ovarian failure, depending on age of the patient and total dose administered.

Existing data on pregnancy outcome do not indicate an excessive risk of congenital or genetic problems following chemotherapy in the mother or father.

6. How often is cancer associated with pregnancy?

Rarely. Normally, pregnant women are in an age range with a low incidence of all malignancies. This may change as women delay childbearing until their late thirties and early forties. The most common malignancies associated with pregnancy are those that occur more frequently at a younger age—i.e., breast cancer, leukemia, lymphomas, melanomas, gynecologic malignancies (especially cervical carcinoma), and bone tumors.

7. What is the incidence of invasive carcinoma of the cervix associated with pregnancy? Of carcinoma in situ?

Carcinoma of the cervix: 1 of 2000–2500 pregnancies.

Carcinoma in situ: 1 of 750 pregnancies.

8. What are the symptoms of cervical carcinoma associated with pregnancy?

Abnormal vaginal bleeding	Postcoital bleeding
Vaginal discharge	Pelvic pain

9. How is the diagnosis of cervical neoplasia made in pregnant women?

The same as in nonpregnant women—by cervical biopsy (colposcopically directed or cone biopsy, as indicated). Most importantly, the clinician must do a speculum examination in pregnant women with vaginal bleeding and biopsy any gross lesion.

10. What is the treatment for cervical carcinoma associated with pregnancy?

The same indications for therapy of cervical carcinoma apply in pregnant as in nonpregnant patients: primary surgery or radiation for early stage disease (stages IB–IIA) and primary radiation therapy for more advanced stages.

11. Does the pregnancy need to be terminated for treatment of cervical carcinoma?

Yes. If the disease is diagnosed in the first or second trimesters, pregnancy termination is advised to allow treatment. If radiation therapy is to be used, the pelvic radiation may induce a spontaneous abortion. If the pregnancy is in the third trimester, one must consider waiting for fetal lung maturation, with delivery before initiating therapy.

The option of delaying therapy until fetal viability exists, and recent retrospective studies suggest no increased maternal risk with treatment delay in patients with early stage disease. Caution must be used, however, because the number of patients and duration of follow-up are limited. The majority of patients have very early disease. Delays up to 30 weeks have been reported without adverse outcomes.

12. Does the mode of delivery affect the course of cervical carcinoma?

No. The major indication for cesarean section is a large cervical lesion that may cause excessive bleeding if vaginal delivery is attempted. If the primary therapy is surgical, a cesarean section is done at the time of radical hysterectomy. Vaginal delivery does not increase the incidence of metastatic disease or adversely affect the prognosis, when corrected for stage of disease.

13. How should an ovarian cyst be managed in pregnancy?

Most ovarian cysts diagnosed in pregnancy disappear by the second trimester. If they persist or increase in size, an exploratory laparotomy in the second trimester is indicated. About 2–5% of such cysts are malignant. Masses > 8 cm should be explored immediately because of the increased number of complications associated with pregnancy. The most frequent complication is torsion.

If ultrasound characteristics of the ovarian cyst are totally cystic, with no internal echos, the need for surgery should be based more on size of the lesion. Now that ultrasounds are more common in pregnancy, more cystic lesions are being found.

14. What treatment is indicated for ovarian carcinoma diagnosed during pregnancy?

Essentially the same treatment as in nonpregnant patients. Adequate staging is essential. Germ cell tumors are more common in patients of childbearing age than epithelial ovarian tumors, but they are aggressive tumors and require immediate adjuvant chemotherapy. In epithelial ovarian malignancies, it may be possible to remove the ovaries and debulk the tumor while leaving the uterus and fetus in place. Chemotherapy can then be initiated after surgery if the fetus is in the second trimester.

15. What is the difference in overall survival rate for breast cancer in nonpregnant and pregnant patients?

The overall survival rate for breast cancer is 50%, but in pregnancy the rate drops to 15–20%, probably because of the more advanced stage at the time of diagnosis. Stage for stage the survival rate for pregnant patients with breast cancer is the same as that for nonpregnant patients. Breast carcinoma is usually diagnosed later in pregnancy because of the physiologic changes in the breast and the rarity of the disease in women of childbearing age.

16. Is therapeutic abortion necessary in pregnant patients with breast cancer?

Not in patients with localized breast cancer. Therapeutic abortion did not affect survival rate despite the theoretical influence of endogenous hormonal production in pregnancy. In advanced breast cancer, therapeutic abortion is indicated for palliative therapy if estrogen receptors are present in the original tumor. If not, the patient may elect to continue the pregnancy and undergo chemotherapy.

Radiation therapy to the breast is contraindicated in pregnant women because of the risk of internal scatter, which cannot be prevented and poses an unacceptable risk to the fetus.

17. Is a subsequent pregnancy contraindicated in a patient who has had a mastectomy for breast cancer?

No. Retrospective studies suggest that subsequent pregnancy does not promote recurrence.

18. Should patients with breast cancer breast-feed their infant?

Most physicians advise against breast-feeding on the theoretical grounds that a possible viral etiology may be passed to the infant and to avoid vascular enrichment of the opposite breast, which may contain a neoplasm. No good data substantiate this position.

19. Is malignant melanoma adversely affected by pregnancy?

The adverse effects of pregnancy on melanoma are unknown but suspected. Theoretically, the level of melanocyte-stimulating hormone (MSH) is increased in pregnancy, and the intrinsic activity of MSH is increased by increased production of adrenocorticotropic hormone (ACTH).

Abortion is not considered therapeutic in the management of melanoma diagnosed during pregnancy. Some data suggest that women who had a pregnancy before the melanoma developed survived longer than women who did not have a previous pregnancy. The theory to account for such data is that exposure to fetal antigen protected against the dissemination of melanoma cells with similar fetal antigens.

20. Do melanomas metastasize to the products of conception (POC) more than other tumors?

Yes. Although metastases to POC are rare, 50% of tumors metastasizing to the placenta are melanomas, and 90% of those metastasizing to the fetus are melanomas.

BIBLIOGRAPHY

1. Bezjian AA: Pelvic masses in pregnancy. Clin Obstet Gynecol 27:402, 1984.
2. Dildy GA, Moise DJ, Carpenter RJ, Kilma T: Maternal malignancy metastatic to the products of conception: A review. Obstet Gynecol Surv 44:535, 1989.
3. Doll DC, Ringenberg QS, Yarbro JW: Management of cancer during pregnancy. Arch Intern Med 148:2058, 1988.
4. Duggan B, Muderspach LI, Roman LD, et al: Cervical cancer in pregnancy: Reporting on planned delay in therapy. Obstet Gynecol 82:598, 1993.
5. Greer BE, Easterling TR, McLennan DA, et al: Fetal and maternal considerations in the management of Stage IB cervical cancer during pregnancy. Gynecol Oncol 34:61, 1989.
6. Hacker NF, et al: Carcinoma of the cervix associated with pregnancy. Obstet Gynecol 39:735, 1982.
7. Nevin J, Soeters R, Dehaeck K, et al: Cervical carcinoma associated with pregnancy. Obstet Gynecol Surv 50:228, 1995.
8. Roberts JA: Management of gynecologic tumors during pregnancy. Clin Perinatol 10:369, 1983.
9. Saunders N, Landon CR: Management problems associated with carcinoma of the cervix diagnosed in the second trimester of pregnancy. Gynecol Oncol 30:120, 1988.
10. Slingluff CL, Seigler HF: Malignant melanoma and pregnancy. Ann Plast Surg 28:95, 1992.
11. van Dessel T, Hameeteman TM, Wagenaar SS: Mucinous cystadenocarcinoma in pregnancy. Case report. Br J Obstet Gynaecol 95:527, 1988.
12. Wong DJ, Strassner HT: Melanoma in pregnancy. Clin Obstet Gynecol 33:782, 1990.
13. Zemlickis D, Lishner M, Degendorfer P, et al: Maternal and fetal outcome after breast cancer in pregnancy. Am J Obstet Gynecol 166:781, 1992.

IV. General Obstetrics

40. PRECONCEPTION COUNSELING

Louise Wilkins-Haug, M.D., Ph.D.

1. Why is preconception counseling important?

Preconception counseling plays two roles. First, interventions to decrease birth defects need to be in place at conception to be effective. By the time of the first prenatal visit, generally at 6–8 weeks' gestation, a portion of the embryologic window for teratogenicity has passed. Secondly, preconception counseling allows assessment and possible alteration of risk factors that may influence pregnancy outcome. Timing of a pregnancy may be altered to occur during optimal health in a woman with a chronic medical condition, early pregnancy interventions such as elective cerclage may need to be considered, and alternative types of care and delivery may be appropriate. In addition, unrecognized risks can be identified and appropriate alterations or treatments pursued.

2. What routine laboratory tests are indicated in preconception counseling?

Hematocrit—iron deficiency anemia, lowered mean corpuscular volume as a screen for hemoglobinopathies if appropriate.

Rubella titer—immunization if nonimmune in the nonpregnant state.

Hepatitis B antigen—women at risk by lifestyle or occupation should consider passive immunization before pregnancy.

Screening for human immunodeficiency virus (HIV)—with appropriate counseling and consent.

Sexually transmitted diseases—in particular, syphilis, which unrecognized can result in fetal complications.

Routine preventative health care—Pap smear, mammogram if appropriate, cholesterol screening should be current.

3. What nutritional disorders should be recognized?

Of risk to the fetus are practices that include pica, bulimia and/or anorexia, strict vegetarianism, and certain vitamin and mineral imbalances (deficiencies as well as excessive use).

4. Why is folate supplementation now suggested before conception?

Folate supplementation for decreasing the risk of neural tube defects (NTD) has been supported by both retrospective and randomized studies. In women with an increased risk for an infant with NTD, high-dose folate (4.0 mg) decreases the risk by 60%. The Medical Research Council vitamin study group also found a 70% reduction in the risk of NTD with a similar dose. In the United States this decreases the risk of recurrence from approximately 2.0% to 1.0%. In 1991 the Centers for Disease Control supported 4.0-mg folate supplementation before conception until 12 weeks' gestation for women who have previously given birth to an infant with a NTD.

For women with no prior history of an infant with NTD, lower doses may also decrease the population risk. In 1992, the CDC recommended that all women of child-bearing age should consume 0.4 mg (400 µg) of folate periconceptionally.

5. How much folate on average do American women consume in their daily diet? How much is available through vitamin supplementation?

In the average diet, 0.2 mg folate is consumed per day. Foods with high folate content include green, leafy vegetables and fortified cereals. Over-the-counter multivitamin preparations generally contain 0.4 mg, whereas most prescription prenatal vitamins contain 0.8 mg.

6. What concerns have been raised about vitamin A and pregnancy?

Vitamin A is an essential vitamin with a recommended daily allowance in pregnancy of 5,000 IU. An average balanced diet supplies 7–8,000 IU per day; thus additional supplementation is usually not needed. Daily vitamin A intakes > 25,000 IU/day, as with diets rich in liver and cod oil as well as supplemental vitamin A intake, increase the risk of birth defects. Recent concern has focused on an increased incidence of cranial neural crest malformations with even lower levels of vitamin A supplementation, > 10,000 IU/day. Vitamin A supplementation should be discontinued; it is not needed and may have harmful fetal effects.

7. What other vitamins, if consumed in excess, can be detrimental to fetal growth?

Other fat-soluble vitamins (D, E, and K) also have been associated with an increased risk of fetal malformations. Specifically vitamin D has been associated with supravalvar aortic stenosis and cranial facial abnormalities. Vitamin K has been associated with skeletal defects in animals.

8. Is caffeine harmful in pregnancy?

Controversial. No standard recommendations currently exist as to caffeine ingestion during pregnancy. Animal studies show an increased rate of birth defects with extremely high amounts of caffeine (at levels greater than reasonably consumed by a person—50 cups/day). In humans, moderate coffee use (< 3 cups/day) has not been associated with adverse pregnancy outcomes. Concern has been raised, however, for an increased rate of spontaneous abortion with even 1–2 cups of coffee/day; more than 3 cups increases the rate further.

9. What is the most common substance of abuse that places pregnancies at risk?

Alcohol. In addition to the well-recognized effects of alcohol on fetal development, growth, and the central nervous system, excessive alcohol consumption is associated in some studies with increased miscarriage and abruption. Several nonthreatening, time-efficient screening tools are available to assess the level of alcohol consumption in the outpatient setting.

T-ACE Questions*

T	How many drinks does it take to make you feel high (tolerance)?
A	Have people annoyed you by criticizing your drinking?
C	Have you felt you ought to cut down on your drinking?
E	Have you ever had a drink first thing in the morning to steady your nerves or get rid of a hangover (eye opener)?

* For the tolerance question, more than 2 drinks is a positive response. A score of 2 is assigned for a positive response to the T question and a score of 1 is assigned for all other positive responses. A score of 2 or greater is considered positive for problem drinking.

10. What is considered a safe level of alcohol consumption in the first trimester?

No proven level of alcohol consumption is considered safe. Even 1 ounce/day has been associated with attention deficit disorders in children. The manifestations of fetal alcohol syndrome are generally seen in women consuming at least 2 oz of alcohol/day.

11. Are other drugs of abuse of concern?

Cocaine has been associated with increased fetal and maternal adverse effects. In the fetus, although reports are conflicting, increased peripheral catecholamine production with resultant vasoconstriction and decreased placental flow may lead to fetal ischemia and increased congenital anomalies, particularly of the genitourinary tract. The incidence of fetal intraventricular hemorrhage is also increased. Pregnancy outcomes include a higher rate of spontaneous abortion, placental abruption, and premature rupture of the membranes. Maternal risks include myocardial infarction, cerebral vascular hemorrhage, hypertension, seizures, and sudden death.

12. Does cigarette smoking affect fertility?

Fertility appears to be adversely affected in women smoking more than 16 cigarettes/day. Both delayed conception and increased ectopic rates have been reported. With cessation of smoking fertility rates return to those of the general population.

13. How much does cigarette smoking lower an infant's birthweight?

The incremental difference in birth weight among smoking vs. nonsmoking populations is on the order of 550 gm.

14. What relatively common medical conditions should be identified and addressed during preconception counseling?

Insulin-dependent diabetes: Poor glucose control is associated with increased birth defects. Assessment of overall health, including blood pressure and renal, cardiac, and retinal evaluation can help to gauge the risk a pregnancy poses to the woman's health and the risk of pregnancy-related complications.

Seizure disorders: The various seizure medications may cause teratogenicity. In conjunction with a neurologist, a trial of a different or possibly no medication may be considered.

Hypertension: Assessment of cardiac and renal function is probably the best gauge for complications during pregnancy. Possible agents to reduce the risk of preeclampsia, such as aspirin and calcium supplementation, warrant discussion. Current medications should be assessed for teratogenicity; acetyl cholinesterase inhibitors and diuretics should be avoided.

Connective tissue disorders (e.g., systemic lupus erythematosus): Current renal function, hypertension, and pericardial/pleural involvement should be evaluated to assess the risk of pregnancy to the underlying disease as well as pregnancy complications. Studies should be undertaken to identify antibodies, including anticardiolipin, lupus anticoagulant, anti-Ro, and anti-La, that may increase the risk of adverse pregnancy outcome and congenital heart block. Possible interventions and alterations in prenatal care can be presented.

15. How should the family history be assessed?

Particular attention should be paid to family members (including the woman and her partner) with recognized Mendelain disorders (either recessive, dominant, or X-linked), multifactorial disorders (neural tube defect, cardiac anomaly, cleft lip or palate), and chromosomal disorders. A first-degree family member, either male or female, or multiple family members with mental retardation of unknown cause may initiate screening for fragile X syndrome. In addition, identification of the patient's race and ethnicity may initiate appropriate population screening for carrier status for such disorders as sickle-cell anemia, thalessemias, Tay-Sach disease, or cystic fibrosis.

17. Are women older than 35 years at increased risk for infertility or miscarriage?

Rates of infertility in women over 35 are 3-fold higher compared with women 20–29 years of age. In addition, chromosomal abnormalities account for a large portion of first-trimester miscarriages; thus the miscarriage rate also increases with maternal age. Miscarriage of chromosomally normal conceptions also may increase with maternal age, although this is less clear.

18. Do nonchromosomal birth defects increase with maternal age?

No. No increase in birth defects that could not be attributed to chromosome abnormalities, single gene defects, maternal diabetes, alcoholism, or teratogen exposure has been found among older women.

19. What other risks are associated with pregnancy after the age of 35?

Preeclampsia—women over the age of 40 have twice the rate of preeclampsia as women under 30

Perinatal demise—women in their late 30s have twice the risk of women in their 20s, and by age 45 this risk is 4-fold. This is due mostly to intrauterine demise.

Fetal growth retardation—suggested by some but not all studies.

20. What effect does maternal age over 35 have on route of delivery?

In historical studies, women over the age of 35 have had a 70% increase in cesarean section rate compared with women in their 20s. However, this increase is partly due to the historical use of advanced maternal age as one indication for primary cesarean section delivery.

21. Are the risks of maternal death greater in pregnant women over the age of 35?

Maternal death rates increase directly with increasing parity and its associated complications. In addition, the higher rate of underlying maternal complications contribute to a higher maternal death rate in older women. Compared with women 25 years old, women 35 years old have twice the maternal death rate; by age 45, this rate is increased 4-fold.

22. For which preconception patient should further cardiac testing be undertaken?

Longstanding diabetes

Chronic hypertension (longer than 15 years, over age 40)

History of repaired cardiac defect as a child

23. What are the absolute contraindications to pregnancy?

Conditions associated with marked maternal mortality include pulmonary hypertension, Marfan syndrome with marked dilation of the aortic root, complicated coarctation of the aorta, and dilated cardiomyopathy.

BIBLIOGRAPHY

1. American College of Obstetricians and Gynecologists: Preconception Care. ACOG Tech Bull 205, 1995.
2. American College of Obstetricians and Gynecologists: Smoking and Reproductive Health. ACOG Tech Bull 180, 1993.
3. Cefalo R, Moos M: Preconception Health Care: A Practical Guide, 2nd ed. St. Louis, Mosby, 1995.
4. Eisenstat S: Preconception counseling and nutrition. In Carlson K, Eisenstat S, Frigolretto F, Schiff I (eds): Primary Care of Women. St. Louis, Mosby, 1995, pp 307–315.
5. Heffner LJ: Pregnancy in the older woman. In Carlson K, Eisenstat S, Frigolretto F, Schiff I (eds): Primary Care of Women. St. Louis, Mosby, 1995, pp 303–306.
6. Sokol R, Martier S, Ager J: The T-ACE questions: Practical prenatal detection of risk-drinking. Am J Obstet Gynecol 160:865, 1990.

41. NORMAL PHYSIOLOGY OF PREGNANCY

Gretchen Frey, M.D.

DIAGNOSIS OF PREGNANCY

1. How soon after fertilization can beta human chorionic gonadotropin (hCG) be detected?

By 7 days after fertilization (4–5 days after implantation), hCG can be found at levels above 25 mIU/ml and thus is detected with the most sensitive test (immunoassay on serum). Levels of hCG peak at about 100,000 mIU by 60 days after conception and then decrease to around 5,000 mIU by 100–130 days.

2. How does the pattern of hCG rise differ in normal and abnormal pregnancies?

In a normal intrauterine gestation, the hCG level should double roughly every 48–60 hours in the first trimester. In an ectopic (tubal or otherwise extrauterine) gestation, the levels may rise abnormally slowly or may plateau. In an impending miscarriage (spontaneous abortion), levels often fall before passage of the fetal tissue.

3. At what hCG level can fetal viability be confirmed by ultrasound?

With modern endovaginal imaging equipment, most experienced technologists can image a fetal pole with cardiac activity at a level of 1,000–1,500 mIU/ml hCG.

4. How accurate are most home pregnancy tests?

Most home pregnancy tests are now nearly as accurate as a laboratory test on serum, with a sensitivity of 25 mIU/ml of hCG.

5. What are the most common causes of false-positive pregnancy tests? False-negative tests?

With current immunoassay methods, only hCG-producing tumors, hemolysis, or lipemia should produce **false-positive** results. Of course, human errors in mislabeling samples or performing the assay are possible. **False-negative** tests generally result when the gestation is below the sensitivity for the test. In most cases, this involves a normal early gestation, although blighted ova and ectopic pregnancies also may cause a false-negative result.

6. What is pseudocyesis?

Increased weight, amenorrhea, and a subjective appreciation of fetal movement lead some women, usually those with an underlying psychiatric disorder, to convince themselves of pregnancy despite negative pregnancy testing.

PHYSIOLOGIC CHANGES OF PREGNANCY

7. By what mechanism is the uterus able to distend to 1,000 times its normal volume?

Stretching and hypertrophy of uterine muscle, not new cell development, are responsible. Estrogen and progesterone initiate changes in the uterine muscle until 14 weeks of pregnancy, after which time the enlarging fetus exerts a direct stretching effect.

8. What is hyperemesis gravidarum? What causes it?

Hyperemesis gravidarum is an extreme manifestation of the common symptom of nausea in early pregnancy ("morning sickness"). It is usually seen in the first trimester. Women with this condition may be unable to keep down even fluids and sometimes require intravenous hydration and/or nutrition for a time. The cause is not well understood and may represent an unusual sensitivity of some individuals to hCG (believed to be the cause of normal first-trimester nausea). Some have also postulated a psychiatric component (ambivalence or hostility toward pregnancy), but this is by no means proven.

9. Why is the uterus often dextrorotated, producing right lower quadrant pain as it enlarges?

The presence of the rectosigmoid colon in the left lower quadrant physically deviates the uterus slightly to the right. This is also the reason why the mild hydroureter of pregnancy (due to the smooth-muscle relaxing effect of progesterone) is often more pronounced on the right, because the mechanical pressure of the uterus at the pelvic brim is greater there.

10. What is the source of the progesterone that maintains the pregnancy during the first weeks?

The corpus luteum of the ovary. After 7–9 weeks, the placenta takes over the main production of progesterone.

11. What is Hartman's sign? How may it confuse the gestational age based on last menstrual period (LMP)?

Some women experience slight spotting as the blastocyst implants into the endometrium. Because this "light period" typically occurs 1 week after ovulation and fertilization (i.e., 3–3.5 weeks after last menses), it is sometimes mistakenly used for calculation of gestational age.

12. What changes typically occur in the pulmonary system as pregnancy progresses?

Mild, compensated, respiratory alkalosis is often present, primarily as a result of increased minute volume.

13. What is characteristic about the cardiovascular system of pregnant women?

Typically a hyperdynamic state is caused by the 50% increase in blood volume, resulting in a slightly increased resting pulse, increased cardiac output, and flow murmurs. A progressive decrease in peripheral vascular resistance accounts for the slight decrease in blood pressure noted in normal second-trimester pregnancies.

14. What produces the inferior vena cava (supine hypotension) syndrome of pregnancy?

Compression of the inferior vena cava by the gravid uterus when the mother is supine can significantly decrease venous blood return to the heart. This effect can be avoided by having the mother lie in the left lateral position. The supine hypotension syndrome is signaled by maternal complaints of dizziness upon lying supine; even fainting may occur.

15. What is physiologic anemia of pregnancy?

The combination of increased plasma volume and slower increase in red blood cell mass produces a dilutional anemia.

16. Can glycosuria be seen in normal pregnancies?

Yes. The glomerular filtration rate is increased during normal pregnancy; as a result, a glucose load may not be reabsorbed sufficiently. For this reason urinary glucose is a poor indicator of control in the pregnant diabetic.

17. How does progesterone affect the gastrointestinal system?

Delayed gastric emptying time, poor esophageal sphincter tone, increased gallbladder stasis, and decreased gut motility are the source of many bothersome but normal complaints of pregnancy.

18. Which hormone has the greatest effect on the ligaments during pregnancy?

Relaxin. In particular, the ligamentous symphysis pubis undergoes softening and partial separation at about 28–32 weeks, often resulting in a dull pain in this area.

19. What are common neurologic complaints during pregnancy?

Carpal tunnel syndrome. Bilateral or unilateral median nerve entrapment, perhaps secondary to fluid retention, may result in pain, decreased sensation, and weakness of predominantly the first three fingers. Splinting provides symptomatic relief, but 15% may require surgical decompression.

Sciatica. Because of shifting of the pelvic bones and their relaxed ligaments, many women have classic sciatic nerve compression pain (felt in one buttock, radiating down the back of the leg to the lateral side of the foot). Fluid retention also may play a role.

20. What are some common skin changes in pregnancy?

Increased pigmentation from increased estrogen and progesterone is seen in the areola, linea nigra, and perineum and also may cause chloasma (the facial pigmentation sometimes referred to as the "mask" of pregnancy). Pruritus gravidarum, or itching without skin changes, is also common (about 15% of pregnant women) and is probably secondary to elevation of bile salts due to changes in liver function. Symptomatic relief (with lotions, topical antipruritic agents, or oral antihistamines) usually suffices. When associated with specific types of skin changes, pruritis may be referred to as pruritic and urticarial papules and plaques of pregnancy (PUPPP). This more severe form usually requires topical or systemic steroids.

21. What is the current maternal mortality rate in the United States? How does it differ from worldwide maternal mortality rates?

From 1979 to 1986, national maternal mortality was recorded as 9.1/100,000 live births. This is five times less than in 1960. Worldwide mortality, however, currently equals one maternal death every minute of every hour, 365 days a year (comparative ratio of 550/100,000 live births). Women in the United States and Europe have about a 1/1,000 lifetime chance of pregnancy-related death, whereas women in areas of Africa face a 1/25 chance of obstetric-related death.

22. What is the most common cause of maternal mortality in the United States?

Pulmonary embolism, followed closely by hypertensive disease, then hemorrhage.

EXERCISE IN PREGNANCY

23. What maximal pulse rate should be observed by exercising pregnant women?

Most would agree that a pulse rate of 140 or below is a conservative target. The underlying issue is to avoid overheating, because high body core temperatures have a small possibility of connection with defects in early fetal development.

24. Are certain types of exercise to be avoided in pregnancy?

Yes. Because of increased ligamentous laxity, pregnant women are more subject to sprains and other ligamentous injury; hence ballistic (jumping or bouncing) types of motion, such as high-impact aerobics or skiing, should be undertaken with caution. This said, many experienced athletes are able to continue their usual exercise routine with appropriate reductions in length and intensity of workout.

25. Does exercise cause miscarriage?

No. Even vigorous exercise (such as daily running) in the first trimester has no effect on the rate of spontaneous abortion.

26. Why are pregnant women told not to exercise in the supine position after 20 weeks gestation?

Because of the supine hypotension effect (see question 14). Even if the woman is asymptomatic, the decrease in placental blood flow due to the combination of (1) caval compression and (2) shunting to the working skeletal muscle is believed to be potentially detrimental to the fetus.

BIBLIOGRAPHY

1. Cunningham PG, McDonald P, Gant N: Maternal adaptations to pregnancy. In Williams Obstetrics, 18th ed. Norwalk, CT, Appleton & Lange, 1989.
2. Grimes D: The morbidity and mortality of pregnancy: Still risky business. Am J Ob Gyn 170:1489–1494, 1994.
3. Maine D: Maternal mortality: Helping women off the road to death. WHO Chron 40:175–183, 1986.
4. Parisi V, Creasy R: Maternal biologic adaptations to pregnancy. In Reece E, Mebbins J, Mahoney M, Petrie R (eds): Philadelphia, J.B. Lippincott, 1992.
5. Rapini R, Jordon R: The skin and pregnancy. In Creasy R, Resnick R (eds): Maternal-Fetal Medicine: Principles and Practice, 3rd ed. Philadelphia, W.B. Saunders, 1994.
6. Yen S: Endocrinology of pregnancy. In Creasy R, Resnick R (eds): Maternal-Fetal Medicine: Principles and Practice, 3rd ed. Philadelphia, W.B. Saunders, 1994.

42. COMPREHENSIVE PRENATAL CARE

John G. McFee, M.D.

1. What does prenatal care encompass?

Prenatal care is the careful, systematic assessment and follow-up of a pregnant patient to ensure the best health of the mother and her fetus. This care is threefold:

1. To prevent, identify, or ameliorate maternal or fetal abnormalities adversely affecting pregnancy outcome, including socioeconomic and emotional as well as medical and obstetric factors.

2. To educate the patient about pregnancy, labor-delivery, parenting, and her overall health.

3. To promote adequate psychological support from her partner, family, and caregivers, especially in the first pregnancy, to adapt successfully to both pregnancy and the challenges of raising a family.

Prenatal care therefore is a continuum from the preconceptional period through the first postpartum year. Prenatal care commences with an extensive initial history and physical examination. Estimated gestational age and estimated date of confinement (EDC) are determined. Routine laboratory tests are drawn. In subsequent visits the physician explores any problems, documents the fetal growth, and identifies potential complications. Assessment for risk factors is done at the initial visit and on each revisit. Weight gain and nutritional well-being are evaluated at the outset and as the pregnancy progresses. Patient education is provided on a timely basis.

2. What are the goals and benefits of prenatal care?

Prenatal care is preventive and has been shown to be beneficial and cost-effective. As a group, women receiving no or inadequate prenatal care have far more complications and poorer outcomes of pregnancy. The costs of care for "no-care" patients are also substantially higher, with increased rates of preeclampsia, low-birthweight infants (both premature and growth-retarded), and perinatal deaths.

3. How often should patients be seen?

The American College of Obstetricians and Gynecologists recommends that pregnant women be seen for an extensive initial visit in early pregnancy and then every 4 weeks until 28 weeks, every 2–3 weeks to 36 weeks, and then weekly until delivery. This may be too many visits for healthy women. For low-risk pregnancies, a national panel has suggested 7 visits for parous women (6–8, 14–16, 24–28, 32, 36, 39, and 41 weeks) and 9 for nulliparas (additional visits at 10–12 and 40 weeks). For high-risk patients, the schedule should be individualized.

4. How should prenatal care be recorded?

Good record keeping is important during pregnancy, and various forms are available. Whichever form is chosen should (1) compel the obtaining of information, examinations, and diagnostic tests at appropriate times and (2) allow easy recognition of risk factors and problems with accompanying management plans. It is important to document all recognized problems legibly both for ease of giving care at future encounters and for medicolegal reasons. During the later months of pregnancy, a copy of the prenatal record should be sent to the obstetrical unit of the anticipated delivery hospital.

5. What historical information should be recorded at the initial visit?

Medical—many chronic medical conditions have an effect, often adverse, on pregnancy outcome; conversely, pregnancy usually has a distinct effect on the course of the condition itself.

Surgical—in particular, any prior surgical or anesthesic complications, the need for prior transfusion

Obstetric gynecologic—some events in the patient's obstetric history often recur in subsequent pregnancies (e.g., fetal and neonatal deaths, low birthweight infants, preterm deliveries, intrauterine growth retardation, fetal macrosomia [> 4000 gm at birth], birth defects, abruptio placentae, preeclampsia or hypertension, and postpartum hemorrhage). A history of recent infertility treatment, pelvic inflammatory disease, or ectopic pregnancy is also important for identifying early pregnancy complications such as tubal pregnancy or multiple gestations. A history for past sexually transmitted diseases should also be taken.

Family history—delving into inherited disease is important because, with time, progressively more of these conditions are becoming amenable to prenatal diagnosis. The history should focus on family members and relatives with cerebral palsy, mental retardation, neural tube defects and other congenital malformations as well as specific conditions such as cystic fibrosis, muscular dystrophy, and hemophilia.

Social—psychosocial background and lifestyle are also important because they frequently affect pregnancy and neonatal outcome. Questions need to be asked about smoking, use of alcohol and illicit drugs, use of prescription and over-the-counter medications, employment, and problems at home, such as domestic violence.

6. What history should be obtained at revisits?

A brief interval history for all patients at each revisit will uncover any new problems as well as provide follow-up for existing problems. Every patient should be asked about pain, contractions or cramping, pelvic pressure, bleeding, discharge, dysuria, gastrointestinal problems, presence and adequacy of fetal movements, and whether any new or other problems have arisen since the last visit. Patients with medical conditions or known complications should be asked specific questions about those problems. Women desiring sterilization should be counseled well ahead of delivery.

7. What findings should be noted on physical examination at the initial visit?

A general physical examination should be carried out on all prenatal patients. For many women, this exam may be the only one over a several year period and thus is important for health maintenance. Recording blood pressure and weight, listening to the heart and lungs, and palpating the breasts and abdomen are the principal components.

Examination of the pregnant uterus is vital. The fundal height is measured in centimeters from the symphysis pubis to the top of the uterus. Serial measurements over the course of pregnancy provide an excellent assessment of fetal growth with a rough approximation between centimeters and weeks of gestation from 18–34 weeks in patients with a normal body habitus. Fetal heart tones should be auscultated either with electronic Doppler or by a head fetal stethoscope. Lastly, uterine contractions can be easily palpated during a routine exam and, if frequent and many weeks before term, may point to the possibility of preterm labor.

A routine pelvic examination can detect abnormalities of the vulva, vagina, cervix, uterus, and adnexae. It is important to estimate the size of the early gravid uterus in weeks and to assess the cervix for length. A Pap smear is taken, and cultures for sexually transmitted infections and wet preparations for any vaginal discharge can be done. Finally, clinical pelvimetry should be carried out to determine pelvic adequacy in first pregnancies and in multiparas who have experienced a previous abnormal labor or difficult delivery.

8. What are Leopold's maneuvers?

In the third trimester the uterus should be examined in four steps for fetal lie, presenting part, and position: (1) What fetal part lies in the fundus? (2) On which side is the fetal back? (3) What fetal pole is headed toward the pelvis? Is it engaged? (4) How far has the fetal presenting part descended into the pelvis?

9. What is important in the physical exam on revisits?

At each revisit the patient's weight and blood pressure should be taken and recorded. Then the gravid uterus should be examined and fundal height measured, fetal position determined by

Leopold's maneuvers (last trimester), fetal weight estimated, and fetal heart tones auscultated. The importance of this exam is illustrated by the following examples: (1) failure of the fundal height growth may indicate intrauterine growth retardation and require extra fetal surveillance until delivery, and (2) recognition of a breech presentation at 36 weeks may require external version to vertex if spontaneous version does not occur by 37–38 weeks. Other examinations, including vaginal, are done as indicated by the patient's interval history of problems. In addition, fetal weight should be estimated to differentiate small-for-date from large-for-date babies.

10. How is gestational age determined?

An accurate last menstrual period (LMP) should be recorded at the first prenatal visit, along with the woman's normal menstrual cycle length and recent use of oral contraceptives. Careful determination of the EDC is needed so that therapeutic decisions at each stage of pregnancy are appropriately made. The EDC is initially calculated on the basis of the first day of the LMP: subtract 3 months, and add 1 year and 7 days. This assumes that a term gestation is 280 days or 40 weeks from the start of the past period and that menstruation is regular, occurring once every 28 days. Frequently, however, variations in the cycle and the timing of ovulation, use of oral contraception in the month preceding the LMP, and the appearance of menstrual-like bleeding during early pregnancy render the calculated EDC inaccurate.

Other parameters that confirm or indicate a different EDC are (1) date of a positive urine (about 5 weeks after the LMP) or serum (8th–10th postconceptional day) pregnancy test; (2) uterine size during the first half of pregnancy; (3) time of quickening (16–20 weeks); (4) time that fetal heart tones are first heard with electronic Doppler equipment (10–12 weeks) and nonelectronic fetoscope (18–20 weeks); and (5) ultrasound, using the crown-rump length in the first trimester (error of 7 days) and the biparietal diameter, femur length, and other measurements later (error of 10 days up to about 22 weeks). Ultrasonic estimates of gestational age are much less accurate in the third trimester.

11. Which laboratory tests should be ordered at the initial visit?

The number of laboratory determinations considered routine has increased over the past 25 years. Generally, the tests listed below as routine should be done in all cases. Additional tests at the initial prenatal visit are done for certain at-risk women only or at a later revisit.

Routine laboratory tests	Additional tests for at-risk patients
Hematocrit or hemoglobin	Glucose screen
Urinalysis and screen for bacteriuria	Maternal serum alpha-fetoprotein or multiple
Blood type and RH; antibody	marker test
screen	Gonorrhea culture
Serologic test for syphilis	Chlamydia test
Rubella hemagglutination-inhibition	Tuberculin skin test
(HI) titer	Sickledex
Hepatitis B surface antigen	HIV antibody
Pap smear	Group B streptococcus culture

12. How are hematocrit determinations useful during pregnancy?

An adequate red blood cell (RBC) volume is of importance, especially after delivery when moderate (500–1000 cc) blood loss normally occurs. Patients who are anemic need to be identified well ahead of delivery so that therapy can improve the hematocrit. Of equal importance is identification of patients with unusually high hematocrits (over 40%), who are apt to have an inadequate plasma volume expansion and thus may be at risk for preeclampsia and other conditions.

13. How is the urinalysis best used?

All patients should have a complete urinalysis, including microscopic testing, and some means of screening for infection on the first visit. Testing for nitrites and leukocyte esterase, usually included in most urinalysis dipsticks, is a cost-effective way of screening for bacteriuria. A urine culture need be done only on positive screens to determine the organism and its antibiotic sensitivities. Detection of the approximately 5% of patients with asymptomatic bacteriuria can prevent progression to pyelonephritis.

14. What is the importance of the blood type and antibody screening test?

Rh-negative women need to be identified and given Rh immune globulin (RhoGAM) at 28–30 weeks and within 72 hours of delivery to prevent Rh sensitization. The antibody screening test is done to detect antibodies, both Rh and other less common types (e.g., lesser Rh, Kell, Duffy, Lewis), some of which have the potential of causing hemolytic disease in the fetus and newborn infant.

15. Is serologic testing for syphilis (STS) still important?

In many areas of the country, both primary-secondary and congenital syphilis have increased in recent years. Women who are STS-positive are further tested with a fluorescent treponemal antibody (FTA) test; if the FTA is also positive, syphilis is diagnosed. If there is no history or treatment is inadequate or unknown, the patient is assumed to have syphilis and is treated with penicillin. The status of past treatment anywhere in the U.S can usually be ascertained by contacting the state health department's division of disease control. Follow-up of both mother and baby with serial Venereal Disease Research Laboratory (VDRL) titers is mandatory.

16. What is the purpose of the rubella hemagglutination-inhibition titer?

Because of vaccination of susceptible individuals, especially children, over the last 20 years, congenital rubella syndrome is now rare. However, substantial numbers of adults (10–15%) continue to show susceptibility by serology. Therefore, to keep this highly contagious infection under control, continued surveillance and vaccination of susceptible individuals are indicated. Mothers who are seronegative should be immunized postpartum. In addition, the test is helpful for advising and for following a patient exposed to someone with a rash or mild febrile illness suggestive of rubella.

17. Why test for hepatitis B?

Mothers who are chronic carriers for the hepatitis B virus transmit this infection to a substantial proportion of their infants during or after birth. Many of these babies also become carriers and can develop various forms of chronic hepatitis; approximately 25% of those affected eventually die from cirrhosis or hepatocellular carcinoma. The Centers for Disease Control (CDC) recommends that all gravidas be screened for the hepatitis B surface antigen and that all newborn infants receive vaccination against hepatitis B. Infants delivered of antigen-positive mothers should be given hepatitis B immunoglobulin as well as the vaccine, both within the first 12 hours of life.

18. Are Pap smears interpreted any differently in pregnant women?

No. A Pap smear should be taken if one has not been done in the previous 6–12 months. Abnormal smears should be managed and followed as for nonpregnant women. Women with smears suggestive of inflammation or infection should be evaluated and treated for specific vaginal or cervical infection. Most reports of low-grade (including koilocytosis and cervical intraepithelial neoplasia 1) and all high-grade squamous intraepithelial lesions (including cervical intraepithelial neoplasia 2-3 and carcinoma in situ), as well as smears positive for carcinoma, require colposcopy and biopsy for further diagnosis. The only difference during pregnancy is avoidance of endocervical curettage.

19. Of what benefit are other tests for sexually transmitted disease?

A cervical culture for gonorrhea and enzyme immunoassay for chlamydia should be done in at-risk patients—i.e., those under age 25, unmarried, and with multiple sexual partners. Many authorities recommend both as routine tests for all pregnant women; some also urge that the tests be repeated at 36 weeks' gestation. In earlier times, gonorrheal transmission at birth caused eventual blindness in many newborn infants (gonococcal ophthalmia neonatorum). State laws mandate neonatal eye prophylaxis, usually with an antibiotic. In addition, the gonococcus can cause chorioamnionitis after preterm rupture of membranes, resulting in a high rate of prematurity and infant morbidity. Pregnant women with a positive culture and their partners should be treated. Once treated, cervical cultures should be obtained for test of cure and repeated at 36 weeks' gestation.

Neonatal chlamydial infection occurs in 60–70% of babies passing through an infected birth canal. Conjunctivitis develops in 25–50% and chronic pneumonia in 10–20% of exposed infants. Whether this infection adversely affects the pregnancy in utero is controversial. Women who are positive must be treated with erythromycin (tetracycline for partners), followed up with a test of cure, and retested at 36 weeks' gestation. Amoxicillin or azithromycin can be given to patients with substantial side effects from erythromycin.

20. Should pregnant women be screened for tuberculosis?

A tuberculin skin test (purified protein derivate [PPD]) is a good idea for women who have immigrated from Asia, Africa, or Latin America, where the infection is not under good control. The same applies to certain crowded inner city areas of the U.S. The newborn infant is especially susceptible to tuberculosis. Thus, women who are PPD-positive should be investigated for active disease, including a chest-x-ray, and, if tuberculosis is found, treated with isoniazid (INH) and other appropriate therapy during pregnancy. If there is no evidence of active disease, the PPD-positive mother is usually treated with INH after delivery, especially if she is a recent PPD convertor or if other family members have active tuberculosis.

21. Why perform a Sickledex in pregnant black women?

This test is done to detect hemoglobin S, the predominant hemoglobin responsible for sickling of red blood cells in patients with sickle cell, sickle cell-hemoglobin C disease, sickle cell thalassemia, and others. Because of different solubilities, blood containing hemoglobin S added to the Sickledex solution results in turbidity and red-cell lysis; this does not occur with hemoglobin A. Women with sickle cell trait, seen in 8.5% of blacks, are well, have normal hematocrit levels, and do not have a chronic disabling condition like patients with full-blown sickle cell anemia. However, under certain circumstances (e.g., physical stress, shock, dehydration, hypoxia) sickling can occur and result in thrombosis. Such women are also prone to urinary tract infections that are believed to be due to minor degrees of sickling in small renal vessels and may lead to infarction of surrounding renal parenchyma. If the partner also has the sickle trait, the risk of sickle cell anemia in the offspring is 25%; it is now possible with prenatal diagnosis to identify fetuses with this condition.

22. Should pregnant women be screened for acquired immunodeficiency syndrome (AIDS)?

Transmission of the human immunodeficiency virus (HIV) to the fetus is well established, and it is currently estimated that 30% of offspring delivered of HIV-infected mothers are HIV-positive. AIDS develops rapidly in many of these infants. The American College of Obstetricians and Gynecologists (ACOG) has recently recommended offering HIV screening to all prenatal patients, given the lack of sensitivity of previously recognized risk factors. Positive results should be confirmed by Western blot analysis. Diagnosed women should be counseled about the spread of HIV infection and how transmission can be prevented. Prescription of oral zidovudine (AZT) to HIV-positive gravidas, coupled with intravenous AZT during labor and oral medication to the newborn, has been recently shown to decrease perinatal transmission by two-thirds.

23. Should screening for group B streptococci be done during pregnancy?

Group B streptococcal (GBS) infection is a common cause of neonatal sepsis and carries a high mortality and morbidity, especially in premature neonates. Although GBS is commonly cultured in mothers (5–30%), actual newborn sepsis occurs in only 0.1–0.5% of all births.

Eradicating the organism with an antibiotic at the time of delivery is the best means of preventing neonatal GBS sepsis, although this approach is costly and encourages the development of antibiotic resistance. Treatment of the neonate is less effective once bacteremia is established.

The Centers for Disease Control currently recommends one of two approaches to prevent early-onset GBS infection: (1) routine screening of all mothers for GBS at 35–37 weeks and treating positives during labor; or (2) giving intrapartum treatment for patients with known risk factors for neonatal GBS sepsis (e.g., < 37 weeks' gestation, ruptured membranes > 18 hours, or maternal fever in labor). In addition, intrapartum prophylaxis should be given to all patients with GBS bacteriuria or a history of a previous infant with GBS disease, and to those managed with the first preventive approach who have these risk factors when culture results are not known at the time of labor (e.g., cases of preterm delivery). For some situations (e.g., preterm PROM) there is often time before labor to make a definite diagnosis by taking a GBS culture on admission. Rapid tests for GBS, although available, are not highly sensitive to light colonization.

24. Who should be screened for diabetes?

Pregnancy poses a diabetogenic stress, and about 2% of gravidas develop gestational diabetes. Of the latter, roughly 30–50% become diabetic (adult onset) later in life. The following are risk factors for gestational diabetes: past macrosomic infant or stillbirth, maternal obesity, strong family history, and glucosuria. However, a substantial number of women with gestational diabetes have no risk factors. Therefore, a glucose screen—a 1-hour blood sugar analysis following 50 gm of oral glucose load—should be done on all gravidas at 24–28 weeks' gestation. A glucose screen should also be done at the initial visit if risk factors for gestational diabetes exist. Upper limits of normal are 140 mg/dl (plasma glucose). Women with elevated values should have a 3-hour glucose tolerance test. Those with risk factors and negative screens at 24–28 weeks should be rescreened at 32 weeks.

25. What is the purpose of maternal serum alpha-fetoprotein (MSAFP) or multiple biologic marker testing?

The MSAFP test is offered to all pregnant women between 15 and 19 weeks' gestation. Originally, MSAFP was used to identify fetuses with neural tube defects, but it also has been found to be a good screening test for a number of other abnormalities. Elevated levels (> 2.5 multiples of the median, MOM) are seen with some congenital malformations (neural tube defects, abdominal wall defects, esophageal and duodenal atresia, some renal and urinary tract anomalies), chromosomal abnormalities (Turner syndrome), and other poor pregnancy outcomes (feto-maternal hemorrhage, some low birthweight fetuses, and fetal death). Low MSAFP levels indicate an increased risk for Down syndrome.

Historically, amniocentesis or chorionic villus sampling for fetal karyotype in women 35 years or older identified about 20% of babies with Down syndrome. Performing amniocentesis on younger patients with low MSAFP values, which gave a risk for Down syndrome of 1:270 or higher, increased the antenatal diagnosis to 40–45%. Use of human chorionic gonadotropin (high levels) and estriol (low levels) along with MSAFP—the current triple marker test—substantially increases the yield to 60–65% of fetuses with Down syndrome. Using these three markers and age, a risk for Down syndrome is computed and amniocentesis is recommended if this is > 1:270. In the future, additional markers, both in serum and on ultrasound, will no doubt contribute further to the sensitivity of identifying fetuses with Down syndrome. At present, this testing does not match the sensitivity of genetic amniocentesis for karyotype of women age 35 or older at delivery.

26. Should a routine prenatal ultrasound scan be done?

Performing an ultrasound scan of the fetus as a routine part of prenatal care is controversial. A recent large American multicentered randomized study of routine scans in low-risk women, with known LMPs and early prenatal care, showed that routine sonography did not improve pregnancy outcome over ultrasound used for specific indications only. On the other hand, in populations who have higher overall risk or who usually enroll in prenatal care during late mid-pregnancy, after many gestational milestones have passed, routine screening may be valid for dating alone. In addition, although uncommon, serious congenital abnormalities can be identified early, with the option of pregnancy termination for some and time for future planning for others. Whether these advantages of universal ultrasonography have significant cost savings has not yet been determined.

27. Which laboratory tests are repeated during the prenatal course?

Hematocrit is generally repeated in the third trimester, or more frequently in at-risk women, to identify anemia (Hct ≤ 32%) or hemoconcentration (Hct ≥ 40%).

Urine dipstick for protein and sugar is done on each revisit; presence of significant protein-uria mandates investigation for preeclampsia, urinary tract infection and renal disease; glucosuria can point to gestational diabetes, although it may reflect normal decreased renal glucose absorbance during pregnancy.

Antibody screening test is repeated at 28 weeks' gestation in Rh-negative women and, if negative, Rh immunoglobulin (RhoGAM) should be given.

Sexually transmitted disease testing, including serologic test for syphilis (STS), gonorrhea culture, and test for chlamydia, is repeated at 28 or 36 weeks' gestation in many offices caring for indigent women, in whom the prevalence of these infections is relatively high.

Glucose screen is often repeated at 32 weeks' gestation in women with risk factors for diabetes but normal values at weeks 24–28.

28. How is a patient determined to be at high risk?

At the conclusion of the initial prenatal exam, the patient needs to be evaluated for overall risk. Scoring systems for risk assessment have evolved in recent years and are available in the literature. Significant problems should be noted and a plan for management and follow-up proposed. Such high-risk charts should be easily identifiable by outpatient careproviders and labor-delivery personnel. On each revisit, risks need to be reassessed; old problems need to be reviewed; problems that have been resolved should be removed; and any new problems should be added to the patient's record.

29. What role should the obstetrician play if he or she suspects that a pregnant patient is a victim of domestic violence?

Domestic violence is a major public health problem in the U.S. It is estimated to involve 2–4 million women annually and pervades all socioeconomic strata. Furthermore, it is the most common cause of trauma to women, accounting for about one-third of all visits by women to an emergency department. Most importantly, spousal abuse is responsible for about one-third of homicides in women aged 15–45. Several reports have found that on average 8–10% of pregnant women are battered by their spouses or partners. In some cases there is a detrimental impact on the fetus with the potential of increased rates of low birthweight, prematurity, and perinatal mortality. Although common, much domestic violence goes unrecognized by health professionals, and finding solutions for each family is difficult. Identification of a battered woman is important because her life and the lives of her children are in danger from further injury, sometimes leading to death. History-taking at the initial prenatal visit should include inquiry into the existence and extent of domestic violence. For trauma not related to other obvious causes, this is even more important. In less acute circumstances, initial clues may involve various, often vague, somatic symptoms, such as headache, insomnia, hyperventilation, choking sensation, gastrointestinal symptoms, and pain in the chest, pelvis, or back.

Most battered women need prompt help from resources available in many communities. Depending on the urgency of the situation, the woman should be referred to family crisis centers, shelters for battered women, the local police department, hospital emergency departments, legal aid services, and social service departments. These resources usually have expertise in providing urgent help for the woman and her children in dealing with the male batterer and in planning for the future. In addition, if the patient cannot or does not wish to leave home, she should formulate a plan of exit from her house for when the need arises. Long-term counseling is usually necessary by a social worker, psychologist, psychiatrist, or others who are experts in the management of battered women. The woman's children also require help, as many are also abused.

30. What advice should be given to pregnant women about work outside the house?

Overall, in the U.S., there has been little to incriminate regular employment at one's usual occupation as a contributory factor to adverse pregnancy outcome. Obviously, some women with specific medical or obstetric conditions who are at high risk for poor outcomes will need to discontinue work early for therapy and rest. In addition, bodily changes that accompany pregnancy—weight gain, fatigue, difficulty in breathing, balance problems, backache, especially in late pregnancy—may make it difficult for some women to continue working, depending on the job and each patient's adjustment to it.

In general, low-risk pregnant women can continue working at their regular jobs as long as the job is not dangerous (physically or environmentally) or overly strenuous and does not cause physical or mental exhaustion. Many women want to take leave or reduce their hours as the demands of pregnancy increase in the last trimester. Often, job requirements can be modified to reduce the physical workload or the woman can be transferred to less strenuous work. Frequent breaks, elevation of legs, and changes in position are good ideas for all working gravidas.

It is important for the patient to find out if maternity benefits are offered by her employer and to plan for maternal leave. By federal law, employers offering medical disability compensation must treat pregnancy-related disabilities in the same way as temporary disabilities due to illness or injury in nonpregnant employees. Such temporary disability can be due to pregnancy per se, complications of pregnancy, or hazardous occupational exposure during pregnancy. If the employer has such coverage, a pregnant employee can apply for benefits if the disability is certified by her obstetrician. If such employee disability coverage is not available, the patient may be eligible for state unemployment benefits, or she must use sick leave or vacation time or take an unpaid leave of absence. A recent congressional act provides that any pregnant woman working for a government or a company of over 50 employees is allowed up to 12 weeks of nonpaid maternal leave, during which time the employer must continue her benefits and seniority and retain her job position or equivalent when she returns after delivery.

31. What kind of education should the pregnant patient receive?

Educating the pregnant woman about pregnancy, labor, and delivery; care of her infant and parenting; common complications of pregnancy; and general improvement in health is an integral part of prenatal care. Various aspects should be discussed at each visit in a logical sequence. Such information can be presented on a one-to-one basis by the physician or nurse, via small group sessions, by videotape or posters (while the patient is sitting in the waiting room), and in books and handouts to be read at home. It is vital that the content of any reading material be written in a manner appropriate for the patient's level of education; otherwise, it will provide little or no benefit. Finally, Lamaze and other childbirth preparation classes are an excellent source of information about pregnancy and labor.

32. What recommendations should be given for exercise during pregnancy?

Most women can continue some form of exercise during pregnancy, although special consideration should be given to women with medical or obstetric complications. In otherwise healthy women, regular exercise (3 times/week) should be encouraged over intermittent exertions. Supine positions (after the first trimester due to vena caval obstruction by the enlarging uterus) should be avoided. Duration and intensity of exercise should be self-monitored; cessation of exercise at early signs of fatigue should be encouraged rather than attainment of rigid goals based on the nonpregnant state. Exercises requiring balance should be avoided during the third trimester in particular, and careful fluid-dietary supplementation and heat dissipation should be encouraged.

32. Of what danger signs should the patient be made aware?
- Abdominal or pelvic pain or cramping
- Frequent uterine contractions or painless tightening from weeks 20–36
- Vaginal bleeding
- Passage of watery discharge
- Significant decrease in fetal movements
- Severe headache or blurring of vision
- Persistent vomiting
- Chills or fever

33. Which common complications of pregnancy can be prevented or minimized by good prenatal care?
- Anemia due to iron or folic acid deficiency
- Urinary tract infections and pyelonephritis
- Pregnancy-induced hypertension (preeclampsia)
- Preterm labor and delivery
- Intrauterine growth retardation
- Sexually transmitted diseases and their effect on the newborn infant
- Rh isoimmunization
- Fetal macrosomia
- Breech presentation at term
- Hypoxia or fetal death from postterm birth

BIBLIOGRAPHY

1. American College of Obstetricians and Gynecologists: The battered woman. Technical Bulletin No. 124. Washington, DC, 1989.
2. American College of Obstetricians and Gynecologists: Ultrasonography in pregnancy. ACOG Technical Bulletin No. 187. Washington, DC, 1993.
3. American College of Obstetricians and Gynecologists: Down syndrome screening. Committee Opinion No. 141. Washington, DC, 1994.
4. American College of Obstetricians and Gynecologists: Exercise during pregnancy and the postpartum period. ACOG Technical Bulletin No. 189, Washington, DC, 1994.
5. American Diabetes Association: Position statement on gestational diabetes mellitus. Am J Obstet Gynecol 156:488, 1987.
6. Centers for Disease Control: Hepatitis B virus: A comprehensive strategy for eliminating transmission in the United States through universal childhood vaccination. MMWR 40(No. RR-13), 1991.
7. Centers for Disease Control: Summary of notifiable diseases, United States, 1993. MMWR 42, No. 53, 1994.
8. Centers for Disease Control: Zidovudine for the prevention of HIV transmission from mother to infant. MMWR 43:285, 1994.
9. Centers for Disease Control: Rubella and congenital rubella syndrome—United States, January 1, 1991–May 7, 1994. MMWR 43:391, 1994.
10. Cunningham FG, McDonald PC, Gant NF, et al: Williams Obstetrics, 19th ed. Norwalk, CT, Appleton & Lange, 1993, p 247–271.
11. Ewigman BG, Crane JP, Frigoletto FD, et al: Effect of prenatal ultrasound screening on perinatal outcome. N Engl J Med 329:821, 1993.
12. Gibbs RS, Sweet RL: Maternal and fetal infections—clinical disorders. In Creasy RK, Resnick R (eds): Maternal-Fetal Medicine: Principles and Practice, 3rd ed. Philadelphia, W.B. Saunders, 1994.
13. Goodlin RC, Dobry CA, Anderson JC, et al: Clinical signs of normal plasma volume expansion during pregnancy. Am J Obstet Gynecol 145:1001, 1983.
14. Moore TR, Origel W, Key TC, et al: The perinatal and economic impact of prenatal care in a low socioeconomic population. Am J Obstet Gynecol 154:29, 1986.
15. Newberger EH, Barkan SE, Lieberman ES, et al: Abuse of pregnant women and adverse birth outcome. JAMA 267:2370, 1992.
16. Robertson AW, Duff P: The nitrite and leukocyte esterase tests for the evaluation of asymptomatic bacteriuria in obstetric patients. Obstet Gynecol 71:878, 1988.
17. U.S. Public Health Service Expert Panel on the Content of Prenatal Care: Caring for Our Future—The Content of Prenatal Care. USPHS, Department of Health and Human Services, 1989.
18. Weinstein L: Irregular antibodies causing hemolytic disease of the newborn. Obstet Gynecol Surv 31:581, 1976.

43. NUTRITION IN PREGNANCY

Miriam Erick, M.S., R.D., C.D.E.

1. How does prepregnant maternal weight affect pregnancy outcome?

Underweight women more frequently deliver small-for-gestational-age (SGA) infants than moderate or overweight women. Placental size is often reduced in smaller women. Women who are < 90% desirable body weight are often underconsuming important nutrients for their own health maintenance, notably iron, calcium, and folate.

Underweight women with financial constraints should be referred to a perinatal nutritionist who can advise dietary quality and connect the client to the Women's, Infant's and Children's (WIC) supplemental feeding program. When financial constraints are not the issue, underweight women with an obsessive focus on overall weight or gestational weight gain and women who continue an intensive exercise program may have eating disorders. Such women may benefit from approaches directed at these issues.

The combination of underweight and inadequate weight gain has a positive association with premature deliveries and growth retardation. A portion of smaller babies have difficulty in later years with cognition and psychomotor skills. The potential neonatal consequence of inadequate nutrition is not confined solely to low income.

2. How should maternal weight and gestational weight gain be assessed?

Use of the prepregnant body mass index (BMI = weight in grams/height in centimeters squared) is favored by many, including the American College of Obstetricians and Gynecologists (ACOG). BMI may be more predictive of body fat distribution than weight alone. Based on the National Institute of Health study in 1990, guidelines for total weight gain in pregnancy are based on prepregnant BMI.

Recommendations for Total Weight Gain in Pregnancy

PREPREGNANCY STATUS	RECOMMENDED TOTAL GAIN (lbs)
Underweight: BMI < 19.8 or < 90% IBW	28–40
Normal weight: BMI 19.8–26.0 or 90–120% IBW	25–35
Overweight: BMI 26.0–29.0 or 120–135% IBW	15–25
Obese: BMI > 29.0 or > 135% IBW	15

IBW = ideal body weight.

3. Should a woman who is obese diet during pregnancy?

Prepregnancy obesity is associated with several obstetric complications, including hypertension, diabetes, increased cesarean rate, and increased postoperative complications (wound infection). Although few practitioners advocate no weight gain for the morbidly obese, incremental increases in weight lead to greater risk of complications. One management tool is to establish a formal written calorie level, follow hunger status, and evaluate urine for ketones. If the calorie level is appropriate for the client, the urine should be ketone-free and the client should not lose weight. Caloric computation in morbidly obese women is difficult, and no standards exist for accurately predicting maintenance kilocalories.

4. How much weight should be gained each gestational week?

Rate of weight gain varies by gestational age and prepregnant weight. For a woman of average weight, one guideline is an average of 5–10 pounds during the first 20 weeks of pregnancy, followed by 1 pound per week thereafter.

5. What information should be given to women with poor or no weight gain?

The reason for the poor weight gain first needs to be assessed:

1. Inadequate intake, either food or fluid
2. Chronic and ongoing nausea
3. Adequate intake but output losses (undiagnosed glycosuria, increased stool output)
4. Increased metabolic demands beyond the normal aspects of pregnancy (undiagnosed HIV infection, cancer, disturbed sleep patterns)
5. High-energy expenditure (athletic activities)
6. Lack of finances or lack of nutrition knowledge
7. Crowded living conditions and shared food
8. Body image issues
9. New food intolerances of pregnancy
10. Undiagnosed multiple gestations

The cause of poor weight gain often dictates the needed services, which may include nutrition, social work, psychiatry, and GI and endocrinologic studies.

6. How much of the total maternal weight gain can be attributed to the various components of pregnancy?

28 lbs, which includes average fetal weight at term, amniotic fluid, placenta, breast enlargement, increased volume expansion, and appropriate fat stores

7. What are the basic nutritional requirements of pregnancy?

Calorically, the allowance has been to add 300 calories and 10 gm/day to the normal diet, starting in the second trimester. Overall vitamin and mineral needs increase approximately 15% or comparably to the overall caloric increase. Nutrient needs can be met by a varied diet:

- 5 servings of fruits and five of fresh leafy green and deep yellow vegetables
- 8 servings of complex carbohydrates (breads, rice, noodles, cereals, grains)
- 4–5 servings of dairy products
- 2 three-ounce portions of protein (meat, tofu, legumes, fish, cheese, eggs)
- 2–5 teaspoons of fats/oils, preferably 50% monounsaturated

This list provides 2200 calories and 60 gm of protein and meets the nutrient needs of most women with a singleton pregnancy.

8. Are the nutritional requirements for multiple gestations different?

Yes, although the exact caloric requirement for twins and higher-order gestations has not been ascertained. Many variations have been suggested, although the tendency is to add 300 calories and 10 gm of protein for each additional fetus beyond the singleton. The optimal weight gain for twins has been suggested as 44 lbs. However, optimal nutrient intake to achieve this weight gain is unknown. For triplets, an additional 500 calories/day has been advocated. Consideration should be given to the amount of additional food recommended, because gastric space is frequently reduced and heartburn is common.

9. Can good nutrition be maintained in the first trimester when morning sickness is often a problem?

It may be difficult for women who are experiencing nausea and vomiting of pregnancy (NVP) to find anything to eat during a crisis. Not surprisingly, among women with hyperemesis gravidarum, mean dietary intakes of most nutrients fall below 50% of the RDA. Suboptimal intake includes thiamin, riboflavin, vitamin B6, vitamin A, and protein. Although a prenatal supplement theoretically would correct these deficiencies, its size often evokes gastrointestinal distress. One children's chewable vitamin with extra iron and folate may be a reasonable solution. Caution must be taken not to exceed the RDA for vitamin A.

10. What suggestions are available for women with nausea and vomiting of pregnancy?
Guidelines for an oral hyperemesis diet favor small frequent meals. Reasons include early satiety, visual overload, and the potential for increased olfactory insult. Often women experience a waxing and waning course with nausea and tend to eat rapidly in periods of remission. Although perhaps a compensatory mechanism, this pattern may precipitate a set-back. Slowly ingested mini meals, taking 20 minutes to complete, can reduce transient overeating. Foods and beverages containing ginger may be tolerated by some women, but tablets of concentrated ginger have been inadequately studied; the major concern is potential testosterone binding.
There is no reason to restrict high-fat foods if tolerance is not a problem. A distinction should be made between nausea generated from eating high-fat foods and nausea from smelling a high-fat food. Recommendations promoting very high-protein diets are ill advised if fluid intake is not appropriate.
The basis for an antiemetic diet is highly personal, revolving around organoleptic properties of food with cultural and psychosocial considerations. Women with NVP should be referred to a Registered Dietitian specializing in perinatal nutrition.

11. What are the guidelines for fluid requirements during pregnancy?
The average woman needs about 2 L/day or approximately 1 ml of fluid for each calorie burned. Allowances for fluid losses due to extreme heat and humidity and high altitudes are additive. Respiratory insensible losses average 300–500 ml/day in women with surface evaporation and sweat averaging 400–600 ml/day. Markedly obese persons have an increased insensible water loss.
In one study, encouraging maternal hydration above 2 L/day increased amniotic fluid indexes (AFI) in women with low AFIs. In women with normal AFI, hydration above 2 L increased AFI by 16%, whereas fluid restriction decreased AFI by 8%. The clinical significance of these AFI alterations remains unstudied. Foods such as watermelon provide 80–90% water by weight (1 cup of watermelon = ¾ fluid; 1 orange, ⅓ cup fluid; crackers, about 5% fluid).

12. Do all pregnant women need additional iron?
Women who eat carefully planned daily diets with maximal dietary iron probably do not need supplemental iron. However, numerous dietary surveys indicate that iron intake is suboptimal in a high percentage of the population. The heart-healthy move to less red meat has much to do with this change. Absorption of iron from heme sources has been shown to be 10%, whereas from nonheme sources, it is approximately 2%. Thus large portions of nonheme foods are required to compensate. Iron-deficient persons, however, generally absorb twice as much iron from a meal as those without iron deficiency. Additionally, in a small study, iron absorption was observed to increase with gestational age: 7% at week 12, 36% at week 24, and 66% by week 36.

13. What sorts of foods should be encouraged to increase iron in the diet?
    High sources: oysters; lean red meats, especially liver; in vegetarian diets, tofu, legumes, and beans when consumed with an acidic beverage such as orange, grapefruit, or tomato juice.
    Moderate sources: enriched grain products and cereals
    Low sources: light and white meats, including chicken, salmon, and pork; dairy products
Iron, whether dietary or supplemented, should not be consumed within 1 hour of calcium intake. An insoluble complex can result in reduced iron absorption. Antacids taken for heartburn can also interfere with iron absorption. Tea and coffee can cut absorption of nonheme iron by more than half compared with water.

14. Are vitamin and mineral supplements necessary during pregnancy?
The overall quality of a woman's diet affects her need for supplementation. If all the necessary nutrients can be consumed in the daily diet, the answer is no. However, women with special needs should be addressed separately. Various categories of special need for vitamin and mineral supplementation include:

1. **Dilantin therapy.** Animal studies have shown more favorable fetal outcomes when folate, vitamins, and amino acids are supplemented. Favorable outcomes include greater fetal weight and length, decreased subcutaneous bleeding, more ossification centers and fewer malformations.

2. **Increased risk of lead exposure.** Women working in manufacturing plants, recent immigrants from countries where lead-free gasoline is not mandated, and residents of old buildings undergoing renovations may benefit from supplementation with vitamins C and E. These antioxidant vitamins may play a role in the reduction of potentially adverse effects of lead during pregnancy, including protection of the fetus against lead toxicity and/or free radical change.

3. **Multiple gestations.** Although the exact amount is not known, supplemental folate is recommended, given the increased red blood cell production.

4. **HIV infection.** Supplemental selenium has been shown to inhibit reverse transcriptase activity in RNA virus-infected animals. Selenium with antioxidant vitamins has been speculated as a measure to reduce the probability of placental transmission of HIV.

5. **Alcohol consumption.** Moderate-to-high alcohol intake may deplete many nutrients, notably B complex, and should be repleted.

6. **Hemoglobinopathies** may benefit by supplemental folate given the increased red blood cell turnover.

7. **Hypertension** may benefit from calcium supplementation.

15. What vitamin supplements are appropriate periconceptionally?

Recently, periconception folate administration to reduce the risk of neural tube defects (NTD) has undergone extensive study. One study evaluating the risk of NTD in first pregnancies suggests intakes of 0.4 mg folate/day. The dose most commonly found in over-the-counter multivitamins reduces the NTD risk by approximately 60%. The timing of folate ingestion for reduction of risk was 28 days before through 28 days after the last menstrual period.

16. What problems are associated with megadose vitamin and mineral therapy?

Large intakes of fat-soluble vitamins such as vitamin A and D have been shown to cause birth defects in both humans and animals. Megadoses of selenium have a similar risk. Large doses of zinc suppress the immune system. Large amounts of fluoride during pregnancy have been associated with mottled teeth. Dolomite from harvested clam shells is often used for calcium supplementation. At one point dolomite was found to contain heavy minerals such as lead after shell contamination with industrial wastes. Many small manufacturers of vitamin and mineral supplements may not use the same quality control standards as large firms.

There are also issues of nutrient displacement. For example, excessive vitamin C appears to interfere with copper metabolism. Additionally, zinc competes with iron for absorption, and iron deficiency anemia may result.

Another problem with megadose vitamin therapy is the source of distribution. Health food stores frequently advocate various herbal remedies and supplements for complaints ranging from headache to heartburn. Some of these may be dangerous during pregnancy. Remedies marketed as calmatives or nervines may contain large amounts of alkaloids, shown to cause hepatic damage. Mate, a tealike infusion commonly found in health food stores, has been reported to increase the risk of digestive tract cancers. An herbal tea, pleurisy root, has been shown to have digoxinlike factors. "Pregnancy tea," containing chamomile, mint, and raspberry leaves, appears to be safe when consumed in moderation.

17. What special considerations apply to women with unusual diets due either to cultural diversity or food fads?

Most obstetric practices are multicultural, which makes it difficult to assess dietary adequacy without a trained perinatal nutritionist. In addition to the various ethnic foods that may make up a daily diet, some cultures have pregnancy taboos that alter nutritional intake. One example is the prohibition in some cultures against consumption of eggs by pregnant women.

Asian women may have diets based on raw fish, which can reduce thiamin status as raw fish contain thiaminases. Raw fish also present danger from parasites and are a potential source of food poisoning.

18. What are the nutritional concerns for the pregnant vegetarian?

The specific restrictions of vegetarian diets should be explored. Ovolactovegetarians consuming milk products, eggs, fish, and poultry generally meet the suggested guidelines without further supplementation. More restrictive diets (lactovegetarians with no fish, eggs, or poultry and vegans, who eat plants only) should consider vitamin B complex which includes B12, calcium, and additional iron supplementation. Highly restrictive diets (only fruits, Zen macrobiotic diets) are best avoided during pregnancy.

19. What role does a perinatal nutritionist play?

Perinatal nutritionists, a subgroup of the American Dietetic Association, specialize in the science of food and nutrition, from source to processing, digestion, and metabolism. In addition to assessing nutritional contribution, they are qualified to advise the obstetric client in various situations of nutritional risk. To obtain a list of perinatal nutritionists in a given area, call the American Dietetic Association at 800-877-1600.

BIBLIOGRAPHY

1. Allen LH: Iron-deficiency anemia increases the risk of preterm delivery. Nutr Rev 51:49–52, 1993.
2. American College of Obstetricians and Gynecologists: Nutrition during pregnancy. ACOG Tech Bull 179, 1993.
3. Backton J: Ginger in preventing nausea and vomiting in pregnancy: A caveat to its thromboxane synthetase activity and effect on testosterone binding. Eur J Obstet Reprod Biol 42:163–164, 1991.
4. Barrett JF, Whittaker PQ, Williams JG, Lind T: Absorption of non-heme iron from food during normal pregnancy. BMJ 309:79–82, 1994.
5. Czeikel AE: Nutritional supplementation and prevention of congenital abnormalities. Curr Opin Obstet Gynecol 92:88–94, 1995.
6. Erick M: Vitamin B6, ginger in morning sickness. J Am Diet Assoc 95:416, 1995.
7. Franko DL, Walton BE: Pregnancy and eating disorders: A review and clinical implications. Int J Eat Disord 13:41–47, 1993.
8. Kilpatrick SJ, Safford KL: Maternal hydration and amniotic fluid index in women with normal amniotic fluid. Obstet Gynecol 81:49–52, 1993.
9. Wada L, King JC: Trace elements and nutrition in pregnancy. Clin Obstet Gynecol 37:754–786, 1994.
10. Worthington-Roberts B: Perinatal nutrition: General issues. In Worthington-Roberts B (ed): Nutrition in Pregnancy and Lactation, 6th ed. Madison, WI, Brown & Benchmark Publishers, 1997.

V. Maternal Complications

44. HYPERTENSION IN PREGNANCY

L. *Dorine Day*, M.D.

1. What are the types of hypertension during pregnancy?

Four categories are now recognized for hypertension in pregnancy: chronic hypertension, preeclampsia, chronic hypertension with superimposed preeclampsia, and transient hypertension.

2. What is the definition of chronic hypertension in pregnancy?

Chronic hypertension antedates the pregnancy or is characterized by blood pressure readings consistently above 140/90 prior to 20 weeks' gestation.

3. What is the classic definition of preeclampsia?

The diagnosis of preeclampsia consists of a triad of elevated blood pressure, proteinuria, and edema in the third trimester. Blood pressure is considered elevated if the systolic reading is > 140 mmHg or the diastolic reading is > 90 mmHg. Of less diagnostic value is a rise in systolic pressure > 30 mmHg or diastolic pressure > 15 mmHg over the patient's baseline blood pressure (preferably a first-trimester reading). Proteinuria is defined as > 300 mg/24 hr.

4. What is the definition of chronic hypertension with superimposed preeclampsia?

The definition is preeclampsia in a patient with known chronic hypertension. Sometimes it is clinically hard to diagnose worsening of the patient's chronic hypertension as opposed to development of preeclampsia.

5. What is the definition of transient hypertension?

Transient hypertension is a diagnosis of exclusion. The actual definition is third-trimester elevation of blood pressure without evidence of preeclampsia in a patient known to be normotensive when nonpregnant. Often transient hypertension is diagnosed only in hindsight.

6. What is pregnancy-induced hypertension? How does it differ from transient hypertension?

Pregnancy-induced hypertension is not a recognized term by the National Workshop on Hypertension in Pregnancy. However, clinicians often use the term to refer to patients with preeclampsia, patients in whom they suspect preeclampsia will develop, or patients with transient hypertension.

7. Are women with chronic hypertension considered high risk pregnancies?

Yes. Because of poor placental vascular development and ongoing elevations of blood pressure, the pregnancy is at risk for intrauterine growth restriction, abruption, and stillbirth. From a maternal perspective, the patient may develop superimposed preeclampsia and all of the associated consequences. Many clinicians believe that superimposed preeclampsia is more serious clinically than simple preeclampsia.

8. Can anything be done to prevent complications in patients with chronic hypertension?

A number of things can be done. Patients with chronic hypertension should have their blood pressure under control when they conceive and continue blood pressure medications when they are pregnant, even when blood pressure drops to normal range in the second trimester. The exception is any hypertensive medication associated with congenital anomalies or adverse fetal outcomes, which should be discontinued; another medication should be substituted. The class of antihypertensives that should not be used in pregnant patients (some clinicians believe it should not be used even in reproductive-aged women) are the angiotensin-converting enzyme (ACE) inhibitors. Low-dose aspirin therapy begun during the second trimester of pregnancy has been shown to decrease the risk of superimposed preeclampsia. Most clinicians follow these pregnancies with serial ultrasounds for fetal growth. Last but not least, surveillance of fetal well-being is recommended, beginning in the third trimester. In general, these pregnancies are not allowed to continue past 40 weeks.

9. How often does preeclampsia occur? Which women are at greater risk?

Preeclampsia occurs in 6–8% of all live births. Risk factors include nulliparity, extremes of reproductive age (< 15 and > 35 years of age), black race, history of preeclampsia in a first-degree female relative, diabetes, chronic hypertension, multiple gestations, and hydrops (isoimmunized or nonimmune). Any process associated with an enlarged placenta increases the patient's risk for preeclampsia.

Risk Factors for Preeclampsia

FACTOR	RELATIVE RISK RATIO
Chronic renal disease	20:1
Chronic hypertension	10:1
Antiphospholipid syndrome	10:1
Family history of pregnancy-induced hypertension	5:1
Twin gestation	4:1
Nulliparity	3:1
Age > 40 yr	3:1
Diabetes mellitus	2:1
African-American race	1.5:1
Angiotensinogen gene T235	
Homozygous	20:1
Heterozygous	4:1

From American College of Obstetricians and Gynecologists: Hypertension in Pregnancy. ACOG Tech Bull 219, 1996, with permission.

10. How is preeclampsia classified?

Preeclampsia is classified as mild and severe. The definition of severe preeclampsia is systolic blood pressure > 160 mmHg and/or diastolic blood pressure > 110 mmHg on two occasions at least 6 hours apart, proteinuria > 5 gm/24 hr, oliguria < 500 cc/24 hr, cerebral or visual symptoms, epigastric pain, pulmonary edema, low platelets, increased liver function tests, or intrauterine growth restriction. The definition of mild preeclampsia is any preeclampsia that is not considered severe. There is no category of moderate preeclampsia.

11. Do we know what causes preeclampsia?

No. Preeclampsia has been described since the time of the ancient Greeks. However, the cause remains unknown. We know that hypertension, proteinuria, and edema are merely the signs and symptoms required for diagnosis of a systemic illness characterized by vasoconstriction and hypovolemia. All organs, including the fetoplacental unit, show evidence of poor perfusion.

12. What are some of the theories of the cause of preeclampsia?

Immunologic response. Inadequate maternal antibody response to the fetal allograft results in vascular damage from the circulating immune complexes. This theory is supported by an increased prevalence of the disease in pregnancies with limited prior antigen exposure (young nulliparas) and in situations with increased fetal antigen (twins, molar pregnancy, hydropic pregnancies, and diabetics with large placentas). Actual measurement of immune complexes has been inconsistent.

Circulating toxins. Vasoconstrictive substances reportedly have been extracted from blood, amniotic fluid, and the placenta in women with preeclampsia. Symptoms have been reproduced in some but not all animal studies.

Endogenous vasoconstrictors. Increased sensitivity to vasopressin, epinephrine, and norepinephrine have all been reported. Loss of normal third-trimester resistance to angiotensin II has also been noted.

Endothelial damage. Primary endothelial damage results in a decrease in prostacyclin production (potent vasodilator) and a relative increase in thromboxane A_2 (relative vasoconstrictor). Low-dose heparin or baby aspirin may play a role in prevention, but the cause of the endothelial damage and prostaglandin change is unclear.

Primary disseminated intravascular coagulation (DIC). Microvascular thrombin formation and deposition have been noted, producing vessel damage especially in the kidney and in the placenta.

13. What fetal and maternal risks are associated with preeclampsia?

Fetal	Maternal
In utero growth restriction	Central nervous system manifestations,
Placental infarcts	including seizures and stroke
Oligohydramnios	DIC and its complications
Abruption	Increase in cesarean section delivery
Consequences of prematurity (when	Renal failure
maternal disease necessitates	Hepatic failure or rupture
delivery remote from term)	Death
Uteroplacental insufficiency	

Preeclampsia is a leading cause of maternal mortality. In most patients who survive, including even those experiencing strokes, problems are reversible, although exceptions have been reported.

14. Does preeclampsia recur in subsequent pregnancies?

Yes. Preeclampsia in the first pregnancy may recur in up to 25% of patients in subsequent pregnancies. The recurrence rate appears to be affected by gestational age at onset in the first pregnancy, severity, underlying maternal diseases, and underlying obstetric diseases. Multiparous patients who have had preeclampsia have a recurrence rate of up to 50% with subsequent pregnancies.

15. Does preeclampsia have ramifications later in life?

No. Preeclampsia does not increase the risk of hypertension later in life. Some exceptions may exist in women who have recurrent preeclampsia, which may suggest unrecognized chronic hypertension or other underlying maternal diseases.

16. Can women who have a pregnancy complicated by preeclampsia take birth control pills after delivery?

Yes. Preeclampsia, especially in a primiparous patient, does not contraindicate the use of oral contraceptives 2 weeks after delivery.

17. What is the "cure" for preeclampsia?

Delivery of the pregnancy "cures" preeclampsia. With delivery, signs and symptoms of preeclampsia resolve, although the time required for resolution is variable. The difficulty in therapy is when to deliver the infant. Obviously, at term the decision is easy to make, whether the preeclampsia is mild or severe. The difficulty arises when preeclampsia is remote from term. The degree of severity and the fetal gestational age are taken into consideration, and either the pregnancy is delivered or the patient is placed at bed rest. With bed rest therapy, close maternal and fetal surveillance is performed until the pregnancy reaches term or the degree of severity worsens, dictating the need to deliver.

18. How should delivery be accomplished in patients with preeclampsia?
There is no advantage to cesarean delivery over vaginal delivery for preeclampsia. Therefore, delivery route should be based on obstetric indications. An indication for cesarean section may be the inability to accomplish a vaginal delivery within a fixed, specified time, governed by maternal condition.

19. What special medicines are used in the delivery process?
A prophylactic agent against overt seizure activity is generally given during the labor process and for the first 24 or so hours of the postpartum period. The drug of choice in the United States is magnesium sulfate ($MgSO_4$). The usual dosing is a 4–6-gm bolus, followed by a 2-gm continuous infusion. If magnesium levels are monitored, the usual goal is a level in the 4–6 range. Unfortunately, magnesium sulfate does not prevent all seizure activity. However, studies using more recognized antiepileptic medications such as phenytoin have not shown an improvement in seizure control over $MgSO_4$. Diazepam is used extensively in Europe for preeclamptic seizure prophylaxis, but it is not used in the U.S. because of neonatal depression.

20. What is the role of antihypertensives, including diuretics, in preeclampsia?
Diuretics are generally not used as a first-line treatment because preeclampsia is characterized by vasoconstriction and intravascular depletion, which are worsened by diuretics. As for other antihypertensive agents, work has shown that treatment of patients with mild-to-moderate hypertension (i.e., 90–110 mmHg diastolic pressure) does not decrease perinatal morbidity or mortality. Therefore, antihypertensive therapy is not usually used. Severe hypertension (> 110 mmHg diastolic pressure) is associated with severe preeclampsia. More than likely, delivery needs to be undertaken, and rapid-acting antihypertensive agents (i.e., intravenous hydralazine or labetalol) are used to control severe hypertension during labor. This therapy, however, is withheld until after initiation of $MgSO_4$, because blood pressure may decrease with bed rest and $MgSO_4$ therapy. In a patient with known chronic hypertension whose elevated blood pressure is believed to be due to underlying disease rather than preeclampsia, an increase in antihypertensive therapy may be appropriate. Note that therapy is for maternal disease, not preeclampsia. In general, antihypertensives are not used for preeclampsia except acutely during the labor process.

21. What is eclampsia?
Eclampsia is the clinical diagnosis given to patients who have seizure activity due to preeclampsia. Eclampsia is considered one of the most severe forms of preeclampsia, and delivery is undertaken after a seizure. About 1% of patients with preeclampsia have eclampsia. There are no recognized clinical determinants of who will experience seizure activity. Because we cannot predict which preeclamptic patients will have seizure activity, the majority (if not all) of these patients are treated with medicine for seizure prophylaxis.

22. How is delivery accomplished in eclamptic patients?
As with preeclamptics, obstetric indications are used to determine route of delivery. It is not unusual to encounter fetal distress in eclamptic patients, but this is not necessarily an indication for cesarean delivery. In general, fetal resuscitation is best accomplished in utero by controlling the maternal state. Stabilizing the patient (i.e., airway, oxygen, circulation, and control of seizure activity) improves fetal outcome and subsequently neonatal outcome. Labor can then be initiated and vaginal delivery accomplished, assuming no obstetric indications for a cesarean delivery.

23. Is MgSO₄ used for eclamptic patients?

Some authorities suggest that phenytoin may be a better choice in patients who have already experienced seizure activity. However, a recent large study clearly favors $MgSO_4$ over phenytoin for recurrent seizure prophylaxis. Most U.S. clinicians continue to use $MgSO_4$ as their first drug of choice in these patients. Most treat the patient for 48 rather than 24 hours in the postpartum period.

24. What is HELLP syndrome?

Most clinicians believe that HELLP syndrome is a subcategory of preeclampsia. Patients present with hemolysis, elevated liver function, and/or low platelets. Patients may or may not have other signs of preeclampsia. HELLP syndrome often has a rapidly accelerating downhill course. Most clinicians deliver infants, with the route determined by obstetric indications.

25. What causes midepigastric pain in HELLP syndrome?

Liver capsule distention produces midepigastric pain, often with associated nausea and vomiting. Liver capsule distention can lead to hepatic rupture, with poor maternal and fetal outcomes.

26. What diagnoses should be considered in the patient who presents at 18 weeks' gestation with increased blood pressure?

Hydatidiform mole. Increased blood pressure, hyperemesis, and fetal size greater than dates are characteristic clinical findings. Hyperthyroidism and distant metastases may be associated with the clinical picture. Hydropic changes in the placenta can be seen on ultrasound.

Chronic hypertension. In some instances, chronic hypertension may have been previously diagnosed and treated. When previous evaluation has not been undertaken, care should be exercised to exclude secondary causes such as renal disease, pheochromocytoma, Cushing syndrome, or coarctation of the aorta.

Drug use. Cocaine use has been associated with increased blood pressure as well as poor perinatal outcome. In some cases, drug withdrawal (i.e., from heroin) has also been associated with hypertension.

Chromosomal abnormalities in the fetus. Triploidy is known to present with preeclampsia in the second trimester.

BIBLIOGRAPHY

1. American College of Obstetricians and Gynecologists: Hypertension in Pregnancy. ACOG Tech Bull 219, 1996.
2. Lubbe WF: Low-dose aspirin in prevention of toxemia of pregnancy: Does it have a place? Drugs 34:515, 1987.
3. Repke JT: Preeclampsia and eclampsia. In Repke JT (ed): Intrapartum Obstetrics, New York, Churchill Livingstone, 1996.
4. Roberts JM: Pregnancy-related hypertension. In Creasy R, Resnik R (eds): Maternal-Fetal Medicine: Principles and Practice, 3rd ed. Philadelphia, W.B. Saunders, 1994, pp 804–843.
5. Schiffe, Peleg E, Goldenberg M, et al: The use of aspirin to prevent pregnancy-induced hypertension and lower the ratio of thromboxane A_2 to prostacyclin in relatively high risk pregnancies. N Engl J Med 321:351, 1989.
6. Sibai BM, Spinnato JA, Watson DL: Pregnancy outcome in 303 cases with severe preeclampsia. Obstet Gynecol 64:319, 1984.
7. Sibai BM, Mercer BM, Schiff E, Friedman SA: Aggressive versus expectant management of severe preeclampsia at 28–32 weeks gestation: A randomized controlled trial. Am J Obstet Gynecol 171:818, 1994.
8. Weinstein L: Preeclampsia/eclampsia with hemolysis, elevated liver enzymes, and thrombocytopenia. Obstet Gynecol 66:657, 1985.

45. GESTATIONAL DIABETES MELLITUS

Shailini Singh, M.D.

1. What is gestational diabetes (GDM)?

GDM is defined as the state of carbohydrate intolerance that has its onset or first recognition during pregnancy.

2. Does the definition vary with severity?

No. The definition applies regardless of severity or whether insulin is required for treatment or the condition persists after pregnancy.

3. Does GDM include type I and type II patients?

Yes. GDM may include a small group of women with previously unrecognized overt diabetes mellitus type I or type II. However, usually the glucose intolerance is mild before pregnancy.

4. How is true GDM differentiated from unrecognized overt type I or type II diabetes mellitus?

1. In GDM the glycosylated hemoglobin (HbA1C) is normal.
2. At 6 weeks after delivery, evaluation with 75-gm oral glucose tolerance test reveals reversion to normal, nonpregnant carbohydrate tolerance.

5. What are the similarities between GDM and non–insulin-dependent diabetes (NIDDM)?

1. The endocrine (impaired insulin secretion) and metabolic (insulin resistance) abnormalities that characterize both disease states are virtually identical.
2. The risk factors for development of NIDDM are similar to those for development of GDM.
3. In people with normal glucose tolerance, the metabolic abnormalities that indicate a high risk for developing NIDDM are similar for increased risk for GDM. Furthermore, women with GDM are at a markedly increased risk for developing NIDDM. GDM thus may represent an early stage in the natural history of NIDDM.

6. What is the importance of diagnosis of GDM?

1. GDM identifies patients in whom aggressive glycemic control will prevent perinatal complications.
2. Diagnosis of GDM identifies patients who may benefit from early therapeutic interventions such as improved nutrition, weight loss (if obese), and regular exercise program to prevent development of NIDDM and associated complications later in life.

7. What are the incidence and prevalence of GDM?

Incidence varies from 0.15–15% of all pregnancies. Because GDM is such a heterogeneous entity, estimates of occurrence vary with ethnic diversity of the population under study, geographic area, screening frequency, and diagnostic criteria.

8. What are the effects of GDM on pregnant women?

Pregnant women with GDM have an increased incidence of short-term maternal complications such as pregnancy-induced hypertension, preterm labor, pyelonephritis, polyhydramnios, and cesarean section. In the long term, such patients are at higher risk of developing NIDDM and associated complications, especially cardiovascular.

9. What are the effects of GDM on the fetus?

Short-term effects include increased perinatal morbidity and mortality. In addition, the incidence of fetal macrosomia, shoulder dystocia, operative delivery, stillbirth, and metabolic problems is similar to that in infants of an insulin-dependent diabetic mother. Long-term effects include an increased incidence of childhood obesity, early adulthood type II diabetes mellitus, and intellectual-motor impairment.

10. Is a patient with well-managed GDM and glucose in the recommended range of fasting plasma glucose of < 105 mg/dl and 2-hr postprandial glucose of < 120 mg/dl at the same risk for developing obstetric complications as the general population?

No. The fetal complications are still significantly higher with a tendency for macrosomia and associated complications because other metabolic fuels are implicated as a cause of hyperalimentation in the fetus.

11. Is there an increased rate of congenital malformations in women with GDM?

No. True GDM usually develops late, in the second or early in the third trimester when organogenesis is already complete. If GDM is diagnosed in the first trimester, then it is imperative to confirm with the help of HbA1C whether it may be overt type I or type II diabetes, which may affect the incidence of congenital malformation.

12. What are the recommendations of the American College of Obstetricians and Gynecologists (ACOG) for GDM screening?

The ACOG recommends selective screening of women 30 years of age and older with 50-gm oral glucose load between 24–28 weeks' gestation. ACOG acknowledges that some populations may benefit from earlier or universal screening. Patients whose plasma glucose levels equal or exceed 140 mg/dl should be evaluated with a diagnostic 3-hr oral glucose tolerance test (OGTT).

13. What patients are at high risk for developing GDM?

The following patients are at high risk for GDM and should be screened at the first prenatal visit and each trimester thereafter:

1. Previous history of GDM
2. History of recurrent spontaneous abortions
3. History of unexplained intrauterine fetal death
4. Previous infant with major congenital anomalies (e.g., of the central nervous, cardiac, or skeletal systems)
5. Previous macrosomic infant (> 4000 gm)
6. History of recurrent preeclampsia
7. History of recurrent moniliasis
8. Family history of DM in first-degree relatives
9. History of polyuria, polydipsia, or glycosuria
10. Fasting plasma glucose of 105 mg/dl or 2-hr plasma protein > 120 mg/dl on two separate occasions
11. Maternal obesity (pregnancy weight > 150 lb or body mass index of > 27 kg/m^2)
12. Development of polyhydramnios and/or fetal macrosomia in present pregnancy
13. Excessive weight gain (> 40 lb) during pregnancy
14. Maternal age over 30 years

14. When can a 50-gm glucose load be administered?

Randomly (i.e., either fasting or in fed state).

15. Can a reflectance meter be used for screening after 50-gm glucose load?

No, because capillary values tend to be variable.

16. What is the rationale for recommending a particular threshold for screening?

The rationale is based on population studies, desired levels of sensitivity and specificity, and maintaining a favorable cost:benefit ratio. Using 130-mg/dl venous plasma levels by hexokinase method of glucose analysis, the sensitivity for diagnosis of GDM is probably 100%, whereas if a screening test threshold > 140 mg/dl is used, sensitivity is 79% and specificity is 87% for all pregnant patients.

17. What diagnostic test is recommended for GDM?

The recommended test varies among countries and institutions. At present, the 3-hour OGTT is the definitive diagnostic test for GDM.

18. What testing methodology is used for the 3-hour OGTT?

In the United States, the test is conducted with a 100-gm glucose load. To standardize testing conditions, an overnight fast should be conducted for at least 8 hours but not more than 14 hours. Adequate pretest loading with 150 gm/day of carbohydrate for 3 days before testing is necessary to avoid false-positive responses. The patient should rest for approximately 30 minutes before starting the test and not smoke for 12 hours before the test. During the test the woman should not smoke and should remain seated with minimal physical exertion. After the fasting sample is drawn, the patient drinks 100 gm of a glucose solution within 5 minutes. For consistency, the timing clock is started the moment the patient begins to drink. Subsequent blood samples are taken at 1, 2, and 3 hours. After the test, the patient may eat whole wheat bread and protein snacks to minimize rebound hypoglycemia.

19. What are the cut-off levels used for the diagnosis of GDM in a 3-hour OGTT?

The most widely used parameters in the United States for the diagnosis of GDM are those of O'Sullivan and Mahan, with modifications for plasma values by the National Diabetes Data Group in 1979. Stricter criteria have been proposed by Coustan and Carpenter.

Three-hour Oral Glucose Tolerance Test: Plasma Glucose Criteria for Diagnosis of GDM after 100-gm Glucose Load*

TIME	NATIONAL DIABETES DATA GROUP	CARPENTER AND COUSTAN
Fasting	≥ 105 mg/dl (5.8 mmol/L)	≥ 95 mg/dl (5.3 mmol/L)
1 hour	≥ 190 mg/dl (10.6 mmol/L)	≥ 180 mg/dl (10.0 mmol/L)
2 hour	≥ 165 mg/dl (9.2 mmol/L)	≥ 155 mg/dl (8.6 mmol/L)
3 hour	≥ 145 mg/dl (8.1 mmol/L)	≥ 140 mg/dl (7.7 mmol/L)

* Positive result for diagnosis of GDM requires two values to be equal to or greater than the cutoff value.

20. What factors regulate blood glucose levels?
- Stress: physical and emotional stress, infection, inflammation, hormonal imbalance of pregnancy, growth
- Time and type of insulin taken
- Diet: type and timing
- Exercise: type and duration

21. What are the dietary recommendations in GDM?

We prescribe 30–35 kcal/kg of ideal body weight per day, with no patients receiving < 1,800 or > 2,800 calories/day. There is some controversy regarding use of hypocaloric diets in markedly obese women because of the hypothetical risks to the fetus from ketonemia due to starvation.

22. What role does exercise play in the management of GDM?

Exercise plays an important role in the management of GDM. Glucose utilization is increased by large skeletal muscles, depending on the type of exercise. The effects may be immediate, as with aerobic exercises, or sustained for a few hours, as after swimming. The Third International Workshop Conference on GDM advocated exercise as a treatment modality in women who do not have a medical or obstetric contradiction. Upper body cardiovascular training has resulted in lower levels of glycemia than in women treated with diet only. The effects of exercise on glucose metabolism may become apparent after 4 weeks of training and involve both hepatic glucose output and glucose clearance. A cardiovascular conditioning program may obviate insulin treatment in some women with GDM.

23. What are the recommendations for timing and frequency of blood glucose monitoring?

The recommendations are controversial. Usually it is recommended that fasting, preprandial, and bedtime plasma glucose levels should be monitored with a reflectance meter at home. But there is evidence that monitoring of fasting and 1-hour plasma glucose level < 140 mg/dl decreases the risk of neonatal hypoglycemia, macrosomia, and cesarean delivery.

24. Describe the management of patients with one abnormal value on the 3-hour OGTT.

Management is controversial, and recommendations vary based on when the test value is obtained. If the test value is obtained before 28 weeks' gestation, the 3-hour OGTT should be repeated 4 weeks later and managed appropriately. If the test value is obtained after 34 weeks, management depends on the level and timing of hyperglycemia (i.e., fasting or postprandial). Our recommendation is to introduce visual home glucose monitoring and appropriate dietary strategies to maintain euglycemia with fasting values < 105 mg/dl and 2-hour postprandial values < 120 mg/dl. This approach should help to decrease the incidence of maternal hyperglycemia, but it is not a universally accepted management plan.

25. Why are oral hypoglycemic agents not used in pregnancy?

Oral hypoglycemic agents cross the placenta and can be teratogenic in the first trimester. In the second trimester they can increase fetal insulin production, leading to fetal growth abnormalities and severe neonatal hypoglycemia.

26. When is insulin recommended in the management of GDM?

The use of insulin in GDM is rather arbitrary. If euglycemia is not achieved with an appropriate diet within 1–2 weeks, use of subcutaneous human insulin is recommended. The type of insulin to be used is controversial. Some authorities recommend intermediate insulin such as NPH (human insulin isophane suspension) or Lente (insulin zinc suspension) forms in the evening or morning or both, whereas others recommend using a mixture of short-acting and intermediate-acting in both the evening and morning (mixture of regular with NPH or Lente). Either regimen is fine as long as euglycemia is achieved. Patients treated with insulin should be reminded about the importance of diet at the time of initiation of therapy, especially the consistency with which the diet is followed. Several studies show the benefits of prophylactic insulin therapy.

27. Describe the management of preterm labor in patients with GDM.

Intravenous magnesium sulfate is used most commonly because beta adrenergic agonists can cause maternal hyperglycemia. Steroid therapy to accelerate fetal lung maturity should be used with caution because it may double the insulin requirement.

28. Are women receiving terbutaline for preterm labor at higher risk for developing GDM?

Yes. Studies indicate that dose-independent, terbutaline-induced glucose intolerance is mediated by glucagon and caused by diminished insulin sensitivity. Body mass index directly correlated with postchallenge measures of insulin, insulin:glucose ratio, and pancreatic polypeptide, but not with other parameters.

29. When and how often should antepartum fetal surveillance be done in women with GDM?

Weekly biophysical assessment should begin between 38–40 weeks' gestation. But if GDM is complicated with fetal macrosomia, polyhydramnios, pregnancy-induced hypertension, or insulin requirement, antepartum surveillance should begin at 32 weeks' gestation.

30. When and how should a patient with GDM be delivered?

Delivery is recommended at no later than 40 weeks' gestation in patients requiring insulin therapy and at 42 weeks for diet-controlled patients. No elective delivery should be performed without establishing lung maturity because of the possibility that even mild GDM can delay lung maturity. GDM is not an absolute indication for cesarean section but its complications may be. For example, if estimated fetal weight exceeds 4,500 gm, elective cesarean section is a viable option to avoid dystocia. At lower estimated weights, previous obstetric history and clinical pelvimetry are useful tools in obstetric management.

31. Describe the management of labor in patients with GDM.

Attempts should be made to avoid maternal hyperglycemia during labor, because acute fetal hyperglycemia and hyperinsulinemia may be associated with neonatal hypoglycemia. Maternal glucose levels should be checked every 1–2 hours during labor, and a constant insulin infusion may be started if values exceed 100–120 mg/dl.

32. How should a woman with GDM be followed after delivery?

Between 5–20% of women with GDM continue to have diabetes or impaired glucose tolerance after they have delivered; presumably the same problem existed before pregnancy. Thus we suggest a 75-gm, 2-hour OGTT 6 weeks after delivery.

33. What percentage of women with GDM become diabetic later in life?

The incidence is variable based on the course of GDM and whether intervention such as weight loss was introduced. O'Sullivan has found that 40% of women diagnosed with GDM in an index pregnancy are diagnosed as diabetic within 20 years.

34. Once a woman has GDM, what specific risk factors increase her risk for GDM in subsequent pregnancies?

In general, patients with GDM have recurrence risks of 60–70%. But recurrence risk based on prepregnant body mass index and fasting plasma glucose level (from pregnant OGTT) plus time since the index pregnancy can predict the likelihood of subsequent glucose tolerance test abnormality.

$$\text{Estimated risk} = 1 / (1 + e - (-10.37 + 0.04 \text{ [fasting plasma glucose]}) + 0.08$$
(body mass index) + 0.03 (months since delivery).

35. What types of contraception are recommended for a patient with GDM?

No contraindications to the usual choices.

36. What are the rules of 15?

15% of the obstetric population have abnormal glucose load test (GLT); 15% of patients with abnormal GLT have abnormal OGTT; 15% of patients with abnormal OGTT require insulin; 15% of all patients with GDM have infants > 4000 gm; and after meals capillary levels are about 15% higher than plasma levels.

BIBLIOGRAPHY

1. American College of Obstetricians and Gynecologists: Diabetes and pregnancy. ACOG Tech Bull 3200, 1994.
2. American Diabetes Association: Position statement. Diabetes Care 12:588, 1989.

3. Coustan DR, Carpenter MW, O'Sullivan PS, Carr SR: Gestational diabetes: Precursors of subsequent disordered glucose metabolism. Am J Obstet Gyecol 168:1139–1144; discussion, 1144–1145, 1993.
4. Coustan DR, Nelson C, Carpenter MW, et al: Maternal age and screening for gestational diabetes: A population-based study. Obstet Gynecol 73:557, 1989.
5. Dickinson JE, Palmer SM: Gestational diabetes: Pathophysiology and diagnosis. Semin Perinatol 14:211, 1990.
6. Durak EP, Jovanovic-Peterson L, Peterson CM: Comparative evaluation of uterine response to exercise on five aerobic machines. Am J Obstet Gynecol 162:754–756, 1990.
7. Foley MR, Landon MB, Gabbe SG, et al: Effect of prolonged oral terbutaline therapy on glucose tolerance in pregnancy. Am J Obstet Gynecol 168(Pt 1):100–105, 1993.
8. Harlass FE, McClure GB, Read JA, Brady K: Use of a standard preparatory diet for the oral glucose tolerance test: Is it necessary? J Reprod Med 36:147–150, 1991.
9. Jovanovic-Peterson L, Durak EP: Randomized trial of diet versus diet plus cardiovascular conditioning on glucose levels in gestational diabetes. Am J Obstet Gynecol 161:415–419, 1989.
10. Jovanovic-Peterson L, Peterson CM: Gestational diabetic women? Diabetes 40(Suppl 2):179–181, 1991.
11. Second International Workshop Conference on Gestational Diabetes: Summary and recommendations. Diabetes 34(Suppl 2):123, 1986.

46. INSULIN-DEPENDENT DIABETES

Michael F. Greene, M.D.

1. What changes in energy metabolism occur during the first trimester?

The hormonal milieu of the first trimester is dominated by estrogen and progesterone production by the corpus luteum and early placenta. Maternal serum amino acid levels go down, including the level of alanine, which is the amino acid chiefly used for gluconeogenesis. Hepatic glucose production decreases, whereas tissue glycogen storage and peripheral glucose utilization increase. These changes combine to decrease maternal fasting plasma glucose levels.

2. What are the practical implications of the first-trimester physiologic changes for women with insulin-treated diabetes mellitus?

Some degree of anorexia, nausea, and vomiting is quite common, if not universal, in the first trimester. Nondiabetic women respond to the resulting decrease in metabolic fuel intake by decreasing insulin production. Diabetic women taking a fixed amount of insulin daily are at increased risk for hypoglycemia. Insulin reactions are common in early pregnancy, and many diabetic women first recognize that they are pregnant when reactions begin to occur for no obvious reason—most commonly, in the morning. The appropriate response is to decrease the patient's insulin dose. Dietary manipulations, such as eating small meals frequently (every 2–3 hours), avoiding caffeineated beverages and fatty and spicy foods, and drinking fluids between meals rather than with meals, may also be helpful.

3. How does energy metabolism change as pregnancy advances?

Estrogen and progesterone production continue to rise throughout pregnancy, but during the second trimester prolactin and human placental lactogen (hPL) (also known as human chorionic somatomammotropin [hCS]) of placental origin begin to appear in the maternal circulation. Both free and total cortisol levels also begin to rise during the second trimester. These hormones antagonize the actions of insulin, producing insulin resistance. Compared with the nonpregnant state, fasting glucose levels remain somewhat lower during later pregnancy. Conversely, postprandial glucose levels are higher and require more insulin to bring them down.

Pregnant diabetic women in good metabolic control respond to hypoglycemia less well than nonpregnant women. The counterregulatory hormones, glucagon and epinephrine, do not begin to rise until maternal glucose levels have fallen lower; they rise less quickly and to lower peaks than in nonpregnant women. These changes combine to produce wider excursions in blood glucose throughout the day with higher highs and lower lows.

7. Are there any prophylactic measures that can prevent malformations among infants of diabetic mothers?

The only measure known to be effective in preventing malformations is good metabolic control during organogenesis. The vast majority of major malformations arise between 2 weeks of fertilization age and 7 weeks (9 weeks from last menstrual period). Because many women do not recognize their pregnancies and first visit their obstetricians 8 or more weeks after their last menstrual periods, and because it may take several weeks of work to achieve good metabolic control, it is really necessary for diabetic women to plan their pregnancies and conceive in good metabolic control. Prophylactic dietary supplementation with folic acid has been shown to reduce the incidence of neural tube defects in the general population. Although folic acid dietary supplementation is prudent and appropriate for diabetic women, too, it has not been shown to protect effectively against neural tube defects specifically in this population.

8. Given their increased risk for occurrence of major malformations, what is an appropriate strategy for screening diabetic patients for malformations?

Maternal serum alpha-fetoprotein (MSAFP) screening should be offered to diabetic patients as to any other patients. MSAFP levels tend to be about 20% lower for women with insulin-treated diabetes mellitus than for nondiabetic women; thus, it is important for the laboratory to know the patient's history of diabetes to interpret correctly the results of the assay. Most physicians who care for diabetic patients recommend an ultrasound examination, including careful study of cardiac anatomy, at approximately 18 weeks' gestation to screen for major malformations. The success rate for diagnosing major malformations varies considerably among laboratories from 17% to virtually 100%. The response to an elevated MSAFP and the decision to perform an amniocentesis depend on both the degree of elevation and the confidence of the sonographer in ruling out major malformations.

9. What is the White classification of diabetes during pregnancy? How is it used?

Nearly 50 years ago Dr. Priscilla White proposed a classification system for women with diabetes prior to pregnancy based on factors that could be identified at the first prenatal visit. It was hoped that this classification could be used both to prognosticate how women would do during pregnancy and to provide guidance for treatment according to the degree of severity of the disease. Although treatment of patients in the various classes without nephropathy is not significantly different, the risks of hypertension and prematurity do vary by class. Most centers continue to use this classification for statistical purposes and to compare their outcomes with other centers.

White Classification

Class A	Diet controlled
Class B	Onset at age 20 or older and duration < 10 years
Class C	Onset at age 10–19 years and/or duration of 10–19 years
Class D	Onset before age 10 years or duration > 19 years
Class R	Proliferative retinopathy
Class F	Diabetic nephropathy
Class RF	Retinopathy and nephropathy
Class H	Clinically manifest coronary artery disease
Class T*	With renal transplant
Gestational diabetes*	Onset or first recognition during pregnancy

* Classes added later by others.

10. Should patients be switched to continuous subcutaneous insulin infusion (CSII) pumps to obtain optimal metabolic control during pregnancy?

The single most important intervention to optimize metabolic control is undoubtedly home capillary blood glucose monitoring. Frequent self-monitoring of capillary blood glucose values with adjustments of diet, insulin, and exercise as necessary are the keys to good metabolic control. The types of insulin used (long-acting vs. intermediate-acting) and mode of delivery (standard injections vs. CSII pump) are less important. Although anecdotally some patients have a difficult time achieving adequate control with standard insulin therapy and succeed with CSII pumps, there are no demonstrable benefits to the routine use of pumps.

11. What are the goals of metabolic therapy in pregnancy?

The risks for spontaneous abortion and major malformation depend on the degree of control in the first trimester, whereas the risks for macrosomia and stillbirth are related to control in the second and third trimesters. To minimize the risks for major malformations and spontaneous abortions requires only fair-to-good control, whereas control must be nearly perfect to avoid macrosomia. The blood glucose goals should be fasting values < 105 mg/dl and 2-hour postprandial values < 130 mg/dl.

12. How should an insulin reaction be treated?

Ideally, treatment for an insulin reaction should restore a normal blood glucose level without resulting in hyperglycemia. If the reaction is mild to moderate and the patient is awake and alert enough to take something by mouth, any glucose-containing solution can be given. Four to six ounces of fruit juice or a soft drink should be adequate; more will cause hyperglycemia. If the patient is comatose or poorly arousable, a dose of glucagon can easily be administered by a friend or relative on the scene. All insulin-requiring diabetic patients should be given a prescription for glucagon to be filled and kept in the refrigerator for just such a possible circumstance.

13. What are the most important complications of late pregnancy among diabetic women?

Hypertension, prematurity, macrosomia, and late fetal demise occur with increased frequency among diabetic women compared with the general population. The incidence of pregnancy-induced hypertension has been reported to be 20–40% in series of diabetic women and as high as 60% among women with diabetic nephropathy. Prematurity is approximately twice as common among diabetic women and is due mostly to the development of hypertension. As many as 25% of infants of diabetic mothers are larger than 4,000 gm, and 60% may be larger than the 90th centile for gestational age. This results in a higher incidence of operative delivery and an increased risk for birth trauma. Late near-term fetal demise has become much less common in the past 20 years but is still a risk to be kept in mind and avoided.

14. What is the mechanism of late fetal demise? How can it be avoided?

Glycosylated hemoglobin carries less oxygen, molecule for molecule, than native hemoglobin. It also binds oxygen more avidly and releases it less readily in areas of low oxygen tension, such as the placental bed. Acute maternal hyperglycemia causes fetal hyperglycemia, which stimulates the fetal pancreas to secrete more insulin. Fetal hyperinsulinemia causes an increased demand for oxygen in fetal tissues, beyond the ability of the placenta to supply. Thus, both chronic and acute hyperglycemia contribute to a physiologic state that can result in a lethal degree of hypoxemia. The best prophylaxis is to keep the patient's diabetes in the best possible control at all times.

15. What fetal surveillance is indicated in late pregnancy?

The optimal scheme for routine antepartum surveillance of women with diabetes has not been established in a scientifically rigorous fashion. Nonetheless, most practitioners begin routine surveillance on a weekly basis at 32 weeks' gestation, using nonstress testing. At 36 weeks, the frequency is usually increased to twice weekly. Nonreactive nonstress tests can be followed with either oxytocin challenge tests or biophysical profiles for reassurance of fetal well-being.

16. How should delivery be timed?

The decision about the timing of delivery should take into consideration the risk for respiratory distress syndrome (RDS), favorability of the cervix for labor, the size of the fetus, and ongoing exposure to the risk of stillbirth. RDS is more common among infants of diabetic mothers at relatively late gestational ages than among other infants. Generally, lung maturity studies should be obtained for any fetus to be delivered electively before 39 completed weeks of gestation. After 39 weeks, the risk is so small that it can be ignored. Patients with poorly controlled diabetes and macrosomic fetuses are at greater risk for stillbirth and, generally, should be delivered somewhat earlier (37–38 weeks) if lung maturity can be assured. Patients with well-controlled diabetes and normal-size fetuses are at lower risk for stillbirth and may be allowed to wait later into their pregnancies for cervical maturity. Most obstetricians in the U.S. do not like to allow diabetic patients to go beyond 40 weeks under any circumstances.

17. How should the route of delivery be determined?

Macrosomic infants of diabetic mothers are at greater risk for shoulder dystocia during pelvic delivery than either nonmacrosomic infants or similar-weight infants of nondiabetic women. Most shoulder dystocias do not result in birth injury, and most birth injuries do not result in permanent disability. Nonetheless, the risk for traumatic birth injury is intimidating. It is difficult to predict accurately which fetuses are macrosomic or which are likely to suffer significant birth injury. Despite this imprecision, most obstetricians give serious consideration to cesarean delivery for any infant of a diabetic mother estimated to be larger than 4,500 gm. Fetuses less than 4,000 gm deserve a trial of labor. Fetuses estimated to weigh 4,000–4,500 gm may be delivered either way at the discretion of the physician and patient. Diabetes per se is not an indication for cesarean section.

18. How should the metabolic control of diabetes be managed during labor?

During labor, insulin requirements are generally relatively low because of reduced caloric intake and probably the work of labor. A patient scheduled for induction should receive a modest dose of intermediate-acting insulin (one-half to one-third of her usual morning dose) before beginning the induction. During labor she should receive a glucose-containing solution (D_5 in a solution of one-half normal saline) at approximately 125 ml/hr, strictly controlled on an infusion pump. Capillary blood glucose values should be monitored hourly. If the blood glucose rises above 120 mg/dl, the patient should receive a continuous intravenous infusion of regular insulin at a rate sufficient to bring the blood glucose down to 80–120 mg/dl.

BIBLIOGRAPHY

1. Brown FM, Hare JW. Diabetes complicating pregnancy. The Joslin Clinic Method, 2nd ed. New York, Wiley-Liss, 1995.
2. Combs CA, Gunderson E, Kitzmiller JL, et al: Relationship of fetal macrosomia to maternal postprandial glucose control during pregnancy. Diabetes Care 15:1251–1257, 1992.
3. Greene MF, Benacerraf BR: Prenatal diagnosis in diabetic gravidas: Utility of ultrasound and maternal serum alpha-fetoprotein screening. Obstet Gynecol 77:520–524, 1991.
4. Greene MF, Hare JW, Krache M, et al: Prematurity among insulin-requiring diabetic gravid women. Am J Obstet Gynecol 161:106–111, 1989.
5. Kitzmiller JL, Buchanan TA, Kjos S, et al: Pre-conception care of diabetes, congenital malformations, and spontaneous abortions. Diabetes Care 19:514–541, 1996.
6. Kitzmiller JL, Younger D, Hare JW, et al: Continuous subcutaneous insulin therapy during early pregnancy. Obstet Gynecol 66:606–611, 1985.
7. McFarland LV, Raskin M, Daling JR, Benedetti TJ: Erb/Duchenne's palsy: A consequence of fetal macrosomia and method of delivery. Obstet Gynecol 68:784–788, 1986.

47. HYPEREMESIS GRAVIDARUM

Miriam Erick, M.S., R.D., C.D.E.

1. How is hyperemesis gravidarum distinguished from ordinary nausea and vomiting of pregnancy?

The true definition of hyperemesis gravidarum (HG), once called pernicious vomiting, is based on the International Classification of Diseases (ICD)-9 parameters formulated by the American Council of Chemistry and Pharmacy in 1956. Clinical symptoms include intractable vomiting and disturbed nutrition, ketosis, weight loss > 5%, acetonuria with ultimate neurologic disturbance, liver damage, retinal hemorrhage, and renal damage. Many, but not all, cases with these characteristics present for hospitalization. Various researchers note that nausea and vomiting, without the criteria of HG, affect 50–90% of all pregnant women. As women are seen in outpatient offices for the treatment of severe nausea and vomiting of pregnancy (NVP), these data are currently not reported. Therefore, the incidence of NVP—an outpatient definition—is an estimate.

2. How often does HG occur?

Based on ICD-9 statistics, approximately 50,000–55,000 women annually in the United States are admitted to hospitals for medical management of dehydration and semistarvation related to severe NVP. As the annual birth rate fluctuates between 3.2–3.9 million infants, approximately 1.3–1.5% of pregnant women (1 in 77) are admitted with HG. In addition, an unclear number in fact may be as disabled but for various reasons remain out of the hospital.

In addition, it is difficult to collect data about the incidence and severity of NVP from different cultures. The incidence of HG in Kuala Lumpur is 2.3%, whereas in the Mori tribes of New Zealand, the incidence is 2.6%. These figures are higher than previously suggested in less industrialized countries. The overall incidence of NVP in South Africa shows a disparity between ethnic groups: 56–57% of black women compared with 64–68% of Indian and white women.

3. Is the etiology understood?

No, although alterations in hormones are more likely than the psychogenic theories popular in the past. A significant number of hormones are necessary to support pregnancy; five are suspected to be involved in NVP.

1. Human chorionic gonadotropin (hCG)—implicated because its rise parallels the onset of NVP.

2. Progesterone—because of its role in relaxing smooth muscles, including the stomach and GI tract, with delayed peristalsis

3. Prostaglandins—released from decidual cells and macrophages of the decidua basalis; may suppress maternal levels of progesterone and cortisol, influencing the pattern of NVP. Supporting data have not yet demonstrated this relationship.

4. Estrogen—with its many derivatives, cited as mildly toxic in and of itself, with a noted side effect of nausea and vomiting. Estrogen has been found to enhance olfaction and in the past has been implicated in increasing nausea. Interest in this relationship has been renewed.

5. Cortisol—whether increases are solely attributable to HG versus stress, lack of sleep, and/or starvation has not yet been determined.

4. How long during pregnancy does NVP usually last?

Although NVP has been presented typically as a first trimester problem, the majority of cases do not attenuate until 17.3 weeks. At 35 weeks, 5% of the population still experiences vomiting and still reports nausea. Data from Australia suggest that 20% of women are sick to term. Because women with NVP are notably anxious about outcome and desperate for relief, they should be directed to available resources that may provide some degree of self-help to control contributing aggravators, such as smells, motion, noise, and fatigue.

5. Does HG have an adverse effect on fetal outcome?

In general, no. In older literature, various complications were ascribed to NVP. However, agents used for management were impressively severe and bizarre, and it is difficult to sort out causal associations. Among the various drugs, vitamins, and minerals used were injections of the husband's blood, intravenous honey, and conductive therapy.

The potential adverse effects of weight loss, electrolyte imbalances and fluid abnormalities versus side effects from treatment are, of course, difficult to separate. In a study of two groups of women with HG, more small-for-gestational-age infants were found in the group with more severe NVP. However, this group also had more reputed incidents of hypokalemia and a lower weight gain. In another study designed to evaluate fetal outcome, investigators examined male and female infants whose mothers had HG. The infants were born between weeks 39 and 42 with the females an average of 97 gm heavier and the males 61 gm heavier than controls. However, the morphologic maturity score was decreased in the HG group.

6. Is there an increase in malformations among infants of mothers with HG?

Currently the answer is no. Regarding medication, however, it is important to keep in mind that none of the drugs currently used has been studied in large random trials in this specific population. It is prudent to remember the unfortunate side effects of one prior medication used in NVP. Thalidomide, a glutamic acid derivative, resulted in a syndrome known as phocomelia or shortened limb syndrome. Reports from early research suggested that the drug irritated nerves in adult rabbits and could stunt growth and produce deformities in fetal rabbits. This research prompted pharmacologist Frances Kelsey to stall the process of the drug's entry into the United States. Thalidomide, a highly effective narcoleptic agent with none of the usual residue of sleeping medications, was used more extensively in Europe and England than in the United States. The teratogenic window for thalidomide was proven to be between 45 and 55 days' gestation, with a single dose capable of producing abnormality.

Bendectin, another drug widely used for NVP, was implicated as a teratogen and litogen in over 1800 lawsuits. Bendectin, a formulation of doxylamine (an antihistamine) and pyridoxine hydrochloride (vitamin B6), was withdrawn from the U.S. market in 1988. Scientific evaluation of Bendectin as a teratogen has been lacking. Of note, at the time of the Bendectin defense, the vice president of ACOG protested Merrill-Dow's decision to remove the drug from the market, stating that severe cases of NVP lead to serious maternal nutritional deficiencies, whereas the causality of the medication for the birth defects was not clear. At this time a drug similar to Bendectin, Diclectin, is being marketed and used in Canada for NVP.

7. What are some suggestions for ensuring adequate nutritional intake during early pregnancy compromised by NVP or HG?

Women with NVP are often unable to eat or drink adequately or to ingest prenatal vitamins. A simple and practical solution is to prescribe one children's chewable vitamins with extra folate, alternating with iron and vitamin C fortification. Care should be taken not to increase vitamin A intake inadvertently. It is highly recommended that women with NVP seek nutritional counseling from a perinatal nutritionist or registered dietitian. Counseling can provide assessment of current intake, computerized dietary analysis, and recommendations for supplementation. Adequate folate intake early in gestation may well reduce the incidence of neural tube defects and some unorthodox foods (i.e., potato chips) provide more of this nutrient than other regularly suggested foods, such as crackers.

8. What does HG involve other than nausea, vomiting, and electrolyte imbalance?

Hyperolfaction or enhanced olfaction seems to to be a major complaint and a negative trigger for the majority of chronic cases. The heightened sense of smell is probably driven by increased estrogen production. Background triggers are common and include brewed coffee, perfume, cologne, tobacco smoke, household garbage, diesel/car fumes, diapers of infants and elders, breath and body odor, and various emanations from work and, in some cases, hospital environments. Hospitalized women in private rooms appear to recover faster if isolated from noisy roommates and family members, unwanted food smells, smoke, alcohol odors, perfume, cologne, and cleaning agents.

Bad mouth taste is another annoyance that may reflect a higher concentration of salivary potassium, as seen in conditions of scant or copious saliva. Magnesium is also lost in excessive saliva. Alterations in saliva production are common and may be due to a progestational surge, dehydration, or concurrent increase in nausea. Increases in saliva are not confined to particular ethnic groups, although disposal of saliva may be different because of social mores and life-time economic conditioning.

Shivering is common, again explained by lack of food, inadequate hydration, or loss of weight. The general response of shivering is often an increase in thermostat setting, which paradoxically facilitates insensible fluid losses from the body. Constipation is common, again due to the general traditional dietary suggestions of bland foods, which are often low in water and fiber content. A "thick tongue" has been reported as a consequence of dehydration; this in itself can make eating dry foods difficult.

Women with NVP often have **difficulty with reading** because the eyeball shape reportedly is altered with dehydration. Wearers of contact lenses often suspend use during this time. Flickering of the television and small busy patterns also may increase nauseous symptoms, probably in relation to the "flickering syndrome." In addition, headaches are common and explained by lack of food, dehydration, or adverse effect of antiemetic therapy.

Delayed gastric emptying has been suspected as a result of progesterone production, although electrolyte depletion, such as hypokalemia and hypomagnesia, also may produce similar effects.

9. Is HG associated with an increased risk of maternal complications?

Some of the more dramatic reported complications are fortunately rare. Examples include spontaneous rupture of the esophagus, Wernicke's encephalopathy, Mallory-Weiss tears, central pontine myelosis, liver and kidney abnormalities, splenic avulsion, and conversion reactions. Anecdotally, ruptured blood vessels in the eyes have been observed as well as fractured ribs.

The largest single maternal complication appears to be altered cognition and emotional exhaustion due to chronic and acute disability. Whether impaired or altered cognition plays a role in elective pregnancy termination is not widely known but bears investigation. One study of women with NVP found that 2.9% of women terminated pregnancy as a result of the NVP.

A higher incidence of cholestasis has been noted during and after NVP. Plausible explanations for predisposing factors to gallstone formation are a high estrogen state and unusually long periods of time between food and fluid intake; constipation has been positively predictive of formation of gallstones and low fat intakes.

10. What are the diagnostic considerations for intractable NVP?

One must always consider more life-threatening conditions such as appendicitis, pancreatitis, cholelithiosis, thyrotoxicosis, hepatitis, brain tumors, intestinal obstructions, gastroenteritis, trophoblastic disease, and Crohn's disease. It is essential to establish an intrauterine pregnancy; 25–30% of women with gestational trophoblast disease present with hyperemesis. Additional laboratory evaluation includes electrolytes, blood urea nitrogen (BUN), creatinine, urinalysis, and complete blood count (CBC). Liver and thyroid function tests should be considered. The cause of any weight changes should be investigated; a loss of 5% over 3 months puts the woman at nutritional risk. The usual parameters used to assess protein-calorie malnutrition in nonpregnant patients are not useful in pregnant women. Total lymphocyte count (TLC) is based on white blood cell count and percent lymphocytes, both of which are altered in pregnancy. Although hypoalbuminemia is usually a good marker for malnutrition, in pregnancy, albumin is generally lower overall.

11. What is treatment?

The immediate treatment is hydration. Lactated Ringer's solution should be used with caution, because persons with undiagnosed anxiety disorders may be affected adversely, with an increase in overall uneasiness, palpitations, and tachycardia. Fluids should always contain a multivitamin preparation with thiamin because of the potential of Wernicke's encephalopathy. In one study, an oral supplement with a combination of 19 vitamins and minerals was shown to reduce the overall incidence of NVP. Although the debate continues about the efficacy of vitamin B6 in 25-mg doses, no overt pyroxidine deficiency has been found.

For hospitalized patients, a private room devoid of aromas and odors is an essential part of therapy, along with immediate hydration. If the patient desires to eat, she should be allowed to eat at will, and her immediate requests should be honored. Food requests may appear unconventional. However, most persons who are ill will not knowingly ingest foods or fluids that aggravate the situation.

12. Does psychotherapy play a role?

Psychotherapy has been suggested based on the supposition that "the woman who vomits in pregnancy is manifesting a subconscious desire to abort her fetus orally." Ambivalence is presumed. However, a more successful approach may be to consider how a sleep-deprived woman with acute or chronic disease would be expected to behave. The woman with chronic and unrelenting NVP is at risk for pregnancy termination as a means to end this poorly understood disability. Psychological counselors and other health care providers need to be aware of the adverse effect of cologne or perfume and breath, body, or incidental odors (coffee cups).

Although historically women with HG have been given derogatory labels such as "pukers," few women obtain secondary gain from nausea and vomiting. Financial and social sacrifices are significant among hyperemetic women. In a reader survey in 1994, 12% of the 307 responders lost over 15 days of work and one nonworking mother on total parenteral nutrition (TPN) at home from weeks 8–18 amassed medical bills over $25,000.

13. What other measures have been tried for relief of symptoms?

Various other agents include seabands, accupressure, hypnosis, ginger, chamomile and raspberry tea. Although several reports discuss reduction of NVP with seabands, data on the optimal torr pressure is lacking. Most bands are "one size fits all" and it is conceivable that a larger woman receives more pressure, whereas a thinner woman receives less. The optimal torr, or pounds per square inch (PSI) is not known. Powdered ginger has been reported successful in some studies at reducing NVP. To date no studies have evaluated the potential fetal side effects of concentrated powdered ginger root. Ginger root contains a potent thromboxane synthetase inhibitor which binds to testosterone binding receptors. Whether fetal development may be altered by administration of concentrated powdered ginger root has not been determined.

14. Which medications are safe to use?

No medications have been approved expressly for the treatment of NVP. In Canada, Diclectin, a reformulation of Bendectin, is used in hospitals. One should keep in mind drug-nutrient interactions. Antacids, for example, have been reported to reduce thiamin status. Compazine and Phenergan affect riboflavin status. The overlap among adverse reactions to antiemetics, sleep deprivation, and symptoms of Wernicke's encephalopathy have not been adequately studied. Symptoms in common include disorientation, nausea, nervousness, vertigo, irritability, lassitude, nystagmus, and tardive dyskinesia.

15. Are tube feedings employed?

There are several reports in the nutrition literature of nasogastric enteral tube feedings for HG. The lack of wholesale popularity and patient acceptance can be explained by the lack of antianxiety medication as well as the excessive gag reflex that most patients appear to have. Hyperolfaction to the smell of formula and tubing has been reported. Although their use is infrequent, in some instances jejunostomy tube feedings have been used in the first as well as second trimester. First trimester use carries with it less risk than insertion in mid trimester, which may precipitate premature contractions.

16. Is there a role for total parenteral nutrition?

Yes, when all conventional measures have failed and protein calorie malnutrition is evident. When TPN is used, the patient should not be overfed to make up for weight deficit because metabolic consequences are highly likely to present. Before TPN via a central line is considered, a trial of D10 with multivitamin preparation and extra folate should be allowed along with an at-will diet. It is not uncommon for some women who are rehydrated to be able to increase solid foot intake before adequate fluid intake. The lipid component of TPN may increase the background bad mouth taste by imparting a fishy or metallic taste that has been reported to increase complaints of nausea.

BIBLIOGRAPHY

1. de la Ronde SK: Nausea and vomiting in pregnancy. JSGC 1994:2035–2041, 1994.
2. Depue R, Bernstein L, et al: Hyperemesis gravidarum in relation to estradiol levels, pregnancy outcome, and other maternal factors: A seroepidemiologic study. Am J Obstet Gynecol 156:1137–1141, 1987.
3. Erick M: No More Morning Sickness: A Survival Guide for Pregnant Women. New York, NAL/Plume, 1993.
4. Gadsby R, Barnie-Adshead AM, Jagger C: A prospective study of nausea and vomiting during pregnancy. Br J Gen Pract 43:245–248, 1993.
5. Gross S, et al: Maternal weight loss associated with hyperemesis gravidarum: A predictor of fetal outcome. Am J Obstet Gynecol 160:906–909, 1989.
6. MacBurney M, Wilmore DW: Parenteral nutrition in pregnancy. In Rombeau J, Caldwell M (eds): Clinical Nutrition, Vol. II: Parenteral Nutrition, 2nd ed. Philadelphia, W.B. Saunders, 1993, pp 615–633.
7. Ornstein M: Bendectin/Diclectin for morning sickness: A Canadian follow-up of an American tragedy. Reprod Tox 9:1–6, 1995.

48. SEIZURES IN PREGNANCY

Jeffrey Pickard, M.D.

1. How does pregnancy affect the frequency of seizures?

Unclear. Probably < 20% of women have an increase in seizures during pregnancy. Of the remainder, most have no change in seizure pattern. Higher rates of worsening in older studies may have been due to such factors as poor seizure control before conception, little or no prepregnancy counseling, poor compliance, and lower serum levels of anticonvulsants during pregnancy. Seizure activity during one pregnancy does not predict what will happen in future pregnancies.

2. What is gestational epilepsy?

In a small number of women, seizures occur only during pregnancy. The presence of gestational epilepsy in one pregnancy is not predictive of recurrence in future pregnancies.

3. Does status epilepticus occur more frequently during pregnancy?
No.

4. How does pregnancy affect blood levels of anticonvulsants?
Subtherapeutic medication levels can occur as a result of the increased maternal plasma volume, delayed gastrointestinal absorption, and the increased hepatic clearance associated with pregnancy. Anticonvulsant levels should be monitored monthly.

5. Are obstetric complications more common in women with seizures?
Controversial. Several studies have suggested minor increased risks for a multitude of obstetric complications. However, no one specific entity has been observed to be consistently increased. One exception may be vaginal bleeding, probably secondary to anticonvulsant therapy-induced vitamin K deficiency.

6. Is breastfeeding contraindicated for women taking anticonvulsants?
No. Anticonvulsants are excreted minimally in breast milk and generally do not harm the infant. However, accumulation of phenobarbital (and primidone, which is metabolized to phenobarbital) can cause lethargy, poor feeding, and inadequate weight gain. If this occurs, bottle feeding may need to be substituted. Breastfeeding does not increase the frequency of seizures.

7. Are infants of mothers with epilepsy at increased risk for congenital malformations?
Yes. The risk of congenital anomalies is 2–3 times greater than for the general population. Antiseizure medications with monotherapy present the lowest risks. The possibility of an increased rate of congenital malformations in epileptic women not on seizure medication continues to be explored.

8. Is there any risk of congenital anomalies in children of epileptic fathers?
Yes. Several studies have shown an increased relative risk (1.7–3.0) for congenital malformations among children of epileptic fathers.

9. What is the risk of epilepsy in the child if a parent has seizures?
In general, the child has a 3% risk of epilepsy. The risk may be higher if the parental seizure etiology is unknown, the mother is the affected parent, or the child has febrile seizures.

10. Which anticonvulsants are safe during pregnancy?
Anticonvulsants in general should not be considered "safe" during pregnancy. Nevertheless, uncontrolled seizures are dangerous for both the woman and the fetus, supporting their judicious use when needed.

11. Should a woman with seizures stop her medications when she becomes pregnant?
Controversial. Stopping anticonvulsant therapy during the first trimester can result in uncontrolled seizures which may be more harmful to the fetus. Some suggest a trial off anticonvulsants prior to pregnancy if the woman has been seizure-free for at least 2 years. Once successfully withdrawn from her medication, a woman may be followed expectantly during her pregnancy.

12. Are any anticonvulsants absolutely contraindicated during pregnancy?
Most physicians would avoid trimethadione and valproic acid. "Trimethadione syndrome" consists of developmental delay, low-set ears, palate anomalies, irregular teeth, speech disturbances, and V-shaped eyebrows. IUGR, short stature, cardiac anomalies, ocular defects, simian creases, hypospadias, and microcephaly are also often present.

Valproic acid is teratogenic in animals, although data in humans are not as clear. It has been implicated in cardiac, orofacial, and limb abnormalities, but the major concern is with neural tube defects. Women exposed during pregnancy should be closely screened with ultrasound and amniotic fluid alpha-fetoprotein.

13. Which anticonvulsants are commonly used during pregnancy?

Anticonvulsant Drugs Used for Epilepsy in Pregnancy

DRUG	DOSAGE	SIDE EFFECTS	TOXICITY	TYPES OF SEIZURES*		
				Tonic-Clonic	Absence	Complex Partial
Phenytoin (Dilantin)	Average, 400 mg/day Range, 300–1200 mg/day Therapeutic level, 10–20 µg/ml	Ataxia, drowsiness, gum hyperplasia, hypertrichosis, nystagmus	Rash, serum sickness, pseudolymphoma, Stevens-Johnson syndrome, lupus erythematosus, macrocytic anemia, rare hepatic or marrow toxicity, cerebellar degeneration, peripheral neuropathy	+	–	+
Phenobarbital	Average, 120 mg/day Range, 30–210 mg/day Therapeutic level, 10–35 µg/ml	Drowsiness, ataxia nystagmus	Rare: rash, possibly teratogenic	+	–	+
Primidone (Mysoline)	Average, 1000 mg/day Range, 500–2000 mg/day Therapeutic level, 4–12 µg/ml	Drowsiness, nausea, ataxia, nystagmus (tachyphylaxis usual)	Rash, adenopathy, lupus erythematosus, macrocytic anemia, arthritis, edema	+	–	+
Carbamazepine (Tegretol)	Average, 600 mg/day Range, 200–1200 mg/day Therapeutic level, 4–8 µg/ml	Drowsiness, dizziness, blurred vision, ataxia, gastrointestinal disturbance	Blood dyscrasia (rare)	+	–	+
Ethosuximide (Zarontin)	Average, 1000 mg/day Range, 500–2000 mg/day Therapeutic level, 40–100 µg/ml	Nausea, abdominal pain, drowsiness, personality change, headache	Rash, nephropathy, marrow depression	–	+	–
Clonazepam (Klonopin)	Average, 3 mg/day Range, 1.5–20 mg/day Therapeutic level, 0.01–0.07 µg/ml	Drowsiness, dizziness, ataxia	Coma	+	+	+

From Dalessio DJ: Current concepts: Seizure disorders and pregnancy. N Engl J Med 312:561, 1985, with permission.
* A plus sign denotes that the drug is useful in the indicated form of seizure, and a minus sign that it is not.

14. What neonatal complications have been associated with phenytoin? Phenobarbital? Carbamazepine?

The **fetal hydantoin syndrome** (craniofacial malformations, distal phalangeal hypoplasia, growth retardation, and mental deficiency) is probably a misnomer because these effects do not appear to be drug-specific. Both phenytoin and phenobarbital may produce hemorrhagic disease of the newborn. Phenobarbital may cause neonatal addiction and withdrawal syndrome. Carbamazepine used to be considered among the safest anticonvulsants for use during pregnancy. However, more recent data suggest that carbamazepine may be associated with an increased incidence of neural tube defects as well as other anomalies.

15. What role does epoxide hydrolase play in the development of congenital malformations?

Epoxide hydrolase is an enzyme within a metabolic pathway common to many anticonvulsant medications. Genetic heterogeneity within this enzyme can affect its overall efficacy. Homozygosity in the fetus for the genes producing lowered efficacy of this enzyme has been shown to be associated with the highest rate of development of the features of congenital phenytoin syndrome.

16. What other metabolic abnormalities associated with anticonvulsant therapy should be corrected during pregnancy?

Women should receive supplemental folic acid, especially with phenytoin use, throughout the pregnancy.

BIBLIOGRAPHY

1. Brodie MJ: Management of epilepsy during pregnancy and lactation. Lancet 336:426–427, 1990.
2. Buehler BA, Delimont D, Van Waes M, Finnel RH: Prenatal prediction of the fetal hydantoin syndrome. N Engl J Med 332:1567–1572, 1990.
3. Cantrell DC, Cunningham FG: Epilepsy complicating pregnancy. In Cunningham FG, MacDonald, Gant, et al (eds): Williams' Obstetrics, 19th ed. Norwalk, CT, Appleton-Lange, 1994.
4. Rosa F: Spina Bifida in infants of women treated with carbamazepine during pregnancy. N Engl J Med 324:674–677, 1991.
5. Shuster EA: Seizures in pregnancy. Emerg Med Clin North Am 12:1013–1025, 1994.

49. THYROID DISEASE IN PREGNANCY

Jolene Johnson, M.D.

1. How do thyroid function tests change during a normal pregnancy?

Test	Changes
Thyroid-stimulating hormone (TSH)	None*
Total thyroxine (T_4)	Increases
Tri-iodothyronine (T_3)	Increases
T3 total resin uptake (T_3RU)	Decreases
Free T_4	None*

* In early pregnancy, when levels of human chorionic gonadotropin are at their peak, free T_4 increases and TSH decreases.

2. What causes the increases in T4 and T3 seen during normal pregnancies?

These increased values reflect estrogen-induced increases in thyroid-binding globulin. A similar increase is observed when oral contraceptives are used. Although increased globulin elevates total T3 and T4, the free thyroid levels remain unchanged.

3. How common is hyperthyroidism during pregnancy? What are the most frequent causes?

0.2% of pregnancies are complicated by maternal hyperthyroidism with the majority of diagnoses made before pregnancy. Common etiologies include Graves' disease (85%), gestational trophoblastic disease, and injudicious exogenous thyroid supplementation.

4. What is Graves' disease? How does it affect the fetus? The newborn infant? The mother?

Graves' disease results in maternal hyperthyroidism secondary to autoantibodies capable of stimulating thyroxine synthesis. Maternal symptoms include weight loss or poor weight gain, tachycardia, and heat intolerance. Laboratory studies reveal increased T4 and T3 levels, an increased free thyroid index, and a low TSH. Untreated maternal hyperthyroidism results in an increased risk of preeclampsia and congestive heart failure.

The thyroid-stimulating antibodies can cross the placenta readily to stimulate the fetal thyroid. Fetal complications include in utero demise, prematurity, intrauterine growth retardation, a widespread fetal autoimmune reaction with lymphatic hypertrophy and thrombocytopenia, fetal goiter, and fetal exophthalmos.

Affected newborns can be expected to have a transient course over 1–5 months as the maternal autoantibodies are slowly cleared from their systems.

5. Should diagnostic iodine studies by done to confirm the diagnosis of Graves' disease during pregnancy?

No. Such iodine studies are performed with radioactive tagging. Radioactive iodine crosses the placenta and is concentrated in the fetal thyroid after 10 weeks' gestation. Iatrogenic fetal hypothyroidism can result.

6. How is the pregnant woman with Graves' disease treated?

Prophylthiouracil (PTU) generally decreases both T4 and the symptoms by 4 weeks after initiating therapy. PTU is gradually decreased thereafter to maintain the mother's T4 at upper limits of normal and to prevent overtreatment and hypothyroidism. Some advocate continuing to decrease PTU and even discontinuing it during the third trimester. Some women experience temporary remission of disease possibly secondary to the relative immunosuppression of pregnancy. The inability of PTU to control hyperthyroidism may necessitate a subtotal thyroidectomy. Radioactive iodine therapy for gland ablation is contraindicated for the same reasons that diagnostic studies with radioactive iodine should not knowingly be undertaken.

7. What are the fetal effects of PTU therapy?

PTU crosses the placenta and iatrogenic fetal hypothyroidism can be produced, with the long-term effects not clearly established. There is some evidence for delayed bone age and central nervous system effects in exposed infants.

8. What other drugs are used in the treatment of Graves' disease?

Methimazole. This medication is generally not used during pregnancy because it has been associated with aplasia cutis and a higher incidence of fetal goiter, but may be used if once-daily dosing is needed. Beta blockers are not contraindicated for the treatment of hypermetabolic symptoms.

9. Can an infant develop neonatal Graves' disease even if the mother's hyperthyroidism is well controlled with PTU?

Yes. Neonatal Graves' disease results from the transplacental passage of thyroid-stimulating antibodies. These remain in the maternal circulation regardless of the treatment of the mother. Even mothers with hypothyroidism secondary to subtotal thyroidectomy or radiation therapy for Graves' disease are at risk for a fetus with thyrotoxicosis. Neonatal Graves' disease occurs in about 10% of women with Graves' disease regardless of their history of treatment. Treatment of the mother who has had a subtotal thyroidectomy and is on thyroid replacement therapy may be necessary and require PTU for the sole purpose of treating fetal hyperthyroidism caused by autoantibodies.

10. How does pregnancy affect Graves' disease?

Patients tend to have remissions during pregnancy and postpartum exacerbations. This is thought to be due to the relative immunosuppression of pregnancy.

11. Can women who are taking PTU breastfeed?

Yes, with some reservations. PTU is excreted in small quantities in breast milk and can theoretically suppress the infant's thyroid function. However, because the amount excreted is small, with monitoring of the newborn's thyroid function breastfeeding is generally permitted.

12. When does thyroid storm usually present?

Characterized by a hypermetabolic state, fever, and change in mental status, this life-threatening complication can occur during labor or cesarean section, or in conjunction with an antepartum or postpartum infection. Thyroid storm can also occur in patients with gestational trophoblastic disease. Most often it manifests itself in the woman with unrecognized hyperthyroidism.

13. How is thyroid storm managed?

Symptomatic and supportive treatment of the pyrexia, tachycardia, and severe dehydration is essential. Thionamides, PTU, beta-blocking agents, steroids, iodines, or ipodate (to block thyroid hormone release) are the mainstays of therapy.

14. What are the common causes of maternal hypothyroidism?

• Hashimoto's thyroiditis
• Previous treatment of Graves' disease by radioactive iodine or subtotal thyroidectomy
• Excessive doses of PTU for the treatment of Graves' symptomatology.

15. Which complications of pregnancy are associated with untreated hypothyroidism?

Marked hypothyroidism usually results in increased prolactin levels (secondary to increased TRH), anovulation, and infertility. In women with overt hypothyroidism who do become pregnant, there is a significantly higher incidence of anemia, preeclampsia, abruption, postpartum hemorrhage, and cardiac dysfunction. Likewise, fetal complications, including low birth weight and perinatal demise, are increased. Lesser degrees of untreated hypothyroidism may be associated with pregnancy loss and prolonged gestation. Women with subclinical disease (increased TSH but normal T4) and women who have adequate replacement therapy have better outcomes.

16. How should the hypothyroid mother be treated?

Treatment consists of 1.6 μg/kg of Synthroid, Levothroid, or Levoxyl, with variation on an individual basis. Assessment of TSH in the first trimester seems reasonable, because up to 45% of treated women with hypothyroidism require higher doses during pregnancy. Post partum, preconception doses are appropriate, with assessment of TSH 6–12 weeks after delivery.

17. Why should thyroid function be tested in women with hyperemesis gravidarum?

Hyperemesis gravidarum in the presence of a viable gestation has been associated with abnormal values on thyroid studies. The majority of these women have no other clinical signs of hyperthyroidism. In these situations, treatment is not advocated. In a small number of cases, hyperthyroidism exists clinically, and in these women treatment of thyrotoxicosis can help to alleviate hyperemesis gravidarum. Use of free T4 by equilibrium dialysis may help to clarify thyroid status.

18. What is postpartum thyroiditis?

Occurring 3–6 months postpartum, this condition may affect 5% of parturients. Initial hyperthyroidism is followed by hypothyroidism with thyroid antibodies often present. Spontaneous recovery occurs in 90%, but during the intervening period may be misdiagnosed as postpartum depression or psychosis. This disorder tends to recur with subsequent pregnancies.

BIBLIOGRAPHY

1. American College of Obstetricians and Gynecologists: Thyroid Disease in Pregnancy. ACOG Tech Bull 181, 1993.
2. Emerson CH: Thyrotoxicosis in pregnancy. Curr Therapy Endocrinol Metab 5:275–277, 1994.
3. Mestman JH, Goodwin TM, Montoro MM: Thyroid disorders in pregnancy. Endocr Clin North Am 24:41–71, 1995.
4. Roti E, Minelli R, Salvi M: Clinical review 80: Management of hyperthyroidism and hypothyroidism in the pregnant woman. J Clin Endocrinol Metab 81:1679–1682, 1996.

50. CARDIOVASCULAR DISEASE IN PREGNANCY

Heidi Tessler, M.D., and Mervyn L. Lifschitz, M.D.

1. What is responsible for anemia in a normal pregnancy?
It is actually a *relative* anemia. There is a 20–40% increase in the number of erythrocytes but a 50% increase in plasma volume, and thus a change in the red cell/plasma volume ratio.

2. Cardiac output rises during pregnancy. When does the peak occur? What is the mechanism?
The peak rise in cardiac output occurs by the 24th week and can be up to 50% over nonpregnant levels. During labor cardiac output increases 20% during each uterine contraction. The increased cardiac output during pregnancy results primarily from an increase in stroke volume and is probably mediated by estrogens.

3. What are symptoms of a normal pregnancy that may mimic heart disease?
Edema (occurs in up to 80% of normal pregnancies), shortness of breath, easy fatigue, lightheadedness, syncope, and prominent neck veins.

4. What are some normal auscultatory findings in pregnant women?
Prominent S1, split S1 (due to early mitral valve closure), wider split S2, S3 (common in pregnancy), S4 (rarer), and systolic murmurs (90% of pregnant women).

5. What are characteristics of innocent murmurs?
Systolic (early or mid), no louder than III/VI, heard along the left sternal border or throughout the precordium, and buzzing quality if present.

6. Which type of murmur almost always indicates heart disease? What are two exceptions?
Diastolic murmurs. Two exceptions are venous hum and mammary souffle.
Venous hum—continuous murmur throughout diastole and systole heard best over the lateral supraclavicular fossa and obliterated by pressure over the jugular vein.
Mammary souffle—high-pitched sound heard in the supine position in the second or third intercostal space.

7. What is the major nonobstetric cause of maternal death?
Heart disease. Rheumatic valvular disease used to account for 90% of heart disease in pregnancy. Now it represents 60–75%, with the incidence of congenital heart disease rising.

8. What are the effects of maternal heart disease on the fetus?
Possible decreased uterine blood flow and fetal oxygenation, preterm delivery, small for gestational age, and higher rate of spontaneous abortion (proportional to degree of cyanosis).

9. What are the goals of therapy for maternal heart disease?
• Prevent or manage endocarditis, congestive heart failure, serious arrhythmias, and thromboembolism.
• Avoid harming the fetus, who is more susceptible to the side effects of medical therapy than is the mother.

10. Mitral stenosis is aggravated by pregnancy because of the associated increase in heart rate, blood volume, and flow across the valve. Of women with mitral stenosis, 25% will have their first symptoms during pregnancy. What are some anticipated complications of mitral stenosis? How are they managed?

Congestive heart failure/acute pulmonary edema. Mortality of up to 70%. Can be precipitated by atrial fibrillation or by the 300–500 ml autotransfusion from the placental circulation at the time of delivery. Management includes digitalis for atrial fibrillation; if this fails, cardioversion or diuretics are used, with the last resort being operative repair with closed mitral valvulotomy or valve replacement. Management during labor should include a Swan-Ganz catheter, careful fluid management, and vaginal delivery if possible with epidural analgesia and second stage shortened by forceps delivery.

Atrial fibrillation. Predisposes to congestive heart failure as well as thromboembolus. Managed using digitalis, cardioversion, and anticoagulation with heparin.

Thromboembolism. Results from chronic atrial fibrillation and auricular thrombus formation. Heparin should be used for anticoagulation.

Hemoptysis. Results from rupture of endobronchial varicosities. If massive, should consider closed mitral valvulotomy or valve replacement.

11. What is the most common rheumatic valvular lesion in pregnancy? How is it diagnosed?

Mitral stenosis. It is diagnosed by a history of "mitral facies" (plethoric checks), rheumatic fever, unexplained atrial fibrillation, arterial emboli, or pulmonary congestion. Significant findings on physical exam include a diastolic rumbling murmur best heard in the apex with the patient on her left side. This murmur is accentuated in pregnancy. An echocardiogram can also supply diagnostic information.

12. What is the significance of mitral valve prolapse in pregnancy? What are the associated auscultatory findings?

It is well tolerated during pregnancy and is not associated with an increased incidence of complications. The need for antibiotic prophylaxis at delivery in order to prevent bacterial endocarditis is debated. Auscultatory findings are a midsystolic click and a systolic murmur which may disappear during pregnancy.

13. What is the management of aortic stenosis during pregnancy?

Pure aortic stenosis without mitral valve involvement is uncommon in pregnancy. Women should avoid pregnancy until after valve replacement. Management of aortic stenosis during pregnancy includes bed rest, increased fluid intake to increase preload, and avoidance of diuretics, beta blockers, verapamil, and vasodilators. As a last resort, valve replacement should be considered, although it is associated with a high fetal mortality.

14. Which congenital heart diseases are well tolerated during pregnancy?

Atrial septal defects (without pulmonary hypertension)

Ventricular septal defects (without pulmonary hypertension or large left-to-right shunts)

Patent ductus arteriosus (corrected in childhood). If uncorrected or with large left-to-right shunt, pregnancy can result in left ventricular overload and failure.

Pulmonary and tricuspid valvular lesions, unless severely compromised predating pregnancy.

15. Name cardiac conditions in which pregnancy should be avoided, since they carry a 25–50% risk of maternal mortality.

Pulmonary hypertension—maternal mortality greater than 50%

Eisenmenger syndrome

Marfan syndrome with cardiovascular disease—dilation of aorta and myxomatous mitral valve

Cardiomyopathy

16. What is tetralogy of Fallot?

Ventricular septal defect with right-to-left shunt, pulmonic/subpulmonic stenosis, right ventricular hypertrophy, and overriding aorta.

17. What are the consequences of tetralogy of Fallot? When is the mother at highest risk?

Increased rate of spontaneous abortions and retarded growth of fetus. The mother has a poor prognosis in pregnancy if she has a hematocrit greater than 65%, syncopal episodes, or $PO_2 < 70$. The mother is at highest risk during labor and delivery, at which time a drop in systemic vascular resistance may result in increased unoxygenated blood flow across the ventricular septal defect. Maternal hypoxia, syncope, and death can result. The risk for the surgically corrected patient is minimal.

18. What is Eisenmenger syndrome?

A right-to-left shunt (or a bidirectional shunt) at any level, plus pulmonary hypertension.

19. What is the risk of pregnancy in a woman with Eisenmenger syndrome? What is the management?

Maternal mortality is high (50–70%) with sudden death from hypoxemia occurring at any time. These patients should be advised to avoid pregnancy and, if pregnant, a therapeutic abortion for maternal indications should be considered in the first trimester. Management during pregnancy includes anticoagulation, maintenance of preload, and avoidance of excess vasodilation. The cause of death is right ventricular failure and hypotension progressing to cardiogenic shock. Drop in systemic vascular resistance (as during delivery) will increase left-to-right shunt and can result in marked hypoxia. Valsalva during labor can result in decreased cardiac output, leading to syncope and death.

20. What role does coronary artery disease have in pregnancy?

This is uncommon in women of childbearing age. However, those who do have ischemic heart disease during pregnancy will likely have their first symptoms during pregnancy. Insulin-dependent diabetics, in particular, are at an increased risk for coronary artery disease. Mortality is 35–45%, with the highest mortality occurring in the third trimester. Management includes oxygen, vasodilators, analgesia, and shortening of second stage with elective forceps delivery.

21. Which cardiac arrhythmias are significant during pregnancy?

Primarily those associated with an underlying cardiac condition such as mitral stenosis, atrial septal defect, and cardiomyopathy; also those in the setting of a preexisting supraventricular tachyarrhythmia such as Wolff-Parkinson-White syndrome. All can be dangerous. On the other hand, atrial and ventricular premature beats are common and pregnancy will lower the threshold for supraventricular tachycardia, which often responds easily to medication such as digoxin. Digoxin, procainamide, and quinidine can be used when needed even in the first trimester, as they have not been associated with teratogenic effects in humans.

22. What is peripartum cardiomyopathy?

It is a cardiomyopathy of unknown etiology that develops in the last half of gestation or in the early postpartum period. Patients at risk are those who are multiparous, are over age 30, have twins, or have preeclampsia.

23. What are the findings in peripartum cardiomyopathy?

Cardiomegaly, S3, jugular distention, mitral or tricuspid regurgitation, murmurs, and cool extremities.

24. What is the prognosis for peripartum cardiomyopathy?

Poor in the 50% of patients whose cardiac enlargement persists past 6 months post partum. Subsequent pregnancy is contraindicated, as recurrent cardiac failure may occur. Patients whose hearts return to normal size have a good prognosis and future pregnancies are not contraindicated.

THROMBOEMBOLIC DISEASE

25. What is the most common vascular complication of pregnancy? How is it diagnosed?

Deep venous thrombosis. Diagnosis is always difficult. Keep a high index of suspicion when there are signs or symptoms of swelling, pain, erythema, cyanosis, or Homan's sign. Noninvasive vascular studies such as impedance plethysmography, Doppler, or ultrasound are risk free but may miss calf thrombosis or be falsely positive in late pregnancy.

26. What are the risk factors for maternal thromboembolism?

Pregnancy itself, bed rest, obesity, advanced maternal age, previous thromboembolism, mitral stenosis, cesarean section, congestive heart failure, pelvic operations such as tubal ligation, suppression of lactation with estrogen, trauma to the lower extremities, and long travel in a car or airplane.

27. How is pulmonary embolus diagnosed?

Historical features include pleuritic pain, syncope, shortness of breath. The physical exam may find nothing or may reveal crackles or a pleural rub on auscultation of the chest. The electrocardiogram most commonly shows a sinus tachycardia with the classic $S_1Q_3T_3$ (S wave inversion in I, Q wave in III, inverted T wave in III) less commonly seen. Arterial blood gases demonstrate decreased pCO_2 or an increased Aa gradient. Ventilation-perfusion scans are of low risk to the fetus and should be performed when indicated. Angiography is most accurate but exposes the fetus to higher levels of radiation and should be avoided if possible during the first trimester.

28. How do you treat deep venous thrombosis and/or pulmonary embolus?

Coumadin is contraindicated certainly during the first trimester because of its teratogenic effects and in the third trimester because of its disruption of the fetal clotting system. Heparin has been the alternative anticoagulant of choice and is generally used throughout the pregnancy. Complications of heparin include maternal bleeding, thrombocytopenia and osteoporosis.

29. What risks are faced in pregnancy by a woman with a history of thromboembolic disease?

It is unclear what magnitude of additional risk a history of a deep venous thrombosis (DVT) confers for a current pregnancy. Recurrence risks have ranged from 0–15%. In the nonpregnant population, evidence suggests that recurrence for thromboembolic disease in the setting of transient risk factors (after surgery) is lower than for individuals with persistent high-risk factors. This will likely prove to be true for the pregnant population as well. High-risk factors include deficiencies of antithrombin III, proteins S and C, and antiphospholipid antibody syndrome. In addition, recent studies have found activated protein C resistance caused by a factor V Leiden mutation to be possibly the most important risk factor for thromboembolic disease during pregnancy or the postpartum period. Detection by actual gene studies or prolonged activated partial thromboplastin time (aPTT) is possible.

30. How should a woman with a history of thromboembolic disease be followed in a subsequent pregnancy?

Based on a division of transient factors vs. high-risk factors, various prophylactic regimens have been recommended for women with a history of thromboembolic disease. In women with prior DVT associated with transient risk factors, protocols of exercise, compression stockings, and close surveillance with Doppler studies of the lower extremities have been advocated. As the risk of thromboembolic disease is believed by many to be greatest in the peripartum period, low-dose heparin prophylaxis often has been instituted in the peripartum period. For women with a prior history of a pulmonary embolism or with high risk factors in addition to a history of DVT, many advocate antepartum low-dose heparin prophylaxis. Given the changing vascular volumes during pregnancy, the doses of subcutaneous heparin usually need to be increased during the third trimester (heparin 5,000 subcutaneously twice daily to 13 weeks; 7500 subcutaneously twice daily 13–30 weeks; 10,000 subcutaneously twice daily 30–40 weeks; 5,000 subcutaneously twice daily postpartum 4–6 weeks). Conversion to Coumadin for the postpartum period is reasonable even in the breastfeeding mother. Laboratory surveillance with plasma heparin levels is recommended to achieve a level of 0.1–0.2 U/ml. Calcium supplementation of 1.5–2.0 gm/day is suggested.

31. What is the role of low-molecular-weight heparin (LMWH)?

In the nonpregnant population, LMWH has been shown to be as efficacious as unfractionated heparin for both prophylaxis and treatment with the advantages of a longer half-life (once-a-day administration) and lower incidence of heparin-induced thrombocytopenia. The risk of heparin-induced osteoporosis is also thought to be lower. Because of evidence that LMWH, like heparin, does not cross the placenta, its use in pregnancy is being explored. For pregnant women with heparin allergy, LMWH is a reasonable alternative, because there is little cross-reactivity with unfractionated heparin. Studies of the efficacy and risks of LMWH in the pregnant population are underway.

BIBLIOGRAPHY

1. Abrams R, Wexler P (eds): Medical Care of the Pregnant Patient. Boston, Little, Brown, 1983, pp 183–199.
2. American College of Obstetricians and Gynecologists: Cardiac Disease in Pregnancy. ACOG Tech Bull 168, 1992.
3. Burrow GN, Ferris TF (eds): Medical Complications During Pregnancy, 3rd ed. Philadelphia, W.B. Saunders, 1988.
4. Gianopoulous J: Cardiac disease in pregnancy. Med Clin North Am 73:639–641, 1989.
5. Ginsberg JS, Hirsch J: Use of antithrombotic agents during pregnancy. Fourth ACCP consensus conference on antithrombotic therapy. Chest 108:305s–310s, 1995.
6. Hirsch DR, Mikkola KM, Marks PW, et al: Pulmonary embolism and deep venous thrombosis during pregnancy or oral contraceptive use: Prevalence of factor V Leiden. Am Heart J 131:1145–1148, 1996.
7. Sullivan J: Management of medical problems in pregnancy—severe cardiac disease. N Engl J Med 313: 304–309, 1985.

---

51. PULMONARY DISEASE IN PREGNANCY

Elizabeth L. Aronsen, M.D., and Polly E. Parsons, M.D.

---

1. How does normal pregnancy affect pulmonary mechanics?

Throughout pregnancy, the diaphragm is progressively displaced upward (about 4 cm) and the anteroposterior and transverse diameters of the chest increase (about 2 cm). Late in pregnancy, these anatomic changes result in decreased total pulmonary compliance due to decreased chest wall compliance and increased work of breathing.

2. How does normal pregnancy affect pulmonary physiology?

Elevation of the diaphragm results in a decrease in functional reserve capacity (FRC) because of decreases in its component volumes: residual volume (RV) and expiratory reserve volume (ERV). Because inspiratory capacity (IC) actually increases somewhat, vital capacity (VC; VC = IC + ERV) and total lung capacity (TLC; TLC = VC + RV) are preserved. Airflow as measured by forced expiratory volume in 1 second (FEV_1) and forced vital capacity (FVC) are unchanged in normal pregnancy, probably as a result of a delicate balance between bronchodilatory (e.g., cortisol, cyclic adenosine monophosphate, prostaglandins E_1 and E_2) and bronchoconstricting (e.g., estrogen, cyclic guanosine monophosphate, prostaglandin $F_{2\alpha}$) substances elaborated during this time. Respiratory muscle function is also preserved.

3. Define dyspnea of pregnancy.

During pregnancy, dyspnea is a common complaint and is often accompanied by hyperventilation. Respiratory center stimulation, probably by progesterone, increases minute ventilation by as much as 50%. This increase in minute ventilation is due primarily to increases in tidal volume rather than in respiratory rate. Because diaphragm elevation can produce lower lung atelectasis, resulting in crackles on exam and decreased colloid oncotic pressure results in peripheral edema, patients with benign dyspnea of pregnancy must be distinguished from patients with significant pulmonary disease. The differential diagnoses that must be ruled out, either clinically or with further testing, include reactive obstructive airways disease (e.g., asthma), pulmonary infection, pulmonary vascular disease (thromboembolism), pulmonary edema (cardiogenic or noncardiogenic), and acute lung injury.

4. What are the effects of pregnancy on asthma?

About 1% of all pregnancies are complicated by asthma; of these, about 1% have serious enough exacerbations to require hospitalization. Of the patients with asthma who get pregnant, about one-third will experience no change in their disease, slightly more than one-half will worsen during pregnancy, and the rest will improve. The majority (nearly 75%) of asthmatic patients return to their nonpregnant baseline within 3 months after delivery, and two-thirds will experience similar asthma courses in subsequent pregnancies.

5. How should asthma be monitored and treated during pregnancy?

Monitoring. Monitoring generally consists of spirometry and peak flow measurements of maternal airflow and, in the third trimester, fetal surveillance.

Therapy. The primary goal of therapy is to maintain maternal health and thereby fetal oxygenation. Treatment requires patient education to avoid precipitants of asthma, to monitor peak flows, and to seek early medical intervention when peak flow drops below 80% of the usual best. The medications used in asthma exacerbations during pregnancy are essentially the same as those used in the nonpregnant asthmatic patient:

- Bronchodilators (β-agonists, theophylline)
- Antiinflammatory agents (steroids, cromolyn)
- Antihistamines (chlorpheniramine, tripelennamine)
- Decongestants (pseudoephedrine, oxymetazoline)
- Antitussives (guaifenesin, dextromethorphan)
- Antibiotics (amoxicillin)

Although most medications have not been tested in pregnant populations and some are contraindicated because of adverse fetal effects, poorly controlled asthma is clearly associated with maternal (hyperemesis gravidarum, toxemia, labor complications) and fetal (low birth weight, prematurity) morbidity. Patients with well-controlled asthma have no significant morbidity over the general population.

6. What is status asthmaticus?

Status asthmaticus represents one of the most feared complications of asthma during pregnancy. Risk factors include a history of previous intubation for asthma, frequent emergency department visits (3/mo) or hospitalizations (2/yr) for asthma, recent corticosteroid withdrawal, a history of syncope or seizure with an asthma attack, and coexisting psychiatric or psychosocial disease.

7. How should status asthmaticus be managed?

Therapy again is essentially the same as for the nonpregnant patient: oxygen, short-onset β-agonists, terbutaline, methylprednisolone, and aminophylline. Close fetal and maternal monitoring is required, and intubation may be necessary. Once mechanical ventilation is required, difficult choices must be made regarding paralysis and permissive hypercapnea because of potential adverse effects on uterine muscle tone and uterine blood flow.

8. What medication commonly used during labor and delivery should be avoided in asthmatic patients?

Prostaglandin F2α, which is commonly used for control of postpartum hemorrhage, may increase airway resistance and exacerbate asthma.

9. Why is varicella pneumonia a major concern during pregnancy?

Maternal mortality from varicella pneumonia approaches 45% in some studies compared with 15–20% in the general population. Major fetal complications include in utero death, prematurity, neonatal varicella, and placental calcification.

10. What pulmonary complications of HIV disease can contribute to morbidity in pregnancy?

HIV infection carries additional risks to the pregnant patient of unusual infectious and noninfectious complications, including pneumocystis pneumonia (PCP), tuberculosis, toxoplasmosis, and lymphoma. Both therapy and the disease itself can be detrimental to the fetus. For example, PCP is ordinarily treated with trimethoprim/sulfamethoxazole combinations; trimethoprim is a potential teratogen, and sulfonamides have been linked to hyperbilirubinemia and kernicterus. Toxoplasmosis, also treated with sulfas, is linked to blindness when acquired in utero.

11. Describe the diagnosis and management of tuberculosis in pregnant patients.

Tuberculosis represents a public health risk as well as a risk to both mother and fetus. Diagnosis is often delayed because the patient is often asymptomatic and there is a reluctance to expose the fetus to diagnostic radiologic examination. This delay results in an increased incidence of advanced lesions. Inadequate, incomplete, or irregular therapy leads to increased resistance, increased spread of infection to contacts, and increased fetal morbidity, including 2-fold increases in prematurity, small for gestational age, and low birth weight and a 6-fold increase in risk of perinatal death. Therapy should not be delayed following the diagnosis of active tuberculosis, and treatment modifications need not be made in lactating mothers. In the case of a normal chest radiograph (CXR) and recent conversion, isoniazid prophylaxis is started in the third trimester. In the case of a normal CXR and remote conversion or in the case of an abnormal CXR in an asymptomatic patient who is not likely to have active tuberculosis, isoniazid therapy is started after delivery.

12. What organisms cause pneumonia in pregnancy?

The etiology of pneumonia includes pneumococci, *Haemophilus influenzae*, and atypical bacterial organisms (although "unknown" is the third most common etiology listed under bacterial causes), influenza A or varicella pneumonia, and aspiration of oral flora. Less common is fungal or mycobacterial disease.

13. What is Mendelson's pneumonia?

Mendelson's pneumonia refers to two syndromes associated with pulmonary aspiration of gastric contents: (1) the aspiration of acidic liquid gastric contents, which can cause a chemical pneumonitis that may progress to respiratory distress syndrome, and (2) the aspiration of particulates that may cause airway obstruction. Pregnant women are more likely to aspirate because of increased intragastric pressure from compression of the abdominal contents by the uterus and relaxation of the gastroesophageal sphincter by progesterone. In some series, aspiration pneumonia has been found to contribute to 2% of maternal deaths.

14. How should thromboembolic disease be diagnosed and treated during pregnancy?

Although overall diagnosis and therapy of deep venous thrombosis (DVT) and pulmonary thromboembolic (PE) disease have improved outcomes in nonpregnant patients, morbidity and mortality in pregnant patients remain unchanged in recent studies.

Diagnosis. Early diagnosis requires high clinical suspicion, especially in the right setting. Left lower-extremity DVTs are more common than right-sided DVTs because of the location of the inferior vena cava in the abdomen. Patients often present with typical complaints of acute onset of shortness of breath, perhaps with pleuritic chest pain and a pleural rub. Diagnosis is made by duplex ultrasonography, impedance plethysmography, or lung ventilation-perfusion (VQ) scan. VQ scan provides < 0.05 rads to the fetus. If further diagnostic examination is necessary, a limited venography exam with the abdomen shielded or pulmonary angiography using a brachial arterial approach have fetal radiation risks similar to the VQ scan.

Therapy. Heparin is the therapy of choice for thromboembolic disease during pregnancy. Warfarin is associated with fetal abnormalities such as brachydactyly, bone stippling, and nasal cartilage hypoplasia (warfarin embryopathy).

13. What is amniotic fluid embolism?

Amniotic fluid embolism is an unpredictable catastrophic peripartum event with an 80–90% mortality rate that generally occurs during any of the three stages of labor or immediately post-partum. The mechanism is complex and likely involves pulmonary microcirculatory obstruction with capillary leak secondary to vasoactive and inflammatory cytokine release. Risk factors include tumultuous labor, uterine stimulant use, advanced maternal age, multiparity, intrauterine death, meconium amniotic fluid staining, and premature placental separation. Patients present with acute onset of dyspnea, hypoxemia, and hypotension. Maternal morbidity is rated to pulmonary edema or hemorrhage, disseminated intravascular coagulopathy and convulsions. The diagnosis, often made at autopsy, can be confirmed antemortem by finding squamous cells in blood obtained from a pulmonary arterial catheter. Therapy is supportive.

14. What are the causes of pulmonary edema in pregnancy?

The causes of pulmonary edema in pregnancy include all of the causes in nonpregnant patients and may be cardiogenic or noncardiogenic. Unique to the pregnant patient is tocolytic-induced pulmonary edema, which occurs either during or up to 12 hours after cessation of therapy. Other risk factors for pulmonary edema include late gestation infection or concomitant cardiac disease with either left ventricular systolic or diastolic dysfunction. Of note, pulmonary edema is more than twice as common in the postpartum period as it is in preeclampsia. Therapy is the same as for nonpregnant patients and includes stopping tocolytics or starting antibiotics where appropriate, oxygen, diuretics, digoxin, and afterload reduction.

15. What risks do women with cystic fibrosis (CF) face during a pregnancy?

Traditionally women with CF have not been encouraged to become pregnant because of early studies that indicated a 10% maternal and 11% perinatal mortality rate. Recent studies have found a greater variability in outcomes among women with CF who become pregnant. Risks during and after pregnancy reflect more closely the state of the underlying disease process. A baseline vital capacity of < 50% is more often associated with a poor pregnancy outcome. Additionally, chronic hypoxia as reflected by $pCO_2 < 60$ is associated with a higher rate of pulmonary hypertension. Pulmonary hypertension, when faced with the increased volume load of pregnancy, may precipitate further hypoxia. Precautions should be taken to monitor nutritional intake given their pancreatic dysfunction and malabsorption as well as to detect early signs of gestational diabetes secondary to poor pancreatic function.

BIBLIOGRAPHY

1. Chatelain SM, Quirk JG Jr: Amniotic and thromboembolism. Clin Obstet Gynecol 33:473–481, 1990.
2. Elkus R, Popovich J Jr: Respiratory physiology in pregnancy. Clin Chest Med 13:555–565, 1992.
3. Fidler JL, Patz EF Jr, Ravin CE: Cardiopulmonary complications of pregnancy: Radiographic findings. AJR 161:937–942, 1993.
4. Hollingsworth HM, Irwin RS: Acute respiratory failure in pregnancy. Clin Chest Med 13:723–740, 1992.
5. Jana N, Vasishta K, Jindal SK, et al: Perinatal outcome in pregnancies complicated by pulmonary tuberculosis. Int J Gynaecol Obstet 44:119–124, 1994.
6. MacLennan FM: Maternal mortality from Mendelson's syndrome: An explanation? Lancet 1(8481): 587–589, 1986.
7. McColgin SW, Glee L, Brian BA: Pulmonary disorders complicating pregnancy. Obstet Gynecol Clin North Am 19:697–717, 1992.
8. Moore-Gillon J: Asthma in pregnancy. Br J Obstet Gynaecol 101:658–660, 1994.

9. Perlow JH, Montgomery D, Morgan MA, et al: Severity of asthma and perinatal outcome. Am J Obstet Gynecol 167(4 Pt 1):963–967, 1992.
10. Phelan JP: Pulmonary edema in obstetrics. Obstet Gynecol Clin North Am 18:319–331, 1991.
11. Working Group on Asthma and Pregnancy: Management of Asthma during Pregnancy. NIH Publication no. 93-3279, September 1993.
12. Zeldis SM: Dyspnea during pregnancy. Distinguishing cardiac from pulmonary causes. Clin Chest Med 13:567–585, 1992.

52. RENAL DISEASE IN PREGNANCY

Edward Frederickson, M.D.

1. What physiologic changes in glomerular filtration and effective renal plasma flow occur in normal pregnancy?

Extensive studies have been performed to answer these questions. The results are somewhat difficult to interpret because of problems in methodology and differences in posture. Clearance measurements made while patients are in the lateral decubitus position are higher later in pregnancy. These studies suggest that during upright and supine posture, the mass of the pregnant uterus impedes effective renal plasma flow. Glomerular filtration rate and effective renal plasma flow have parallel increases of 25–50% above normal beginning by the 12th week of gestation. The exact mechanism resulting in this increase is unknown.

2. What is the normal response of the renin-angiotensin system in pregnancy?

Renin is a proteolytic enzyme that is secreted by the afferent arteriole. It cleaves angiotensin I, a decapeptide, from angiotensinogen or renin substrate. Angiotensin I then undergoes further cleavage of two additional amino acids to form angiotensin II. Angiotensin II is a potent vasoconstrictor and stimulator of adrenal aldosterone secretion. The pregnant uterus and the placenta also produce renin. Uterine renin has been shown to be inactive as it enters the maternal circulation; however, there is evidence that renin may regulate uterine blood flow. During gestation plasma renin activity, renin substrate, plasma aldosterone, and plasma angiotensin I and II levels all increase. There is a down-regulation of the vasoconstrictive response to angiotensin II, demonstrated by a diminished pressor response to infused angiotensin II. Evidence exists suggesting that the blunted pressor response to infused angiotensin II is related to the marked increase in circulating prostaglandins, specifically prostacyclin of uterine and placental origin.

3. What are the anatomic changes associated with normal pregnancy?

The calyces and renal pelvis dilate and decrease the frequency of peristalsis. These changes occur by the end of the first trimester. The early effects on the collecting system are thought to be secondary to hormonal influence on the smooth muscle. By the third trimester, the enlarging uterus may entrap one or both ureters at the pelvic brim, resulting in partial obstruction during both supine and upright posture. The clinical implication of the physiologic dilation relates possibly to the increase in urinary tract infections in pregnancy and to the proper interpretation of urographic studies.

4. Can females with underlying renal disease who require maintenance hemodialysis conceive?

Most dialysis patients are anovulatory and unable to conceive. Those who do conceive are usually unable to sustain a viable pregnancy. Despite this, on occasion, women with azotemia have become pregnant and have delivered viable fetuses. Early reports indicate that recombinant erythropoietin can correct the anemia associated with end-stage renal disease and can reverse the anovulatory state, normalizing menses and the potential for fertility.

5. What is the most common cause of nephrotic syndrome in nondiabetic pregnant women?

Preeclampsia is the most common cause of nephrotic syndrome in pregnancy, usually presenting in the third trimester. Other causes of the nephrotic syndrome during pregnancy include membranous glomerulonephritis, membranoproliferative glomerulonephritis, minimal change disease, systemic lupus erythematosus, diabetes, and renal vein thrombosis. Nephrotic syndrome is defined by the presence of 3.5 gm/24 hr of proteinuria and denotes the triad of hypoalbuminemia, edema, and hyperlipidemia. The nephrotic syndrome is caused by a constellation of diseases, a few of which respond to corticosteroid therapy. Therefore a histologic diagnosis should be obtained before empirical therapy is instituted. The prognosis for patients with the nephrotic syndrome in pregnancy depends upon the underlying renal pathology. In the absence of hypertension or renal insufficiency, the likelihood of a successful outcome to the pregnancy is very good and a conservative approach is indicated.

6. When is childbirth safe in patients who have had renal transplantation? What adjustments should be made in their immunosuppressive medications?

Renal transplantation represents the only reliable means that a female with end-stage renal disease can reproduce. Regular menses and ovulation usually return within 6 months of a successful transplant. The current recommendation is to wait 1–2 years after the transplant before conceiving. Potential mothers should be informed about possible increased risks for the fetus and counseled against pregnancy if hypertension or renal insufficiency is present. Most centers do not recommend alteration of the immunosuppression regimen. Many women on triple-drug therapy (cyclosporine, azathioprine, and prednisone) have experienced successful pregnancies.

7. What advice should be given to a woman with systemic lupus erythematosus (SLE) considering pregnancy?

A threefold increase in exacerbation of disease during the first 20 weeks of pregnancy and a sevenfold increase postpartum can be seen in patients with active SLE, i.e., those not treated effectively or those who were undiagnosed. A history of SLE does not preclude successful gestation. Patients should be stable for 6 months prior to conception. They should continue on a stable course of immunosuppression throughout the pregnancy. There is no convincing evidence that corticosteroids or cytotoxic agents such as azathioprine or cyclophosphamide taken during pregnancy induce fetal anomalies. Congenital heart block may result in fetuses of patients with high titers of anticardiolipin antibody, representing a specific risk for this group of patients.

8. What advice should be given to women who have a parent with autosomal dominant polycystic kidney disease (ADPCKD) prior to considering pregnancy?

ADPCKD has a prevalence of 1 in 400–1000 individuals. The age of diagnosis is highly variable, with 16% being diagnosed by age 35 and 40% by age 45. Ultrasound is a very sensitive test but may be normal in individuals who will develop the disease later in life. A carrier of the gene has a 50% chance of passing the disease to offspring. Gene-linking studies have located the defective gene responsible for ADPCKD on chromosome 16. Presymptomatic screening and prenatal screening are available at some centers. Genetic counseling of suspected gene carriers is important in the management of these patients.

9. Do females have more frequent urinary tract infections during pregnancy?

Asymptomatic bacteriuria occurs in 4–7% of all pregnant women, which is the same incidence as in all sexually active females; however, 20–40% of women with asymptomatic bacteriuria develop symptomatic infections. *Escherichia coli* is the most common offending organism, and treatment of asymptomatic urinary colonization will prevent symptomatic urinary tract infections.

10. What determines maternal and fetal outcome in patients with chronic renal disease?

The course is largely affected by functional renal status and the presence or severity of hypertension. Superimposed preeclampsia is common in the presence of significant functional impairment (creatinine > 2.0 mg/dl). Proteinuria increases during pregnancy, but the degree of proteinuria appears to have little bearing on outcome. Severe malnutrition, as determined by a low serum albumin, has been associated with low fetal birth weight. There is very little evidence that pregnancy has a negative effect on the course of mild maternal renal disease.

Categories of Prepregnancy Functional Renal Status*

CATEGORY	SERUM CREATININE (mg/100 ml)
Preserved/mildly impaired renal function	< 1.4
Moderate renal insufficiency	> 1.4 to < 2.5
Severe renal insufficiency	> 2.5

Pregnancy and Renal Disease: Functional Renal Status and Prospects*

PROSPECTS	CATEGORY		
	Mild	Moderate	Severe
Pregnancy complications	22%	41%	84%
Successful obstetric outcome	95%	90%	47%
Long-term sequelae	< 5%	25%	53%

Estimates are based on 804 women/1162 pregnancies (1973–1987) and do not include collagen diseases.

Renal Disease and Pregnancy: Improvements in Perinatal Mortality Over 4 Decades*

RENAL DISEASE	PREGNANCY OUTCOME	1950s	1960s	1970s	1980s
Mild	Preterm delivery	8%	10%	19%	25%
	Perinatal mortality	18%	15%	7%	< 5%
Moderate	Preterm delivery	15%	21%	40%	52%
	Perinatal mortality	58%	45%	23%	10%
Severe	Preterm delivery	100%	100%	100%	100%
	Perinatal mortality	100%	91%	58%	53%

Estimates are based on 1778 women/2463 pregnancies (1954–1987) and do not include cases of SLE.

* All three tables from Davidson JM, Lindheimer MD: Renal disease. In Creasy R, Resnik R (eds): Maternal-Fetal Medicine: Principles and Practice, 2nd ed. Philadelphia, W.B. Saunders, 1989, with permission.

11. What is the significance of hypertension in pregnancy?

Hypertension is the most common medical complication of pregnancy; 70% of the time it is associated with preeclampsia, 25% with underlying essential or secondary hypertension, and 5% with underlying renal disease. The perinatal mortality trial showed in a prospective study that women with a diastolic blood pressure greater than 85 mmHg have a perinatal mortality of 37.9/1,000 births compared with 17.2/1,000 births in normotensive pregnancies.

12. At what level of blood pressure should antihypertensive drugs be prescribed?

This question should be approached on an individual basis. If the woman has baseline mild or moderate hypertension prior to pregnancy, it is reasonable to treat her by the same criteria as nonpregnant patients and employ or continue antihypertensive therapy, attempting to maintain a blood pressure below 140/90 mmHg. Patients with chronic hypertension have a higher incidence of superimposed preecclampsia. Fetal outcome is related to the amount of end-organ damage present prior to conception and the severity of superimposed preeclampsia. Normal pregnancy is associated with a drop in peripheral vascular resistance, resulting in a decrease in blood pressure of 10–15 mmHg by mid-trimester. Blood pressure then increases gradually, approaching non-pregnant values before delivery. Pregnancy-induced hypertension is defined as an increment of 30 mmHg systolic or 15 mmHg diastolic above the nadir established in the first trimester. Conservative management includes hospitalization and bed rest. If this fails, pharmacologic therapy is indicated.

13. Does hypertension in pregnancy more commonly cause hypertensive encephalopathy?

Hypertensive encephalopathy is the result of generalized cerebral edema secondary to forced hyperfusion of the cerebral vasculature. The high perfusion pressures commonly seen in preeclampsia are sufficient to overcome the maximal cerebral autoregulatory vasoconstriction. Chronic hypertensives develop vascular hypertrophy, shifting the autoregulatory curve and protecting against hyperfusion. The sudden increase in blood pressure that may be experienced in pregnancy and also the presence of endogenous humoral vasodilators make hyperfusion and development of hypertensive encephalopathy possible at relatively low pressures by nonpregnant standards. A sudden increase to diastolic blood pressures of 100 mmHg or greater can cause confusion, disorientation, and somnolence in patients who have previously been normotensive.

BIBLIOGRAPHY

1. Barron WM, Murphy MB, Lindheimer MD: Management of hypertension during pregnancy. In Laragh JH, Brenner BM (eds): Hypertension: Pathophysiology, Diagnosis, and Management. New York, Raven Press, 1990.
2. Chapman AB, Johnson AM, Gabow PA: Pregnancy outcome and its relationship to progression of renal failure in autosomal dominant polycystic kidney disease. J Am Soc Nephrol 5:1178–1185, 1994.
3. Davidson JM: Pregnancy in renal allograft recipients: Problems, prognosis and practicalities. Clin Obstet Gynecol 8:501, 1994.
4. Hou S: Frequency and outcome of pregnancy in women on dialysis. Am J Kidney Dis 23:60–63, 1994.
5. Hou S, Orlowski J, Pahl M, et al: Pregnancy in women with end-stage renal disease: Treatment of anemia and premature labor. Am J Kidney Dis 21:16–22, 1993.
6. Jungers P, Houillier P, Forget D, et al: Influence of pregnancy on the course of primary chronic glomerulonephritis. Lancet 346:1122–1124, 1995.
7. Stettler RW, Cunningham FG: Natural history of chronic proteinuria complicating pregnancy. Am J Obstet Gynecol 167:1219–1224, 1992.

53. INFECTIONS DURING PREGNANCY

James A. McGregor, M.D., C.M.

1. Should nonpregnant women infected with the human immunodeficiency virus (HIV) be routinely evaluated and treated for HIV and potential opportunistic infections? What about pregnant women?

Yes, in both cases. Convincing information shows that women with HIV-1 infection should be aggressively treated to reduce virus replication in order to (1) suppress HIV destruction of the immune system and (2) retard rates of HIV mutagenesis. Clinically optimal regimens continue to be investigated but probably include two- or three-drug combinations, including an HIV protease inhibitor plus one or two reverse transcriptase inhibitors (i.e., 3TC or zidovudine). Alternative regimens using 2 or 3 reverse transcriptase inhibitors may also be effective and are less costly. Specific treatments for opportunistic infections, including a single, double-strength trimethoprim/sulfamethoxazole tablet daily, are effective chemoprophylaxis for *Pneumocystis carinii* pneumonia and toxoplasmosis for individuals with CD_4 T-cell counts < 500/ml. Other chemoprophylaxis regimens for mycobacterial and other infections are indicated with more severe immunosuppression.

The safety and efficacy of multidrug regimens during pregnancy requires urgent study. All pregnant women should be treated with zidovudine during pregnancy and in labor (100 mg 5×/day until labor, then 2.0-mg/kg intravenous loading dose followed by 1.0 mg/kg per hour until birth), followed by oral zidovudine or other regimens for the newborn. Pregnant women with > 500 CD_4/cc should receive trimethoprim/sulfamethoxazole for *P. carinii* pneumonia and reemergence of toxoplasmosis.

2. Should pregnant women be routinely screened for HIV infection?

Yes. Screening tests for HIV should be routinely offered to all pregnant women. Rates of HIV infection during pregnancy in general populations approximate 1/500–1,500 women. HIV vertical transmission is more common than syphilis in most U.S. populations. As with syphilis, vertical transmission can be effectively prevented by screening asymptomatic women and providing treatment. The AIDS Clinical Trial Group (ACTG) 076 of the National Institutes of Health demonstrated a more than two-thirds (25% placebo vs. 8% zidovudine) reduction in perinatal HIV transmission with a single-drug, zidovudine-based regimen (100 mg 5×/day after 14 weeks' gestation until the start of labor, then 2.0 mg/kg intravenous loading dose in 1 hour, followed by 1.0 mg/kg until birth). This is followed by oral zidovudine syrup for the neonate for 6 weeks. All women receiving HIV testing should be appropriately consented and counseled. Women who refuse testing should be approached again during pregnancy. Care should be taken not to discriminate against refusers or infected women.

3. Which common urogenital infections should be diagnosed and treated in women obtaining preconceptual counseling?

The same infections that are screened and treated during pregnancy should be identified and effectively treated in women preparing for pregnancy, including gram-negative and group B streptococcal bacteruria (asymptomatic bacteruria), bacterial vaginosis (BV), trichomoniasis, and other prevalent sexually transmitted diseases (STDs). Partners of women with STDs should be treated appropriately. All treated patients and partners should reasonably receive a test of cure (TOC) 3 weeks after treatment.

4. What are the best clinical criteria for diagnosing bacterial vaginosis during pregnancy?

Of the standard Amsell's criteria, the characteristic milky, homogeneous, adherent discharge is most difficult to detect reliably in pregnancy. Many studies of bacterial vaginosis require two of the three remaining Amsell's criteria: vaginal pH > 4.5; amine odor with a drop of KOH (whiff or sniff test); and/or presence of characteristic "clue cells" as evidence of bacterial vaginosis. Alternatively, Gram-stain criteria, such as Nugent's or Speigal's criteria showing diminished lactobacilli and increased *Gardnerella* and *Mobiluncus* species, or alternative chemical tests can be used. Cultures for *Gardnerella vaginalis* are expensive, inaccurate, and unnecessary.

5. What are optimal treatments for bacterial vaginosis in pregnancy?

The most effective regimens for treatment of bacterial vaginosis (BV) during pregnancy utilize either oral metronidazole (500 mg twice daily for 7 days) or clindamycin (300 mg twice daily for 7 days). Each is approximately 85–90% effective in treating symptomatic and asymptomatic BV. Topical regimens are similarly effective for the mother but do not reduce risks of preterm labor or premature rupture of membranes when treatment is initiated in the second trimester. Traditional concerns about metronidazole use in pregnancy and teratogenesis are unfounded. Studies of metronidazole use in pregnancy show no increased risks of birth defects. If concern persists, oral treatment with clindamycin is similarly effective and significantly reduces risk of preterm birth as shown in a large Denver study.

6. Which antibiotic agents are currently recommended by the Centers for Disease Control for intravenous intrapartum antimicrobial prophylaxis of perinatal group B streptococcal disease?

The CDC recommends penicillin G, 5 Mu intravenous loading dose, then 2.5 Mu intravenously every 4 hours until delivery. Alternatively the CDC suggests ampicillin, 2 gm intravenous loading dose followed by 1 gm intravenously every 4 hours until delivery. If the patient is allergic to penicillin, the CDC recommends clindamycin, 900 mg intravenously every 8 hours until delivery or erythromycin, 500 mg intravenously every 6 hours until delivery. Patients treated for chorioamnionitis should receive one of these agents for group B streptococcal coverage in addition to coverage for *Enterobacteriaceae*—i.e., ampicillin and gentamicin or ampicillin/sulbactam intravenously.

7. Describe adjunctive antibiotic treatment in women with preterm premature rupture of membranes or preterm labor, which also covers for group B streptococcus.

Agents that prolong time until labor (latency) and reduce neonatal and maternal morbidity as well as provide antibiotic coverage for group B streptococcus include erythromycin base, clindamycin, or ampicillin. Each of these agents can be given intravenously or orally for a limited (7-day) course. Intravenous treatment with penicillin, ampicillin, or alternative agents should be given when labor ensues.

8. Which common genital infections are implicated in preterm birth?

Multiple studies from many countries associate various common lower reproductive tract infections with increased risks of preterm labor, preterm premature rupture of membrane (PPROM), and preterm birth as well as low birth weight (LBW). The preponderance—but not all—of these studies demonstrate increased risks of preterm birth with asymptomatic maternal bacterial vaginosis (BV). BV should be identified early and treated with oral metronidazole or clindamycin during pregnancy. Treatment of BV is associated with reduced rates of preterm birth, PPROM, and LBW in women deemed to be at high or normal risk for preterm birth. Large prospective studies of initial infection with herpes simplex virus infection, trichomoniasis, and chlamydia cervicitis also demonstrate increased risks of preterm birth.

Sexually transmitted diseases such as trichomoniasis, chlamydia cervicitis, and gonorrhea should be screened and treated at the initial antenatal visit to reduce risks of vertical infection and spread to partners, as well as preterm birth and PPROM. Partners of women with STDs should be effectively diagnosed and treated. Both the pregnant woman and her partner should optimally receive a test of cure (TOC) for STDs to ensure compliance and treatment efficacy in pregnancy. Counseling should be culturally appropriate. Rescreening may be appropriate for pregnant women at clinically perceived risk of STD acquisition during pregnancy.

9. What are some well-tolerated, effective treatments for pregnant women with chlamydial infection?

Alternatives to oral erythromycin-base treatment for chlamydial infection include generic enteric coated erythromycin (333 mg 3×/day for 7 days), ampicillin (500 mg 3×/day for 7 days), and azithromycin (1 gm once). Treatment of chlamydial genital infections in pregnancy is associated with reduced risks of prematurity and PPROM and neonatal conjunctivitis. Primary and secondary partners also should be treated. Patients and partners should be given a TOC approximately 3–4 weeks after treatment to ensure compliance and antibiotic efficacy. New nucleic acid-based techniques, such as polymerase chain reaction or LCR, offer optimal sensitivity and specificity for both screening, diagnosis, and TOCs.

10. Should pregnant women with preterm (< 35 weeks' gestation) premature rupture of membranes (PPROM) be routinely treated with a limited course of an antibiotic?

Three meta-analyses of adjunctive treatment of women with PPROM published in 1995 and 1996 demonstrate (1) significant prolongation of pregnancy duration, (2) increased birth weight, and (3) reduced rates of perinatal morbidity (e.g., sepsis, intraventricular hemorrhage) and maternal morbidity (e.g., chorioamnionitis, febrile morbidity). These analyses of published studies did not identify an optimal treatment regimen. Reasonable regimens should be of defined length (7 days) and ensure coverage for group B streptococcus, i.e., enteric-coated erythromycin (generic 333 mg E-mycin 3×/day for 7 days) or ampicillin (250 mg 3×/day for 7 days).

11. Should women with a history of preterm birth be screened and treated for bacterial vaginosis? What about other common genital infections?

Yes, in both cases. Two well-controlled, placebo-controlled trials demonstrate that identification and treatment of BV in women with prior preterm birth reduces risks of preterm birth (due to preterm labor and/or PPROM) by up to 70%. Screening and treatment of trichomoniasis and other common genitourinary tract infections and STDs is easily accomplished and also associated with reduced risks of preterm birth in less well-controlled studies. Treatment of genital chlamydial infection and gonorrhea greatly reduces risks of neonatal conjunctivitis (opthalmia neonatorum) and may obviate need for neonatal eye chemoprophylaxis in many populations.

12. Should women with preterm labor (< 35 weeks) receive a defined course of adjunctive treatment with systemic antibiotics?

Yes, if macrolides are used. Double-blind, placebo-controlled trials of macrolides and lincosamides, such as erythromycin or clindamycin, demonstrate prolongation of time to delivery (latency), increased birth weight, and decreased morbidity. Alternatively, large studies employing beta-lactam antibiotics (i.e., ampicillin, expanded-coverage penicillins) with or without erythromycin do not show similar benefits. Beta-lactam antibiotics are bacteriocidal and cause bacteria to break apart, thus throwing fuel on the fire of inflammation.

Women with preterm labor should be treated with antibiotics to reduce risks of early onset group B streptococcal infections according to current CDC and ACOG protocols. A defined 7-day course of erythromycin or clindamycin provides for group B streptococcal prophylaxis as well as significant, safe, and cost-saving prolongation of pregnancy.

BIBLIOGRAPHY

1. Alary M, Joly JR, Moutquin JM, et al: Randomized comparison of amoxicillin and erythromycin in treatment of genital chlamydial infections in pregnancy. Lancet 334:1461, 1994.
2. Ho DD, Neuman AU, Perelson AS, et al: Rapid turnover of plasma viron and CD4 lymphocytes in HIV-1 infection. Nature 373:1236–1240, 1995.
3. Bronson BM: Early intervention for persons with Human Immunodeficiency Virus. Clin Infect Dis 20(Suppl 1):S3–S22, 1995.
4. Burtin P, Taddio A, Ariburnu O, et al: Safety of metronidazole in pregnancy: A meta-analysis. Am J Obstet Gynecol 172(2):525–529, 1995.
5. Bush MR, Rosa C: Azithromycin and erythromycin in the treatment of cervical chlamydial infections in pregnancy. Obstet Gynecol 84:61–63, 1994.
6. Centers for Disease Control: HIV testing among women aged 18–44 United States 1991–1993. MMWR 45, 1996.
7. Centers for Disease Control: Prevention of perinatal group B streptococcal disease: A public health perspective. MMWR 45, 1996.
8. Centers for Disease Control/United States Public Health Service recommendation for HIV counseling and voluntary tests for pregnant women. MMWR 44, 1995.
9. Drugs for sexually transmitted diseases. Med Lett 37:117–120, 1995.
10. Hauth JC, Goldenberg RL, Andrews WW, et al: Reduced incidence of preterm delivery with metronidazole and erythromycin in women with bacterial vaginosis. N Engl J Med 333:1732–1736, 1995.
11. Hay PE, Lamont RF, Taylor-Robinson D, et al: Abnormal bacterial colonization of the genital tract and subsequent preterm delivery and late miscarriage. BMJ 308:295–298, 1994.
12. Hillier SL, Nugent RP, Eschenbach DA, et al: Association between bacterial vaginosis and preterm delivery of a low birth weight infant. N Engl J Med 333:1737–1742, 1995.
13. Kaplan JE, Masur H, Holmes KK, et al: USPHS/IDSA Guidelines for the prevention of opportunistic infections in persons infected with human immunodeficiency virus: Introduction. Clin Infect Dis 21(Suppl 1):S1–S11, 1995.
14. Landers DV, Sweet RL: Reducing mother-to-infant transmission of HIV—the door remains open. N Engl J Med 334:1664–1665, 1996.
15. McGregor JR, French JI, Seo K: Adjunctive clindamycin therapy for preterm labor: Results of a double-blind, placebo-controlled trial. Am J Obstet Gynecol 165:867–875, 1991.
16. McGregor JA, French JI, Parker R, et al: Antenatal microbiologic and maternal risk factors associated with prematurity. Am J Obstet Gynecol 163:1465–1473, 1990.
17. McGregor JA, French JI, Parker R, et al: Prevention of premature birth by screening and treatment for common genital tract infections: Results of a prospective controlled evaluation. Am J Obstet Gynecol 173:157–167, 1995.
18. Mercer BM, Arhart KL: Antimicrobial therapy in expectant management of preterm premature rupture of membranes. Lancet 346:1271–1279, 1995.
19. Morales WJ, Schorr S, Albritton J: Effect of metronidazole in patients with preterm birth in preceding pregnancy and bacterial vaginosis: A placebo-controlled, double-blind study. Am J Obstet Gynecol 171:345–349, 1994.

20. O'Donnell L, San Daval A, et al: STD prevention and the challenge of gender and cultural diversity: Knowledge, attitudes and risk behaviors among STD patients. Sex Transm Dis 21:137–148, 1994.
23. Rosenn MF, et al: Randomized trial of erythromycin and azithromycin for treatment of chlamydia infection in pregnancy. Infect Dis Obstet Gynecol 3:241–244, 1995.
24. Ryan GM, Abdoul, DT, McNeely E, et al: *Chlamydia trachomatis* in pregnancy and effect of treatment on outcome. Am J Obstet Gynecol 162:34, 1990.
25. Thomsen AC, Morup L, Hansen KB, et al: Antibiotic elimination of group B streptococci in urine in the prevalence of preterm labor. Lancet 1:591–592, 1987.

54. AUTOIMMUNE DISEASE IN PREGNANCY

Robert Silver, M.D., D. Ware Branch, M.D.

1. What is autoimmune disease? Is it common in pregnant women?

Autoimmune disease refers to various disorders characterized by immune-mediated damage to various tissues. Normally, the immune system discriminates between self and nonself and is tolerant of self-tissues. However, a failure of self-tolerance can lead to severe and debilitating illness. Pregnancy in women with autoimmune disease can be especially risky, because in special circumstances the fetus can be directly affected by maternal autoimmunity. This chapter focuses on antiphospholipid syndrome, an autoimmune condition characterized by pregnancy loss and obstetric complications. Other topics include systemic lupus erythematosus (SLE), autoimmune thrombocytopenia, myasthenia gravis, and rheumatoid arthritis. Autoimmune conditions such as thyroid disease and diabetes are covered in other chapters. Most autoimmune diseases occur primarily in women of reproductive age. Thus, simultaneous pregnancy is common.

2. What are antiphospholipid antibodies? Which ones provide clinically useful assays?

Antiphospholipid antibodies are a heterogeneous group of autoantibodies that recognize epitopes expressed by negatively charged phospholipids. Three are well characterized and generally accepted as having clinical relevance: lupus anticoagulant, anticardiolipin antibodies, and the biologically false-positive serologic test for syphilis. Lupus anticoagulant and anticardiolipin antibodies are most strongly correlated with clinical disorders and are the only two recommended for routine clinical use. Several other antiphospholipid antibodies, such as antiphosphatidylserine or antiphosphatidylcholine antibodies have been described. However, current data are insufficient to recommend testing. Laboratory detection of antiphospholipid antibodies can be confusing because the field is relatively new and the assays are still being perfected. It is important to use a reliable laboratory with a special interest in such testing.

3. What medical and obstetric problems have been associated with antiphospholipid antibodies?

The presence of antiphospholipid antibodies has been associated with various clinical disorders, including recurrent spontaneous abortion, fetal death, recurrent thromboses, and thrombocytopenia. Perhaps the most serious complication is thrombosis, which occurs in 10–60% of individuals with high levels of antiphospholipid antibodies. Thromboses may be arterial or venous, and occlusions in unusual locations are common. Other medical conditions associated with antiphospholipid antibodies include chorea gravidarum, transverse myelitis, livedo reticularis, autoimmune thrombocytopenia, autoimmune hemolytic anemia, and pulmonary hypertension. There is also a relationship between systemic lupus erythematosus (SLE) and antiphospholipid antibodies.

Numerous investigators have established a strong association between recurrent pregnancy loss and lupus anticoagulant and anticardiolipin antibodies. In fact, the rate of pregnancy loss in women with lupus anticoagulant may be higher than 90%. In our experience at the University of

Utah, clinically relevant levels of antiphospholipid antibodies are found in 5% of women with recurrent spontaneous abortion (defined as 3 consecutive losses with no more than 1 live birth). In addition, a relatively large proportion of antiphospholipid antibody-related pregnancy loss occurs during the second or third trimester. Although fetal deaths normally account for only a few percent of all pregnancy losses, 50% of losses were fetal deaths in a cohort of 76 women (333 pregnancies) with antiphospholipid antibodies.

In addition to pregnancy loss, several obstetric disorders have been associated with antiphospholipid antibodies. Successful pregnancies in women with antiphospholipid antibodies are often complicated by preeclampsia, fetal growth impairment, abnormal fetal heart rate tracings, and preterm delivery. In a cohort of 82 pregnancies in 54 women followed prospectively at the University of Utah, one-half were complicated by preeclampsia and abnormal fetal heart rate tracings and one-third by fetal growth impairment and preterm delivery.

4. What is the best test for lupus anticoagulant?

Lupus anticoagulant is a peculiar name for an autoantibody and a double misnomer to boot. It can be detected in plasma by any of several phospholipid-dependent clotting assays. Phospholipids serve as a template on which enzymes and cofactors of the clotting cascade interact. Lupus anticoagulant binds to the phospholipids that form the template, thus interfering with the timely interactions of the clotting factors. This results in a prolonged clotting time, prompting the term *lupus anticoagulant*. This is a classic misnomer, because many individuals with lupus anticoagulant do not have SLE, and lupus anticoagulant is associated with thrombosis, not anticoagulation.

The most commonly used phospholipid-dependent clotting test to screen for lupus anticoagulant is the activated partial thromboplastin time (APTT). Others include the dilute Russel viper venom time, Kaolin clotting time, and plasma clotting time. The sensitivity and specificity of these assays are affected by the types and concentrations of phospholipid reagents used. For these reasons, the most sensitive test may vary among laboratories.

Factors other than lupus anticoagulant, such as clotting factor deficiencies, anticoagulant medications, and improperly processed specimens, also can cause prolonged clotting assays. Thus, plasmas suspected of containing lupus anticoagulant should undergo confirmatory testing. First, the patient's plasma is mixed with normal plasma. If an inhibitory antibody such as lupus anticoagulant is present, the clotting test remains abnormal. In contrast, if a clotting factor deficiency is present, the clotting assay normalizes because the deficient factor is provided by the normal plasma. A second confirmatory test recommended by some authorities is the confirmation that prolongation of clotting is sensitive to phospholipid. The clotting assay is repeated after phospholipid is either added to or removed from the system. Lupus anticoagulant is considered present if reducing the phospholipid increases the clotting time or if adding phospholipid normalizes the clotting time. An example of the second principle is the platelet neutralization test. Regardless of the assay used, lupus anticoagulant cannot be quantified and is reported as present or absent.

5. What is the best test for anticardiolipin antibodies?

Anticardiolipin antibodies are detected by immunoassays. The most common is an enzyme-linked immunosorbent assay that uses cardiolipin as an antigen. An unacceptable degree of interlaboratory variation prompted several international workshops to standardize the assay. Assays using standard sera derived from these workshops are quite reliable and allow semiquantitation of antibody levels. Standard sera have been assigned numeric values, termed GPL and MPL units, for IgG and IgM antibodies, respectively. Results are reported as negative or low, medium, or high positive. Medium or high-positive results correlate well with clinical disorders.

6. What is the relationship between lupus anticoagulant, anticardiolipin antibodies, and other antiphospholipid antibodies?

There is a substantial overlap among all antiphospholipid antibodies, and many individuals with one antiphospholipid antibody have several. However, the correlation is imperfect. More than 70% of persons with lupus anticoagulant also have anticardiolipin antibodies. Fewer individuals with anticardiolipin antibodies have lupus anticoagulant, although the likelihood increases with increasing titers of anticardiolipin antibodies. The recommendation to test for both lupus anticoagulant and anticardiolipin antibodies is based on this imperfect correlation. As many as 50% of women with a false-positive serologic test for syphilis also have anticardiolipin antibodies, as do most women with high levels of other antiphospholipid antibodies (e.g., antiphosphatidylserine). It is unclear whether these antibodies are all members of a family of related antibodies or, less likely, the same antibody detected by different methods.

7. What is the definition of antiphospholipid syndrome?

Antiphospholipid syndrome is a clinical syndrome that requires both characteristic clinical features and confirmatory antibody testing. There are specified criteria for the syndrome, as much as for the diagnosis of systemic lupus erythematosus. The clinical criteria include unexplained arterial or venous thrombosis, recurrent pregnancy loss, or autoimmune thrombocytopenia. Recurrent pregnancy loss has not been strictly defined but (in this setting) is generally considered to indicate 3 or more consecutive first trimester losses or at least 1 mid or third trimester fetal death. The laboratory criteria are either lupus anticoagulant or moderate-to-high levels of IgG anticardiolipin antibodies. Low levels of these antibodies are common (especially after systemic infections), nonspecific, often transient, and not associated with increased risk for disorders associated with antiphospholipid antibodies. Thus, women with only IgM or low levels of IgG anticardiolipin antibodies in the absence of lupus anticoagulant should not be considered to have antiphospholipid syndrome.

8. What are the indications for antiphospholipid antibody testing?

* Three or more consecutive first trimester pregnancy losses
* Unexplained second or third trimester fetal death
* Early-onset (≤ 34 weeks early gestation) severe preeclampsia
* Unexplained severe fetal growth retardation
* SLE or other connective tissue disease
* Unexplained thrombosis
* Unexplained cerebrovascular accident
* Unexplained transient ischemic attack or amaurosis fugax
* Autoimmune thrombocytopenia or hemolytic anemia
* Unexplained prolongation in clotting studies
* False-positive serologic test for syphilis

Testing healthy individuals is ill advised. Antiphospholipid antibodies, especially anticardiolipin antibodies, are present in low levels in some normal individuals. The presence of antiphospholipid antibodies in the absence of pertinent clinical features is likely meaningless.

9. Are antinuclear antibodies part of the evaluation for antiphospholipid syndrome or recurrent pregnancy loss?

Antinuclear antibodies are not part of the evaluation for antiphospholipid syndrome. These antibodies (which recognize antigens other than phospholipids) are characteristic of SLE but are not associated with medical problems associated with antiphospholipid antibodies. Several case-control studies have linked antinuclear antibodies to recurrent pregnancy loss. However, not all studies found such an association. In addition, antinuclear antibody levels do not correlate with subsequent pregnancy outcome; elevations of antinuclear antibodies were only slightly increased (levels that are usually of no clinical significance) in women with pregnancy loss; and elevations of antinuclear antibody levels occur in many healthy pregnant women. Current data do not support clinical testing for antinuclear antibodies in women with recurrent pregnancy loss.

10. Can medical therapy improve pregnancy outcome in women with antiphospholipid syndrome? Which therapies are best?

Although most studies are flawed, nonrandomized, and poorly controlled, most investigators conclude that fetal outcomes are improved in treated pregnancies in women with antiphospholipid syndrome. Therapies include high-dose prednisone (40 mg/day), heparin (prophylactic doses, e.g., 5000–10,000 U twice daily), or intravenous immune globulin (IVIG) (1 gm/kg on 2 consecutive days monthly) in combination with low dose aspirin (80 mg/day). The treatments are based on proposed or theoretical mechanisms of fetal loss. Prednisone and IVIG are logical therapies because they are used to treat other autoimmune conditions. As an anticoagulant, heparin may prevent placental thrombosis and infarction, and low-dose aspirin increases prostacyclin:thromboxane ratios by suppressing platelet production of thromboxane. Therapy is initiated after confirmation of a formed fetus with cardiac activity.

At the University of Utah we have considerable success with both prednisone/aspirin and heparin/aspirin. Both regimens have resulted in a 70% live-birth rate in women with only a 10% success rate in untreated pregnancies. Based on a small randomized trial comparing prednisone and heparin, Cowchock reported that heparin and prednisone were equally efficacious but that heparin had fewer side effects. Because heparin may provide prophylaxis against thrombosis and has fewer side effects, we recommend heparin and low-dose aspirin as primary therapy. Heparin use is also fraught with side effects, including bleeding, osteopenia, and thrombocytopenia. Heparin and high-dose prednisone should not be used simultaneously because both predispose women to osteopenic fractures and combination therapy is no better than either drug alone. IVIG has been quite promising in a small number of cases refractory to heparin or prednisone. However, it cannot be recommended as primary therapy (in the absence of further study) because of its extremely high cost.

Women with antiphospholipid syndrome are at substantial risk (5% at the University of Utah) for developing thromboses during pregnancy or puerperium. Thus, we recommend continuation of low-dose anticoagulation (5,000 units twice daily of heparin or 2 mg daily of coumarin) through the sixth postpartum week. Low-molecular-weight heparin is probably as efficacious as unfractionated heparin, but less experience has been reported.

11. Do women with antiphospholipid syndrome require special care when they are not pregnant?

Yes. They are at substantial risk for all of the medical problems associated with antiphospholipid antibodies. Women with previous thromboses and antiphospholipid syndrome should receive lifelong anticoagulation. Coumarin should be used to achieve an international normalized ratio of 2.5–3.0. Acute thromboses are treated with heparin in doses elevating the APTT to 1.5–2 times normal. Adequate heparin therapy can be difficult to manage in women with lupus anticoagulant. One approach is to adjust the heparin so that the thrombin time is elevated to 100 seconds or greater, while ensuring that the prothrombin time is not elevated. It is unclear whether individuals with no previous thromboses and antiphospholipid syndrome require treatment.

12. How often do tests for antiphospholipid antibodies need to be repeated?

Many authorities recommend confirming high levels of antiphospholipid antibodies with testing at least 6 weeks apart. Although advocated by some, serial testing during pregnancy and titrating medications to suppress antibody levels have no proven benefit. We do not routinely repeat testing once the diagnosis of antiphospholipid syndrome is secure. Some individuals testing negative or low positive for antiphospholipid antibodies develop high levels after incurring new disorders (e.g., thrombosis or pregnancy loss). Thus, it is reasonable to repeat testing in such patients after the development of new disorders associated with antiphospholipid antibodies.

13. How are systemic lupus erythematosus and antiphospholipid syndrome related?

Although many patients have both, SLE and antiphospholipid syndrome are considered distinct autoimmune conditions. Seven to 30% of women with SLE have antiphospholipid antibodies, and approximately 40% of individuals with antiphospholipid syndrome have SLE. Individuals with SLE and antiphospholipid syndrome are considered to have secondary antiphospholipid syndrome, whereas those without SLE have primary antiphospholipid syndrome.

14. Does pregnancy worsen systemic lupus erythematosus?

No consistent evidence indicates that pregnancy worsens the course of SLE. Many older reports suggested that pregnancy exacerbates SLE. However, the majority of recent, well-controlled studies have shown no increase in SLE flares during either pregnancy or the postpartum period.

The one exception may be women with severe lupus nephropathy. Several investigators have noted an increased risk of progression to end-stage renal failure during pregnancy in women with serum creatinine levels > 1.5 mg/dl. Thus pregnancy cannot be advised in women with severe renal insufficiency. However, several women with serum creatinine levels > 2.0 mg/dl have had uncomplicated pregnancies.

Active disease at the time of conception may increase the risk of exacerbation during pregnancy. Similarly, the initial presentation of SLE during pregnancy or puerperium is often associated with severe disease. Despite these trends, termination of pregnancy has not been demonstrated to improve maternal outcome or to alter the risk of exacerbation.

15. What is the effect of systemic lupus erythematosus on pregnancy outcome?

Pregnancy loss, preeclampsia, small-for-gestational-age fetuses, and preterm delivery are more common in women with SLE. The majority of adverse fetal outcomes occur in women with antiphospholipid antibodies, who are treated as outlined above. Other risk factors associated with adverse pregnancy outcome are severe renal disease, active disease at conception, and onset of disease during pregnancy. Women with active SLE should be advised to delay conception until remission is established. Those with renal disease should be offered low-dose aspirin and perhaps calcium supplementation to decrease their chances of developing preeclampsia. Patients in remission and without other risk factors, such as antiphospholipid antibodies, severe renal disease, and hypertension, can be reassured that their likelihood of pregnancy loss is similar to that of the general population.

16. Do women with systemic lupus erythematosus require special care during pregnancy?

Ideally, care of pregnant women with SLE should be provided by obstetricians and rheumatologists working together. Laboratory studies include evaluation of renal function, platelet count, and testing for antiphospholipid antibodies. Although recommended by some investigators, serial testing for antinuclear antibody titers and complement levels has not been shown to be clinically useful in asymptomatic patients. Increased maternal surveillance for the development of lupus flares and preeclampsia (e.g., visits every 2 weeks in the second trimester) as well as fetal surveillance for growth (ultrasound) and well-being (nonstress testing) are also recommended. Caesarean delivery should be reserved for the usual obstetric indications. The use of prednisone in women with SLE during pregnancy should be the same as in non-pregnant patients. Despite serious side effects, the risk-benefit ratio clearly warrants the use of prednisone during pregnancy. As always, doses should be minimized, and patients taking chronically administered steroids should receive peripartum stress doses. Antimalarials, cyclophosphamide, chlorambucil, azathioprine, and nonsteroidal antiinflammatory drugs are best avoided, if possible, because of potential untoward fetal effects.

17. What is neonatal lupus erythematosus?

Neonatal lupus erythematosus (NLE) is an uncommon syndrome of the fetus and neonate. Clinical features include skin lesions reminiscent of adult cutaneous lupus, complete heart block, and hemolytic anemia and thrombocytopenia. This disorder is attributable to immune damage caused by maternal autoantibodies that cross the placenta. Most often these are anti-SSA (Ro) antibodies but anti-SSB (La) and rarely antiribonucleoprotein antibodies have also been associated with NLE. The prospective risk to a patient with SLE for delivering an infant with NLE is uncertain but is estimated to be 1–2%. Many infants with NLE are in fact born to asymptomatic mothers without SLE. Heart block can appear in utero and may be fatal. Steroids that cross the placenta (e.g., dexamethasone) may improve fetal outcome. The presence of anti-SSA is poorly predictive of NLE and should be assessed only in the presence of congenital heart block.

18. What is autoimmune thrombocytopenia? What is incidental thrombocytopenia of pregnancy? What are other common causes of thrombocytopenia during pregnancy?

Autoimmune thrombocytopenia (ATP), also termed idiopathic thrombocytopenia purpura, is characterized by IgG antiplatelet antibodies against antigens on both maternal and fetal platelets. It is most common in women of childbearing age and often encountered during pregnancy. ATP is essentially a diagnosis of exclusion. It is unnecessary to obtain antiplatelet antibodies or to document increased megakaryocytes on bone-marrow aspiration to confirm the diagnosis.

It can be very difficult to distinguish ATP from other causes of thrombocytopenia. The most common cause of thrombocytopenia in pregnancy is incidental thrombocytopenia of pregnancy, a mild (usually > 80,000 cells/µl platelet count), common (up to 5%), asymptomatic thrombocytopenia that is incidentally noted with automated complete blood counts. Women with incidental thrombocytopenia have no history of ATP and are not at risk for maternal or fetal bleeding complications. They do not require additional evaluation or care.

Other causes of maternal thrombocytopenia that should be excluded are preeclampsia, SLE, antiphospholipid syndrome, HIV infection, drug-induced thrombocytopenia, pseudothrombocytopenia (laboratory artifact), disseminated intravascular coagulation, and thrombotic thrombocytopenia.

19. How should autoimmune thrombocytopenia be treated during pregnancy?

Pregnancy does not substantially worsen ATP. However, the risk of hemorrhage associated with pregnancy requires careful attention to the maternal platelet count. Despite some controversy, most experts recommend treatment with high-dose (60-80 mg/day) glucocorticoids when the maternal platelet count drops below 50,000 cells/ml. After a response is noted (typically seen within 3 weeks), the dose is tapered to the lowest that maintains an acceptable platelet count. Refractory cases may be treated with IVIG or splenectomy. Splenectomy is reserved for extreme cases and is best done in the second trimester. Platelet transfusions are helpful to temporize bleeding in acute situations or if a patient requires immediate surgery with a platelet count < 50,000/ml. Women with ATP also should be instructed to avoid trauma and nonsteroidal antiinflammatory drugs.

20. What are the risks of fetal thrombocytopenia in women with autoimmune thrombocytopenia?

Antiplatelet antibodies can cross the placenta, leading to the destruction of fetal platelets and fetal thrombocytopenia. This may lead to fetal bleeding problems such as intracranial hemorrhage and has been a central issue to the obstetric care of women with ATP. Over the past decades, vaginal delivery has been considered to increase the risk of intracranial hemorrhage. This led to recommendations to deliver women with ATP by cesarian section. Based on the observation that bleeding complications are rare with fetal platelet counts > 50,000/µl, abdominal delivery was then reserved for severely (platelet count < 50,000/µl) thrombocytopenic fetuses. This approach required a reliable method to determine which fetuses were thrombocytopenic. Several noninvasive tests, such as maternal platelet count and antiplatelet antibodies, proved unreliable in predicting the fetal platelet count. Thus, obstetricians have used either fetal scalp sampling or cordocentesis to determine directly the fetal platelet count.

Recently, however, it has become apparent that the risk of intracranial hemorrhage is much lower than initially reported. Few cases of fetal intracranial hemorrhage have been documented in women with ATP, and the majority of fetal/neonatal intracranial hemorrhage is instead due to alloimmune, not autoimmune, thrombocytopenia. Furthermore, vaginal delivery has not been proved to cause hemorrhage in fetuses with thrombocytopenia, nor has cesarean delivery been shown to prevent it. Because invasive tests and treatments such as cordocentesis and cesarian delivery are costly, cause morbidity, and are not proven to decrease fetal bleeding problems, they are no longer recommended in the management of ATP.

21. What special considerations are necessary for the management of myasthenia gravis in pregnancy?

Myasthenia gravis is characterized by skeletal muscle weakness and excessive fatigability. It is thought to be mediated by autoantibodies that recognize acetylcholine receptors, leading to the destruction of the postsynaptic portion of the neuromuscular junction. Pregnancy does not consistently worsen or improve the course of myasthenia gravis. Transplacental passage of anti-acetylcholine receptor antibodies can lead to neonatal myasthenia gravis. This disorder is typified by flat facies, respiratory distress, and difficulty in feeding and crying; it affects 10–20% of infants born to women with myasthenia gravis. Rarely symptoms appear in utero as hydramnios, decreased movement, and limb contractures. Symptoms are transient, resolving within 60 days.

The mainstay of therapy for myasthenia gravis is anticholinesterase inhibitors such as pyridostigmine, which can be taken safely during pregnancy. Corticosteroids are also efficacious and can be used during pregnancy as outlined for SLE. Because smooth muscle contractions are not influenced by myasthenia gravis, the first stage of labor is unaffected. Forceps may be necessary to shorten the second stage, but cesarean delivery should be reserved for the usual obstetric indications. During labor, anticholinesterase drugs should be administered parentally to avoid erratic absorption. Certain medications may exacerbate muscle weakness in women with myasthenia gravis and should be avoided, including magnesium sulfate, aminoglycosides, β-mimetics, lithium salts, and several other antibiotics.

22. What special considerations are necessary for the management of rheumatoid arthritis in pregnancy?

Rheumatoid arthritis has been reported to improve in pregnancy in approximately 75% of women. Unfortunately, over 90% of these women have remissions during the 6 months after delivery. Analgesia is best accomplished with acetaminophen or low doses of narcotics; nonsteroidal antiinflammatory agents and salicylates should be avoided. Glucocorticoids are considered safe during pregnancy, but gold salts, cytotoxic agents, penicillamine, and antimalarials may have adverse fetal effects. No special intrapartum care is required in the absence of gross contractures that have the potential to interfere with the mechanics of vaginal birth.

BIBLIOGRAPHY

1. Branch DW, Silver RM, Blackwell JL, et al: Outcome of treated pregnancies in women with antiphospholipid syndrome: An update of the Utah experience. Obstet Gynecol 80:614–20, 1992.
2. George JN, El-Harake MA, Raskob GE: Chronic idiopathic thrombocytopenic purpura. N Engl J Med 331:1207–1211, 1994.
3. Hughes GRV, Harris EN, Gharavi AE: The anticardiolipin syndrome. J Rheumotol 13:486–489, 1989.
4. Lockshin MD: Pregnancy associated with systemic lupus erythematosus. Semi Perinatol 14:130–138, 1990.
5. Lockwood CJ, Romero R, Feinberg RF, et al: The prevalence and biologic significance of lupus anticoagulant and anticardiolipin antibodies in a general obstetric population. Am J Obstet Gynecol 161:369–373, 1989.
6. McCarty DJ, (ed): Arthritis and Allied Conditions, 11th ed. Philadelphia, Lea & Febiger, 1989.
7. Silver RM, Branch DW: Autoimmune disease in pregnancy. Ballieres Clin Obstet Gynecol 6:565–600, 1992.
8. Silver RM, Branch DW, Scott JR: Maternal thrombocytopenia in pregnancy: Time for a reassessment. Am J Obstet Gynecol 173:479–482, 1995.
9. Silver RM, Branch DW: Recurrent miscarriage: Autoimmune considerations. Clin Obstet Gynecol 37:745–760, 1994.
10. Silver RM, Draper ML, Scott JR, et al: Clinical consequences of antiphospholipid antibodies: An historic cohort study. Obstet Gynecol 83:372–377, 1994.
11. Silver RM, Porter TF, van Leeuwen I, et al: Anticardiolipin antibodies: Clinical consequences of "low titers." Obstet Gynecol 87:494–500, 1996.

55. ALCOHOL AND DRUG ABUSE DURING PREGNANCY

Grace Chang, M.D., M.P.H., and Scott Farhart, M.D.

ALCOHOL ABUSE

1. Why is alcohol use during pregnancy of clinical importance?

Maternal alcohol consumption during pregnancy is one of the most common preventable causes of birth defects and childhood disabilities. Varying levels of fetal alcohol exposure can result in a spectrum of alcohol-related disabling conditions, ranging from cognitive and behavioral problems to fetal alcohol syndrome (FAS). According to the latest available data from the Centers for Disease Control, the FAS rate for 1993 (6.7 per 10,000 births) was more than 6-fold higher than that for 1979 (1 per 10,000 births). Alcohol is the most commonly used substance during pregnancy, consumed by as many as 70% of pregnant women.

2. What are the features of fetal alcohol syndrome (FAS)?

Fetal alcohol syndrome includes growth retardation before and after birth, abnormalities of the head and face, and central nervous system anomalies.

3. Is there a "safe" limit of alcohol consumption?

No safe limit of alcohol consumption has been identified. An advisory not to drink alcohol both for women who are pregnant and women attempting conception was issued by the Surgeon General in 1981 and by the Secretary of Health and Human Services in 1990.

4. Is there a dose/response relationship between alcohol consumption and pregnancy outcome?

No. Among women who consume 5 ounces of alcohol daily, about one-third have offspring with FAS, one-third of the infants show some prenatal toxic effects, and the remaining one-third appear to be normal. Alcohol consumption within the social drinking range has been associated with persistent effects on IQ and learning problems in young school-aged children without apparent anatomic abnormalities.

5. How much does a woman have to be drinking to consume 5 oz of alcohol per day?

Beer is generally 5% alcohol; one 12-oz can contains 0.6 oz of absolute alcohol. Wine contains approximately 0.5 oz per glass, as does a shot of liquor. Four to five ounces of alcohol may be reached through various combinations of the above, such as a couple of "mixed" drinks before and after dinner with four glasses of wine at dinner or a six-pack of beer plus four glasses of wine.

6. Does alcohol cross the placenta?

Ethyl alcohol does cross the placenta. Fetal blood alcohol levels approximate those of the mother.

7. Should an alcoholic pregnant woman stop drinking on her own?

A pregnant woman who is physically dependent on alcohol requires medically supervised detoxification. The risk of preterm labor is significantly increased with alcohol withdrawal.

8. When do the signs and symptoms of alcohol withdrawal appear during pregnancy?

Withdrawal symptoms begin when blood alcohol concentrations decline sharply after cessation or reduction, usually within 4–12 hours. However, it is possible that withdrawal symptoms develop even a few days after abstinence. Untreated withdrawal symptoms reach their peak intensity at 48 hours and may persist for up to 3–6 months at lower levels of intensity. Signs and symptoms of alcohol withdrawal include tremulousness, anxiety, increased heart rate, increased blood pressure, sweating, nausea, hyperreflexia, and insomnia, depending on the severity of previous alcohol dependence and the general condition of the patient.

9. Once a pregnancy is recognized, does decreasing alcohol intake affect the rate of fetal abnormalities produced?

In at least one preliminary study, self-reported decreases in alcohol exposure during pregnancy were associated with a lesser degree of fetal damage. Women who stop excessive alcohol use after recognition of pregnancy in either the first or second trimesters had fewer diagnoses of FAS. Cessation after the first trimester or second trimester resulted in a 5% rate of FAS vs. a 30% rate if significant alcohol use continued throughout the gestation.

COCAINE ABUSE

10. What is the prevalence of cocaine abuse in the obstetric population?

The prevalence of cocaine abuse in the obstetric population is estimated to range from 5–15%.

11. How does cocaine affect the pregnant patient?

Cocaine prevents uptake of norepinephrine. The increase in norepinephrine causes vasoconstriction, tachycardia, and rapid rise in maternal and fetal arterial pressure. Uterine and placental blood flow decreases, with resultant fetal tachycardia and increased fetal oxygen consumption. Uterine contractility also increases.

12. What risks are associated with cocaine use during pregnancy?

Pregnancy risks associated with cocaine use include irregularities in placental blood flow, abruptio placentae and premature labor and delivery. Use of cocaine in the third trimester increases the risk of abruption tenfold. Abruption and stillbirth have been documented in 8% of cocaine abusers. Cocaine use in the first trimester results in a spontaneous abortion rate of 40%. In terms of fetal development, reported risks include low birthweight, congenital anomalies, urogenital anomalies, mild neurodysfunction, transient electroencephalographic abnormalities, and cerebral infarction and seizures. Hypertonicity, spasticity and convulsions, hyperreflexia, and irritability have been observed in children exposed to cocaine in utero.

13. How long do cocaine metabolites remain in the urine?

Cocaine use can be detected in a urine sample for up to three days after last use.

HEROIN ABUSE

14. What is the prevalence of opiate abuse or dependence during pregnancy?

The true extent of opiate abuse and dependence by women is unknown. Overall, women account for about one-fourth of all opiate-dependent individuals, and most of the estimated 300,000 women are untreated for their addiction.

15. What risks are incurred by opiate dependence during pregnancy?

A 6-fold increase in maternal obstetric complications, toxemia, third-trimester bleeding, and puerperal morbidity has been reported. There is also an increase in neonatal complications including narcotics withdrawal, postnatal growth deficiency, microcephaly, neurobehavioral problems, and marked increase in sudden infant death syndrome.

16. What is the best treatment for opiate dependence during pregnancy?

Methadone maintenance confers several treatment benefits for the pregnant opiate-dependent woman. It eliminates the need for illicit behavior to support a drug habit, prevents fluctuations in maternal heroin levels, and removes the patient from a drug-seeking environment.

17. Should a woman on methadone be weaned during pregnancy?

No. Although it is desirable to use the lowest possible dose, reduction below 20 mg/day may precipitate in utero withdrawal. Whatever dose is required to prevent symptoms in the mother is also best for the fetus, and no attempt should be made to taper and discontinue methadone until after delivery.

18. Does methadone prevent withdrawal in the newborn period?

No. About 80% of infants exposed to methadone require treatment for neonatal withdrawal in contrast to 100% of infants exposed to heroin. The incidence of withdrawal is reduced in infants of mothers on the lowest methadone doses.

19. What are the symptoms of neonatal withdrawal from heroin or methadone?

The classic symptom complex of neonatal abstinence syndrome (NAS) includes central nervous system hyperirritability, gastrointestinal dysfunction, respiratory distress, tremors, high-pitched cry, poor feeding, and electrolyte imbalance.

20. What is the recommended treatment for neonatal withdrawal?

Paregoric is recommended for opiate withdrawal and phenobarbital for withdrawal from multiple substances. Prophylactic drug therapy is not recommended because not all infants develop the abstinence syndrome.

21. Should patients who abuse drugs breastfeed?

Breastfeeding is not recommended. Alcohol, cocaine, and opiates cross into breast milk to some extent. Because cocaine may cause significant cardiovascular changes in neonates, breastfeeding is absolutely contraindicated.

BIBLIOGRAPHY

1. Centers for Disease Control. Update: Trends in fetal alcohol syndrome–United States, 1979–1993. MMWR 44:249–253, 1995.
2. Chasnoff IJ, Griffith DR, Freier C, Murray J: Cocaine/polydrug use in pregnancy: Two year follow-up. Pediatrics 89:284–289, 1992.
3. Cyr MG, Moulton AW: Substance abuse in women. Obstet Gynecol Clin North Am 17:905–925, 1990.
4. Dombrowski M, Wolfe H, Welch R, Evans M: Cocaine abuse is associated with abruptio placentae and decreased birth weight, but not shorter labor. Obstet Gynecol 77:139, 1991.
5. Finnegan LP, Kandall SR: Maternal and neonatal effects of alcohol and drugs. In Lowinsin JH, Ruiz P, Millman RB, Langrod JG (eds): Substance abuse: A Comprehensive Textbook, 2nd ed. Baltimore, Williams and Wilkins, 1992, pp 628–656.
6. Mastrogiannis D, Decavalas G, Verma U, Tejani N: Perinatal outcome after recent cocaine usage. Obstet Gynecol 76:8, 1990.
7. Streissguth AP, Barr HM, Sampson PD: Moderate alcohol exposure: Effects on child IQ and learning problems at 7½ years. Alcohol Clin Exp Res 14:662–9, 1990.
8. Wiemann CM, Berenson AB, San Miguel VV: Tobacco, alcohol, and illicit drug use among pregnant women. J Reprod Med 39:769–776, 1994.

56. PSYCHIATRIC ISSUES DURING PREGNANCY

Randy Glassman, M.D., and Joanna Bures, M.D.

1. What are the normal reactions and psychological adjustments to a normal pregnancy?

In a healthy woman, adjustment to pregnancy involves a developmental crisis with reworking of old relationships (especially with her mother and father), revisiting issues of attachment and separation, gaining a sense of mastery, and coming to terms with her own femaleness. Normal reactions can also include anxiety, fear, ambivalence, and mixed anticipation. Social, cultural, economic, and emotional factors in the environment mediate many of the responses.

For men, adjustment to pregnancy often involves satisfaction of a narcissistic wish to reproduce and the desire to identify with their offspring and promulgate the family line. It can also be a time of reworking old relationships and gaining a new sense of purposefulness and seriousness. However, normal pregnancy can also stimulate concerns about personal health, finances, job security, and personal freedom. Men may feel left out and resentful of the new mother-child dyad. Once again, social, cultural, economic, and emotional issues mediate these adjustments.

2. What psychiatric symptoms and emotional reactions are associated with infertility, fetal anomalies, pregnancy loss, and high-risk pregnancy–all of which share some elements of loss and uncertainty? How can caregivers help?

Patients and couples who have to deal with these situations are often faced with many different feelings and reactions. Some determinants of such reactions include premorbid adjustment, personality traits, and coping styles. However, many persons share the following cluster of symptoms:

1. Sadness, grief, depression, helplessness, and somatic symptoms
2. Shock, denial, and acceptance
3. Anxiety, guilt, isolation, withdrawal, anger, and shame
4. Narcissistic vulnerability, including difficulties with self-esteem and sense of self
5. Problems with attachment and separation
6. Loss of libido and impaired sexual functioning
7. Symptoms similar to those of chronic illness or disability
8. Symptoms of posttraumatic stress disorder
9. Sense of injustice, envy, and resentment for the healthy
10. Severe stress in the marital/couple relationship
11. Disruption of normal family and social relationships
12. Loss of hope for the future and loss of faith

The realistic and unrealistic expectations associated with such situations can be overwhelming for the women, couples, and people taking care of them. However, when the above reactions and symptoms persist and begin to impact on social functioning and when vegetative symptoms last for more than a few weeks or a month, psychiatric evaluation and treatment may be necessary.

Caregivers can help by allowing the woman or couple to mourn or cope in their own individual ways while keeping watch for serious psychiatric sequelae. Caregivers should be careful not to impose their own values and judgments, should offer supportive assistance, and can help with appropriate referral to counseling and/or psychiatric services. Caring, involvement, and nonabandonment are extremely important.

3. Give examples of psychiatric disorders commonly encountered during pregnancy.

Psychiatric illnesses are important to think about in evaluating pregnant women because (1) they are common, (2) they may be undiagnosed or kept secret, (3) they may worsen during the course of the pregnancy or the puerperium, and (4) if they are not treated, psychiatric and other sequelae may occur. Common disorders include mood disorders (major depression, bipolar [manic-depressive] disorder, and other variants), anxiety disorders (with or without panic symptoms and agoraphobia), obsessive-compulsive disorders, and eating disorders (anorexia nervosa and bulimia).

4. What are the characteristics of the psychiatric disorders commonly encountered during pregnancy?

Mood disorders: symptoms may include changes in mood (depression, euphoria or irritability), energy, sleep, appetite, concentration, and libido. Feelings of hopelessness and guilt or grandiose thoughts may be present. Diagnosis is complicated by moderate changes in mood, cognition, and somatic symptoms that often occur during pregnancy, unrelated to psychiatric illness.

Anxiety disorders: excessive generalized anxiety, irritational fears, panic (sudden onset of intense anxiety without precipitants), autonomic responses (shortness of breath and palpitations), obsessive-compulsive thoughts or actions, and fear of recurrence of symptoms. Diagnosis may be complicated in women who have a history of infertility, prior complicated pregnancy, current high-risk pregnancy, or some other active anxiety-producing situation.

Eating disorders: among the more difficult to diagnose because patients may be secretive about symptoms. Patients with active anorexia nervosa rarely present pregnant because they are markedly underweight (15% below ideal body weight) and have amenorrhea. Patients with bulimia, however, who may be of normal weight or slightly above or below ideal body weight, do present pregnant and are often successful in concealing their problem from obstetricians. Symptoms include binge eating followed by purging behavior–most commonly self-induced vomiting, but also chronic abuse of laxatives, diet pills, and/or excessive exercise. Some patients with hyperemesis may have undiagnosed eating disorders.

5. How are psychiatric disorders best detected?

Diagnosis involves good history taking and nonjudgmental questioning. Important areas include history of psychiatric disorders in the patient herself, a family history of such disorders, postpartum disorders, premenstrual disorders, substance abuse disorders (which can be an indication of self-medication for comorbid psychiatric disorders), and descriptions of psychosocial functioning. Using the patient's desire to protect her pregnancy and baby can be important in building an alliance to gain accurate information for treatment.

6. Can psychiatric disorders be treated during pregnancy?

Psychiatric disorders can and should be treated during pregnancy because of significant risks to both the mother and developing fetus. A depressed or overly anxious woman may be unable to adjust to pregnancy and her new role as a mother, and she may be unable to mobilize needed supports when the baby arrives. More seriously, she may not be able to maintain an adequate weight gain or good physical health during her pregnancy.

Depending on the severity of illness, nonpharmacologic treatments are often used initially, including individual supportive or insight-oriented psychotherapy, couples or family therapy, and/or cognitive behavioral interventions.

Psychopharmacologic treatments are required when responses to other interventions are inadequate and the severity of the illness poses a greater risk to the mother and fetus than the risk of medication exposure to the developing fetus. Such cases require a complicated risk/benefit assessment, considering the severity of the psychiatric illness, the risk of the untreated psychiatric illness in causing increased morbidity to the mother and fetus, and the risk of medication exposure to the fetus.

7. What are the risks of psychopharmacologic medication exposure to the developing fetus? How can these medications be used safely during pregnancy?

The risks that psychopharmacologic medications pose to the fetus fall into three main categories: (1) teratogenicity, (2) neonatal side effects and toxicity and (3) behavioral teratogenicity.

Tricyclic antidepressants are considered relatively safe during all trimesters and are not associated with increased risk of congenital malformations; withdrawal symptoms and feeding difficulties have been reported in infants. Less anticholinergic preparations, such as nortriptyline (Pamelor) and desipramine (Norpramin), should be considered first. Fewer data are available about trazodone (Desyrel), a tetracyclic antidepressant.

Serotonin reuptake inhibitors: Fluoxetine (Prozac) appears relatively safe during pregnancy and has not yet been associated with an increased risk of congenital anomalies according to the manufacturers' register. Fewer data are available about sertraline (Zoloft) and paroxetine (Paxil), and even less is known about the newer agents. However, because these medications are new, caution should still be advised, especially in the first trimester. Irritability in newborns exposed to fluoxetine in utero has been reported.

Mood stabilizers: Lithium has been associated with an increased risk of cardiac malformations–most notably Ebstein's anomaly, with a reported 20 times greater risk (1/1,000 vs. 1/20,000) with first-trimester exposure. Newer data, however, may reveal a lower risk. Hypotonia and cyanosis or "floppy baby" syndrome may occur in exposed newborns. Valproic acid (Depakote) and carbamazepine (Tegretol) are associated with higher rates of neural tube defects (3% and 1%, respectively) and an increased risk of craniofacial defects and possibly growth retardation. Behavioral difficulties have not yet been described.

Benzodiazepines: An increased risk of cleft lip/cleft palate with diazepam (Valium) exposure is currently being reevaluated. Higher-potency agents like clonazepam (Klonopin) and alprazolam (Xanax) are being reevaluated with respect to organ dysgenesis. Lethargy and withdrawal symptoms have been described in neonates.

Antipsychotics: Higher-potency neuroleptics such as haloperidol (Haldol) are recommended over low potency drugs like thioridazine (Thorazine) and are fairly safe to use during pregnancy. Extrapyramidal side effects can be seen in the neonates. Few data are available about newer antipsychotic agents such as clozapine (Clozaril) and risperidone (Risperdal).

In general, behavioral teratogenicity with the use of psychopharmacologic medications is just beginning to be studied. Risks can be minimized with prepregnancy psychiatric evaluations and thorough planning based on the severity of the patient's psychiatric illness. Assessment should include recurrence risk without medications, nonpharmacologic treatments, and available data about the risk of medications. First-trimester exposure should be avoided whenever possible, and patients should be monitored closely on the lowest possible doses.

8. What are the main psychiatric disorders during the postpartum period? How are they treated?

Postpartum or maternity "blues" is very common, occurring in 50–80% of all new mothers. Symptoms include emotional lability, sleep disturbance, and difficulty in concentrating. Symptoms may begin shortly after delivery and usually resolve spontaneously by 2 weeks postpartum. Helpful interventions include education, supportive therapy, and reassurance. If symptoms persist beyond two weeks, other disorders need to be considered.

Postpartum depression is a more serious and clinically significant disorder with a prevalence rate of 8–15%. Symptoms may begin early, immediately following delivery or the blues or anytime during the first year postpartum, peaking at 2–4 months. The hallmarks are depression longer than 2 weeks and neurovegetative signs such as depressed mood, changes in appetite, sleep disturbance, guilt, fatigue, concentration difficulties, and suicidal ideation. Intrusive thoughts about harming the baby may or may not be present. The patient may be unable to care for her infant adequately, and antidepressants are often required. Hospitalization is sometimes necessary.

Postpartum psychosis: The most serious of the postpartum disorders occurs in 1–2 per 1,000 deliveries and may develop within hours or days postpartum. Symptoms often include severe anxiety, agitation, restlessness, insomnia, and, at times, disorganization and confusion. Delusions about the baby and hallucinations about harming one's self or the baby may also be present. This situation can be dangerous because of the risk of suicide and/or infanticide.

Psychiatric hospitalization is nearly always required, as is treatment with antipsychotic or other psychopharmacologic medications.

Postpartum anxiety disorders, including obsessive-compulsive disorders, are now being described. They may be variants of postpartum depression or they may be independent disorders. The incidence rate is still unknown.

9. What risk factors identify women who may be vulnerable to postpartum depression and psychosis?

Risk factors for postpartum depression include (1) a history of depression, (2) a history of a previous postpartum depression, (3) depression during pregnancy, (4) a family history of depression, (5) lack of adequate social supports, and (6) negative life events late in pregnancy. Additional risk factors for postpartum psychosis include (1) a history of bipolar disorder or psychotic disorder, (2) a family history of bipolar disorder or psychosis, (3) previous postpartum psychosis, and (4) primiparity.

10. Does postpartum depression recur?

Yes. Women with a history of postpartum depression have a 50% recurrence rate with the next pregnancy and even higher recurrence rates with each subsequent pregnancy.

11. Do patients with a history of postpartum psychiatric illness benefit from prophylactic treatments?

Yes. Recurrences may be significantly decreased with initiation of peripartum psychopharmacologic medication. Women with bipolar disorder, who are at significant risk for developing postpartum psychosis (50%), are less likely to suffer this serious complication if treated either during the pregnancy or just prior to delivery with mood-stabilizing medications.

12. What is known and recommended about the use of psychopharmacologic medication during lactation?

Facts

1. All psychopharmacologic medications are secreted into breast milk.

2. Lithium is the one drug that most experts agree is absolutely contraindicated in breast-feeding women.

3. True risks to the infant with respect to short- or long-term sequelae are not well-documented or understood.

4. Serum levels of psychopharmacologic agents in infants are often inaccurate.

5. Premature infants may be at more risk from medication exposure because of immature development of their kidneys and liver.

Recommendations

1. Decisions about use of psychopharmacologic medication during breast feeding involve a complicated risk/benefit analysis. The assessment should include the risk to the mother and infant when the psychiatric condition is treated or not treated and an exploration of alternative treatment methods and supports.

2. The pediatrician, obstetrician, internist, and psychiatrist should be involved in the decision-making process for optimal care.

3. If medication is used, care should include (1) careful monitoring of mother and infant, (2) use of lowest possible doses of medication, (3) use of medications with short half-lives and few or no active metabolites, and (4) possible adjustments of feeding schedule relative to peak and trough levels of medications.

13. What do studies show about the psychiatric sequelae of abortion? Which patients are at risk for developing psychiatric problems? What about caregivers?

Without making moral judgments, abortion is a life-changing event for many women. Some are little affected, whereas others may feel the effects for years. Most studies done in the 1970s and 1980s show relatively good psychological adjustment for the majority of women and indicate that serious negative emotions are usually transitory. Patients at risk for psychiatric illness following induced abortion include (1) those with prior psychiatric illness, (2) those pressured or coerced into undergoing the procedure, (3) those markedly ambivalent about the procedure, (4) those with fewer social supports, and (5) those who experience negative attitudes from caregivers. Because of the nature of the procedure, caregivers often have mixed emotions. Acknowledgment of these feelings and of concerns for safety in a politically-charged environment is often helpful.

14. What are the major hypotheses about the psychological reasons for teen-age pregnancy?

1. Some adolescents may consciously wish for a pregnancy to fill their own lives or their family's lives, whereas others may be trying to rebel against their parents and to separate from them.

2. Adolescents who become pregnant may have histories of truancy, running away, or drug and alcohol abuse and often are trying to escape poor social situations at home. Some of those confronted with such problems manage by taking over certain aspects of the household at an early age and becoming competent in the role of caretaker. Having a child fits into this mode of adaptation.

3. From a psychiatric perspective, as many as 8–10% of pregnant teenagers suffer from medically-diagnosable depression and may become pregnant in an effort, however misguided, to alleviate the depression. In addition, special categories of adolescents, victims of abuse, incest, and rape, and those with specific psychiatric illnesses or conditions, (i.e., schizophrenia or mental retardation)—are emotionally and physically vulnerable and at risk for unwanted pregnancies.

15. What is known about domestic violence in pregnancy? How can caregivers help?
   Facts

1. Prevalence rates for domestic violence reported during pregnancy range from 4–17%, with a 10% overall risk in the general population.

2. The most commonly struck area in pregnant women is the abdomen; in non-pregnant women, it is the face and head.

3. Abused patients tend to be younger and unmarried and to have higher rates of smoking, drug abuse, and psychiatric problems.

4. Most women do not tell their caregivers.

5. A history of abuse is a strong predictor of abuse during pregnancy.

6. Adverse effects of abuse include miscarriage, abruptio placentae, fetal loss, premature labor and delivery, and low birth weight.

7. Risk factors for men who abuse are ambivalence about the pregnancy, history of substance abuse, and social, psychological, and financial difficulties.

   How caregivers can help

1. By thoroughly questioning trauma patients about etiology

2. By having an open door and being willing to listen, because patients who initially deny the problem may return at future times for help

3. By having knowledge of community resources and referral systems for domestic violence victims.

16. What issues are involved in a pregnant woman's right to refuse treatment?

Treating pregnant women against their will has been a complicated and controversial issue in the 1980s and 1990s. Doctors, who are used to upholding the sanctity of life, can be put in a bind when they are caught between the fetus's well-being and the mother's health. The invitation of judicial involvement into medical decision-making can be a mixed blessing from both clinical and medicolegal perspectives. While court-ordered decisions should theoretically lend support to medical decisions, they may also raise a new standard of care that could possibly affect future litigation.

In recent years, decisions have gone against doctors who propose relatively invasive procedures such as cesarean sections. In these cases, courts have upheld the woman's right to autonomy over her own body, even at risk to the fetus or baby. Transfusions and less invasive interventions have fallen into a gray area.

17. What are the legal standards that determine competency when pregnant patients make decisions for themselves and their fetuses?

1. The ability to communicate
2. The ability to understand relevant information
3. The ability to appreciate the current situation and the consequences of various actions and interventions
4. The ability to manipulate the medical information in a rational way

Many decisions about competency are clear-cut and never reach court. Physicians often make bedside determinations and may use persuasion, family members, and other means to influence the process. The judicial process should be involved only as a last resort. When psychiatrists are involved at early stages in such cases, they may be able to help mediate decisions, steer cases to more collaborative conclusions, and avoid the adversarial nature of court proceedings.

BIBLIOGRAPHY

1. American Academy of Pediatrics Committee on Drugs: The transfer of drugs and other chemicals into human milk. Pediatrics 93:137–149, 1994.
2. Applebaum P, Grisso T: Assessing patients' capacities to consent to treatment. N Engl J Med 319:1635–1638, 1988.
3. Blumenthal SJ: Psychiatric consequences of abortion: Overview of research findings. In Stotland NL (ed): Psychiatric Aspects of Abortion. Washington, DC, American Psychiatric Press, 1991.
4. Brazleton TB, Cramer BG (eds): The Earliest Relationship: Parents, Infants, and the Drama of Early Attachment. Boston, Addison-Wesley, 1990.
5. Cohen LS, Rosenbaum JF, Heller VH: Psychotropic drug use in pregnancy. In Gelenberg AJ, Bassuk EL, Schoonover SC (eds): The Practitioner's Guide to Psychoactive Drugs. New York, Plenum, 1991.
6. Freedman R, Gladstein B: Surviving Pregnancy Loss. Boston, Little, Brown, 1982.
7. Hamburg B: Subsets of adolescent mothers: Developmental, biomedical, and psychosocial issues. In Lancaster JB (ed): School-Age Pregnancy and Parenthood. New York, Aldine di Gruyter, 1986.
8. Kolder EB, et al: Court ordered obstetrical interventions. N Engl J Med 316:1192–1196, 1987.
9. Mahlstedt P: The psychological component of infertility. Fertil Steril 43:335–346, 1985.
10. Nadelson C: "Normal" and "special" aspects of pregnancy. In Notman M, Nadelson C (eds): A Psychosocial Approach to the Woman Patient, vol. 1. New York, Plenum, 1978.
11. Newberger EH, Barkin S, McCormack M, et al: Abuse of pregnant women and adverse birth outcome. JAMA 17:2370–2372, 1992.
12. Notman MT: Reproduction and pregnancy: A psycho-dynamic developmental perspective. In Stotland NL (ed): Psychiatric Aspects of Reproductive Technology. Washington, DC, American Psychiatric Press, 1990, pp 13–24.
13. O'Hara MW: Postpartum mental disorders. In Sciarra JJ (ed): Gynecology and Obstetrics, vol. 6. New York, Harper and Row, 1991.
14. Rosenthal M: Psychiatric aspects of infertility and the assisted reproductive technologies. In Greenfield D (ed): Infertility and Reproductive Medicine Clinics of North America. Philadelphia, W.B. Saunders, 1993, pp 455–477.
15. Sichel DA: Psychiatric issues of the post partum period: An interview with Deborah A. Sichel, M.D. Curr Affect Ill 11(10):4–12, 1992.
16. Solnit AJ, Stark MH: Mourning and the birth of a defective child. Psychoanalytic Study of the Child 16:523–527, 1961.
17. Stowe ZN, Nemeroff CB: Psychopharmacology during pregnancy and lactation. In The American Psychiatric Press Textbook of Psychopharmacology. Washington, DC, American Psychiatric Press, 1995.
18. Stewart D, Stotland N: Psychological Aspects of Women's Health Care. Washington, DC, American Psychiatric Press, 1993.
19. Stewart D, Cecutti A: Physical abuse in pregnancy. Can Med Assoc 149:1257–1263, 1993.
20. Wolreich MM: Psychiatric aspects of high-risk pregnancy. Psychiatr Clin North Am 10:53–68, 1986.

57. SURGICAL DISEASE IN PREGNANCY

Mark D. Iafrati, M.D., and Craig E. Haug, M.D.

1. Should surgical procedures, especially abdominal operations, be avoided during pregnancy and postponed until the postpartum period?

Yes and no. Certainly elective operations should be postponed to avoid any possible risk of drug teratogenicity, radiation exposure, or anesthetic complications. Potentially semielective conditions (e.g., cholecystitis) should be delayed until the second trimester, if possible. However, acute surgical conditions must be dealt with perhaps even more expeditiously than normally. As many as 2% of pregnant women undergo nonobstetric surgical procedures each year.

2. Why is there often a delay in diagnosing acute abdominal conditions during pregnancy? How does pregnancy change the interpretation of the abdominal exam?

The symptoms of an acute abdominal process often can be mistaken for the numerous gastrointestinal alterations associated with a normal pregnancy (nausea, emesis, epigastric pain, constipation, and lower abdominal cramping). The gravid uterus displaces everything cephalad, placing the appendix in the right mid or upper quadrant rather than the right lower quadrant. Peritonitis is often more subtle, possibly because of stretching of the abdominal wall muscles. Obviously, abdominal distention is masked by the background distention of the uterus.

3. Do older pregnant women have more surgical complications?

No. Important peripartum maternal **surgical** complications are no more frequent in pregnant women aged 35 years or more than in women 20–34 years old. The incidence of **medical** complications, on the other hand, is probably increased in the older parous patient.

4. Should radiologic studies be withheld during pregnancy?

No. The value of the information obtained generally outweighs the relatively small risk associated with diagnostic radiation exposure during any trimester. Precautions should include fetal shielding and minimizing the number of films obtained.

5. What are the relative risks of diagnostic radiation exposure during pregnancy?

Teratogenic risks. Of most concern is first-trimester exposure. Animal and human data agree that < 10 rads to the fetus does not significantly increase the risk of congenital malformation.

Cancer risks. Some studies report a twofold increase in childhood leukemia and some solid tumors in children with in utero radiation exposure.

The following are the fetal exposures:

Chest	0.008 rads	Barium enema	0.80 rads
Abdomen	0.30 rads	Lumbosacral spine	0.3 rads
Upper GI series	0.60 rads	Abdominal/pelvic CT	0.25–2.25 rads
Intravenous pyelography	0.60 rads		

6. Marked changes in maternal physiology mandate certain perioperative precautions. What are they?

Left lateral tilt. A tilt of at least 15° helps to prevent the maternal and fetal hypotension that results when the gravid uterus decreases venous return by compressing the inferior vena cava.

Adequate preoxygenation before intubation. Preoxygenation can compensate for the decreased pulmonary functional residual capacity noted especially during the third trimester.

Elevated minute ventilation. Increased tidal volume and respiratory rate raise minute ventilation by as much as 50% by the 7th–8th month.

Avoidance of vasodilation. Using anesthetic agents that have the least effect on the maternal vascular system can help to ensure a constant placental perfusion.

Perioperative antacids. Pregnancy predisposes to reduced esophageal sphincter tone, increasing the risk of aspiration—the lower the gastric pH, the worse the chemical pneumonitis.

Reduction of thromboembolic risks. Prophylactic heparin 2 hours preoperatively (7,500–10,000 units 2 times/day subcutaneously) or pneumatic compression stockings can help to reduce the risk of deep venous thrombosis exacerbated by bed rest and the hypercoagulability of pregnancy.

7. Does the surgical procedure itself, even an abdominal operation, precipitate labor?

No. Most investigators believe that the severity of the condition requiring operation, maternal cardiovascular collapse, and peritonitis are the major contributors to preterm labor following operative procedures. Although the use of prophylactic tocolytic agents is not recommended by all obstetricians, if preterm labor is a perioperative problem, tocolysis should be instituted.

8. How can fetal well-being be established during a surgical procedure?

In all pregnancies, fetal heart tones should be recorded before the operation, preferably by ultrasound in order to avoid confusion with the maternal pulse. In gestations > 24 weeks, some advocate the intraoperative use of fetal external cardiac monitoring.

9. What is the most common nonobstetric surgical procedure performed during pregnancy?

Appendectomy. This procedure is done with the same frequency in pregnant as in nonpregnant women, and there seems to be no predilection for any trimester. The perforation rate is significantly increased, however, during the third trimester because of delay in diagnosis and the relative immunosuppression of pregnancy.

10. How does the surgical management of appendicitis differ in pregnancy?

Most studies advocate a lower threshold of suspicion and thus an earlier laparotomy because of the relatively low morbidity of a negative laparotomy, even during pregnancy, vs. the 1% maternal mortality and the 35% fetal mortality with perforated appendices (as opposed to 10% fetal mortality for nonperforated appendicitis). The incision of choice is generally muscle splitting over the point of maximal tenderness. Alternatively, a laparoscopic approach may be used. Adjunct cesarean section even for the term infant is not generally recommended.

11. What is Alder's sign? When is it helpful?

Alder's sign seeks to differentiate abdominal from uterine pathology. The maximal point of tenderness is identified with the patient in a supine position. The patient is then placed in a left lateral tilt, effectively displacing the gravid uterus to the far left, and the point of tenderness is again located. Uterine pain, such as from fibroid degeneration or adnexal torsion, tends to move with the uterus, whereas pain from an inflamed appendix more often favors a constant position.

12. Do any abdominal conditions improve during pregnancy?

Peptic ulcer disease often improves during pregnancy secondary to a reduction in gastric acid secretion. Incarceration of inguinal or femoral hernias occurs less commonly during late pregnancy. Although increased abdominal pressure seems to exacerbate this condition, the third-trimester uterus sufficiently fills the lower abdomen, preventing passage of the small bowel into the hernia sac.

13. Which surgical conditions occur more commonly when the uterus is undergoing rapid changes in position and size, such as during the second trimester or after delivery?

Adnexal torsion. This condition is most prevalent when an adnexal mass exists. Peritoneal inflammation can be produced and significant hemorrhage can be concealed.

Intestinal obstruction. Adhesions secondary to previous pelvic surgery (including cesarean section) can incarcerate loops of small bowel as the uterus enlarges.

14. Left upper quadrant (LUQ) pain without associated trauma is an unusual complaint during pregnancy but warrants serious consideration. Which two conditions presenting with LUQ pain occur with increased frequency during pregnancy?

Splenic rupture. Pregnancy is second only to malaria as a predisposing factor for spontaneous splenic rupture. Both hypervolemia and relative anemia contribute to hypersplenism, thus increasing the risk for spontaneous rupture.

Splenic artery aneurysm rupture. 25% of cases of this rare but catastrophic event occur in pregnant women. Both pregnancy-induced hypersplenism and moderate displacement of the spleen by the gravid uterus are believed to compromise already diseased vessels. LUQ tenderness, peritoneal irritation, and shock necessitate immediate operative exploration. However, despite aggressive intervention with splenectomy, fetal and maternal mortality remains high.

15. Right upper quadrant (RUQ) pain is a relatively common complaint during pregnancy and signals a variety of possible diseases. Name two surgical conditions and two medical conditions.

Cholecystitis. Treatment is identical to that in the nonpregnant female. Laparoscopic cholecystectomy, preferably during the second trimester, is the treatment of choice. If common bile duct stones are present, endoscopic retrograde cholangiopancreatography with sphincterotomy is followed by laparoscopic cholecystectomy.

Hepatic capsule rupture. Rarely diagnosed preoperatively, this emergent condition should be considered in patients with severe preeclampsia who experience increasing RUQ pain in association with cardiovascular instability and peritoneal signs.

Hepatitis. Symptoms are similar to those in the nonpregnant female. Supportive analgesia, adequate hydration, and treatment of the infant with gamma globulin and vaccine at delivery are indicated.

Pyelonephritis. Transmission of pain to the RUQ from an inflamed kidney is not unusual during pregnancy. Closer clinical examination usually documents right costovertebral tenderness on percussion. Renal stones also should be considered in the differential of patients with such symptoms.

16. What minimally invasive (laparoscopic) general surgical techniques are currently used in pregnant women?

Cholecystectomy and appendectomy.

17. Has the introduction of the laparoscopic approach to cholecystectomy changed either the indications for or the timing of cholecystectomy during pregnancy?

No and no. The indications for cholecystectomy are not affected by the route of access to the abdomen; they are neither more nor less liberal. Timing is also unaltered; cholecystectomy (laparoscopic or open) is ideally performed in the second trimester (negative fetal effects minimized). Beyond 20 weeks' gestation, as the fundus extends above the umbilicus, a laparoscopic approach becomes increasingly difficult and may necessitate an open cholecystectomy.

18. What are the adverse effects of CO_2 pneumoperitoneum on a pregnant patient? How may these be treated?

Pressure effects: CO_2 insufflation creates a pseudopregnancy from the standpoint of pressure effects (increased vagal tone, decreased venous return, impaired pulmonary mechanics). Obviously, these effects are compounded in someone already experiencing them from a real pregnancy. Reverse Trendelenberg employed during laparoscopic cholecystectomy may further exacerbate decreased venous return. Fortunately, routine positioning also incorporates a left lateral tilt to improve gallbladder visibility. This maneuver rotates not only the intestines off the gallbladder but also the uterus off the vena cava, thereby improving venous return. Further compensatory measures depend on the anesthesiologist.

Chemical effects: Although proper mechanical ventilation can usually control CO_2 excretion, inadvertent hypercarbia and respiratory acidosis either intra- or postoperatively may result in dysrhythmias, increased peripheral resistance, elevated central venous pressure, and catecholamine release. Again, an anesthesiologist alert to such dangers is the best protection. The use of alternative gases such as helium is under study.

Nonpressurized technique: A new technique involving the use of an abdominal wall lifting device ("laparolift") is gaining popularity for use in the pregnant patient. The lifting device maintains a laparoscopic operative field, obviating the need for a pressurized pneumoperitoneum of any kind. This technique could potentially eliminate all pressure and chemical related complications.

19. True or false: Primary hyperparathyroidism during pregnancy is associated with high fetal morbidity and should usually be treated surgically.

True. Maternal hypercalcemia results in fetal hypercalcemia, leading to suppression of fetal parathyroid gland function and neonatal hypocalcemia with tetany after birth when maternal calcium flow is interrupted. Hyperparathyroidism characterized by progressive symptoms should be treated surgically, preferably during the second trimester. Symptom-free patients and patients with mild hypercalcemia diagnosed in the third trimester may be managed medically, postponing operation until after delivery.

20. True or false: Breast cancer in the pregnant patient is more aggressive and mandates a different approach in pregnant and nonpregnant patients.

False. There is no evidence that carcinoma of the breast in pregnant women is biologically different from carcinoma of the breast in other premenopausal women, and recent reports suggest similar long-term survival rates. Preoperative staging (including mammography), operation, and postoperative adjuvant therapy should proceed normally. Some advocate mastectomy over lumpectomy in this setting to avoid the radiotherapy required after breast conservation surgery. Management of the fetus is controversial, with some recommending abortion or induction, depending on how advanced the pregnancy is.

BIBLIOGRAPHY

1. Baillie J, Cairns SR, Putman WS, Cotton PB: Endoscopic management of choledocholithiasis during pregnancy. Surg Gynecol Obstet 171:1–4, 1990.
2. Barnavon Y, Wallack MK: Management of the pregnant patient with carcinoma of the breast. Surg Gynecol Obstet 171:347–352, 1990.
3. Iafrati MD, Yarnell R, Schwaitzberg SD: Gasless laparoscopic cholecystectomy in pregnancy. J Laparoendoscop Surg 5:127–130, 1995.
4. Kort B, Katz VL, Watson WJ: The effect of nonobstetric operation during pregnancy. Surg Gynecol Obstet 177:371–376, 1993.
5. Lowe T, Cunningham I: Surgical diseases complicating pregnancy. In Cunningham FG, et al (eds): Williams Obstetrics and Supplement. Norwalk, CT, Appleton & Lange, 1990.
6. Morrell DG, Mullins JR, Harrison PB: Laparoscopic cholecystectomy during pregnancy in symptomatic patients. Surgery 112:856–859, 1992.
7. Slater G, Aufses A: Surgical aspects of pregnancy. In Cherry S, Berkowitz R, Kase N (eds): Medical Surgical and Gynecologic Complications in Pregnancy. Baltimore, Williams & Wilkins, 1984.

58. TRAUMA IN PREGNANCY

Craig Haug, M.D., and Louise Wilkins-Haug, M.D., Ph.D.

1. Is trauma an important issue in pregnant women?

Yes. Trauma is the leading cause of death in women 15–45 years of age in the United States. Trauma complicates 6–7% of all pregnancies and accounts for about 50% of all maternal mortality compared with about 20% due to complications of pregnancy, labor, and delivery. By the third trimester, minor trauma occurs more often than at any other time during adult life. Perinatal mortality associated with minor trauma is 0.5%, rising to 61% with major trauma and to 80% when shock is part of the presentation.

2. Should the use of seat belts be avoided during pregnancy, especially the third trimester?

No. Both lap belts and shoulder harnesses significantly reduce ejection from the motor vehicle during an accident, thus lowering maternal mortality and subsequent fetal demise. However, concern about lap belts placed improperly across rather than below the third trimester uterus is justified because deceleration injury may compress the fetus against the sacrum. Proper use of a 3-point shoulder harness is advocated.

3. True or false: The obstetrician is a secondary member of the trauma team in the pregnant trauma patient.

False. The obstetrician has unique expertise that plays a vital role in minimizing morbidity and mortality to both mother and fetus.

4. When the trauma patient is pregnant, are initial resuscitation priorities altered?

No. The most common cause of fetal demise is maternal death. Conversely, the best chance for fetal survival is maternal survival by expedient maternal resuscitation (airway, breathing, circulation). Only in the case of an entirely stable mother or a mother who cannot be saved do management priorities revert to the fetus.

5. In hypovolemic shock, is the fetus treated by the maternal system as a vital organ along with the brain and heart?

No. Hemorrhagic shock and catecholamine release cause uterine artery vasoconstriction, putting the fetus squarely in the expendable category along with other peripheral organs. In fact the fetus may serve as a blood reservoir to stave off maternal hypotension. Although seemingly unmaternal, it is nature's recognition that the best chance for fetus survival and species propagation is a mother's survival.

6. From the perspective of the mother, if she is to sustain penetrating trauma, is it advantageous to be pregnant?

Yes. The enlarged uterus acts to shield the abdominal contents, resulting in a decreased injury rate to intraabdominal organs and lower maternal mortality. There have been no reported maternal deaths from gunshot wounds of the uterus since 1912. Conversely, the fetus fares less well, with penetrating trauma resulting in a 60–80% injury rate and a 40–70% mortality rate.

7. What are the mechanisms of fetal demise in blunt trauma? In penetrating trauma?

Fetal demise in blunt trauma may result from placental abruption, uterine rupture, or rupture of membranes with subsequent preterm delivery. In penetrating trauma, uterine perforation with fetal injury, placental laceration, or cord damage may occur. Maternal death is the most common cause of fetal demise in both blunt and penetrating trauma.

WORK-UP

8. Can the pregnant patient be assessed and treated just like any other trauma patient?

No. The gravid uterus is at risk from even seemingly minor trauma necessitating an early aggressive posture. In addition, the pregnant trauma patient has a host of anatomic and physiologic alterations in every organ system that may mimic pathologic conditions or mask the signs of shock.

Anemia. A hematocrit of 35% may appear like blood loss but is physiologic for pregnancy.

Hypervolemia. Patients can lose more blood before hypotension is clinically significant and require more volume to resuscitate.

Anatomy. The gravid uterus bullies everything in its way, displacing abdominal organs and the diaphragm upward, thus changing the interpretation of the exam and the pattern of injuries seen.

9. Should a pregnant trauma patient presenting with seizures be assumed to have an intracranial injury and be sent for a CT scan?

Yes and no. Eclampsia can cause seizures and seizures can lead to automobile accidents. Although an intracranial injury is always possible and should be ruled out, magnesium sulfate therapy for toxemia should be initiated until the diagnosis is established.

10. In addition to the usual work-up for trauma patients, what key additional facts must be established in the pregnant patient?

1. Estimation of fetal age by history, last menstrual period (LMP), clinical exam, and ultrasound.

2. Assessment of fetal cardiac activity (preferably by ultrasound initially, then on external cardiac monitor).

3. Cervical examination for dilation, rupture of membranes, and bleeding.

4. Evaluation for placental abruption with Kleihauer-Betke test, screening for disseminated intravascular coagulation (DIC), and ultrasound looking for a retroplacental clot.

11. What are the most common complications after blunt abdominal trauma? How are they best evaluated?

The two most common complications are premature uterine contractions (67%) and abruptio placentae (11%). Abruptio placentae complicates 1–5% of minor injuries and 40–50% of major injuries. Both uterine rupture and direct fetal injury are uncommon (< 1% each). When used together, external fetal monitoring (EFM) and fetal ultrasound (US) identify most complications within 6 hours of admission.

12. What is the role of diagnostic peritoneal lavage (DPL) in the gravid patient?

Although the issue is controversial, most trauma surgeons respect the 98% accuracy rate of DPL and use DPL in pregnant patients as long as an open supraumbilical technique is used. If the patient is relatively stable, CT is another option. CT is less invasive, provides injury-specific data, is superior for evaluation of retroperitoneal injuries, and provides a simultaneous intravenous pyelogram and C-loop. However, it exposes the patient to radiation, and its sensitivity is still controversial. Ultrasound is increasingly used in the trauma setting, especially in pregnant patients, to avoid exposure to radiation. With advances in technique and equipment, ultrasound may eventually supplant DPL.

MANAGEMENT

13. Maternal left lateral positioning prevents the supine hypotension syndrome of pregnancy and reduced placental perfusion. Should this positioning be attempted only after the maternal cardiovascular status has been stabilized?

No. Fetal hypotension is caused by maternal hypotension secondary to inferior vena cava (IVC) compression. Furthermore, IVC syndrome increases venous pressures in the lower extremities and can exacerbate blood loss in traumatized limbs. If the patient must remain supine (e.g., suspected spinal injury or ongoing CPR), manual deflection of the uterus to the left with a hand and placement of a wedge under the patient's hip usually suffice.

14. Should military antishock trousers (MAST) be used to treat shock in the pregnant trauma patient?

The abdominal portion of the suit should not be inflated, as this may further compress the IVC. The leg portion may be useful, especially in splinting fractures of the lower extremity.

15. Should cardiovascular resuscitation in hypotensive pregnant women include vasopressors to maintain a systolic blood pressure of > 90?

No. Aggressive volume expansion constitutes the mainstay of therapy. Vasopressors are not used in the trauma patient, pregnant or not.

16. Are the indications for laparotomy after blunt abdominal trauma different in pregnant and nonpregnant women?

Yes and no. As in any patient, laparotomy is indicated for overt peritonitis, massive hemoperitoneum, positive DPL, or significant injury on CT (hollow viscus or major solid organ). In pregnant patients additional potential indications include uterine rupture, placental abruption, fetal distress or bloody amniocentesis.

17. How should the uterus be dealt with during a laparotomy?

If the uterus is not injured, it should be left intact and gently packed out of the way. If the uterus is involved, it should be repaired or removed if deemed unsalvageable.

18. Does pregnancy change the management of stab wounds?

Controversial. The standard management protocol limits laparotomy to patients with peritoneal violation and positive DPL. In pregnant trauma patients, some advocate even further restriction of the use of exploratory laparotomy, especially in lower abdominal injury, as the gravid uterus displaces all but the bladder out of the lower abdomen. If the fetus is stable and retrograde cystoscopy is normal, observation may be adequate.

19. What are the indications for cesarean section during trauma laparotomy?
- Uterine damage—vessel or extensive uterine lacerations may threaten the well-being of the fetus and the mother if left unrepaired
- Mechanical limitation of gravid uterus, compromising maternal repair
- Risk of fetal distress exceeds risk of prematurity
- Unstable thoracolumbar spinal injury with fetal maturity
- Persistent maternal shock

Note: Fetal death is *not* an indication for cesarean section.

20. Is penetration of the uterus (with fetal injury or leak of amniotic fluid into the peritoneal cavity) an indication for cesarean section?

Not necessarily. Rupture of membranes due to a penetrating uterine injury may seal over, and infection is not inevitable. Likewise, fetal injury, if not severe and occurring at < 30 weeks' gestation, does not require immediate delivery, as the fetus may heal in utero. If > 30 weeks' gestation, the risks from prematurity are probably lower than those resulting from the complications of unrepaired fetal injury.

21. Is cesarean section indicated in the near-term trauma patient to avoid dehiscence during labor from a fresh midline laparotomy incision?

No. Vaginal delivery is well tolerated even in the early postoperative period.

22. Do pelvic fractures during pregnancy necessitate delivery by cesarean section?

No. However, there are some exceptions, and cases should be individualized. Approximately 10% require operative delivery based on pelvic deformity and instability. Some obstetricians advocate cesarean section when maternal fractures have occurred within 8 weeks of delivery because of inadequate healing time. Fractures involving the symphysis pubis should be closely evaluated for stability, as the bladder and urethra may be at risk of injury by compression from the descending fetal head.

23. What are the indications for trauma hysterectomy?

Uterine repair not only preserves fertility but is usually the quickest and safest route. However, hysterectomy may be indicated when (1) even the empty uterus interferes with exposure and repair of other injuries, (2) there is severe uterine or broad ligament bleeding despite bilateral hypogastric and ovarian artery ligation, or (3) there is severe contamination.

24. What are the indications for perimortem cesarean section?

Maternal death and (1) the fetus has reached a gestational age considered to be viable by the available neonatal nursery and (2) the fetal ultrasound is either positive or indeterminate for cardiac activity.

25. How long after maternal cardiac arrest can perimortem cesarean section be performed?

Within 5 minutes of cardiac arrest, results are very good, but dismal if delayed > 15 minutes. The case may be made for cesarean delivery *for maternal benefit* after 5 minutes in order to facilitate resuscitative efforts.

26. In addition to the usual causes of acute respiratory distress syndrome (ARDS) in trauma patients, what additional factors may play a role in pregnancy?

Amniotic fluid embolism caused by amniotic fluid or trophoblastic debris entering the venous circulation through subplacental sinusoids. Although rare, this complication has a 50% immediate mortality and another 25% delayed mortality. Death is usually secondary to cor pulmonale, and treatment is unsatisfactory.

27. True or false: Consideration should be given to administering Rh D immunoglobulin to all unsensitized, Rh-negative pregnant trauma patients.

True. The incidence of fetal-maternal hemorrhage is raised fivefold with trauma.

BIBLIOGRAPHY

1. Buchsbaum HJ: Accidental injury complicating pregnancy. Am J Obstet Gynecol 102:752–769, 1968.
2. Crosby WM, Costiloe JP: Safety of lap-restraint for pregnant victims of automobile collisions. N Engl J Med 12:632–636, 1971.
3. Drost TF, Rosemurgy AS, Sherman HF, et al: Major trauma in pregnant women: Maternal/fetal outcome. J Trauma 30:574–578, 1990.
4. Hoff WS, D'Amelio LF, Tinkoff GH, et al: Maternal predictors of fetal demise in trauma during pregnancy. Surg Gynecol Obstet 172:175–180, 1991.
5. Katz VL, Dotters DJ, Drogemueller W: Perimortem cesarean delivery. Obstet Gynecol 68:571–576, 1986.
6. McKenney M, Lentz K, Nunez D, et al: Can ultrasound replace diagnostic peritoneal lavage in the assessment of blunt trauma? J Trauma 37:439–441, 1994.
7. Pearlman MD, Tintinalli JE, Lorenz RP: A prospective controlled study of outcome after trauma during pregnancy. Am J Obstet Gynecol 162:1502–1507, 1990.
8. Towery R, English TP, Wisner D: Evaluation of pregnant women after blunt injury. J Trauma 35:731–735; discussion, 735–736, 1993.

VI. The Fetus

59. TWIN PREGNANCY

Nina M. Boe, M.D., and John G. McFee, M.D.

1. How often do twins occur?

Twins occur in 1 of 100 pregnancies among white women, 1 of 80 pregnancies in black women, and in only 1 of 155 pregnancies in Asian women. Monozygotic twins occur in 1 in 250 births and are independent of race, heredity, age, and parity. Dizygotic (DZ) twinning, however, is affected by each of these factors and also by fertility drugs. A woman who is a DZ twin is twice as likely to give birth to DZ twins. Assisted reproductive technologies also increase the rate of multiple gestations, with a 20–40% rate with gonadotropin induction of ovulation and a 7–13% rate with clomiphene (Clomid) therapy. Additionally, women undergoing in vitro fertilization often have multiple embryos replaced into the uterus; of such pregnancies that reach viability, 22% are multiple.

2. What are the mechanisms that lead to identical twins?

Identical or monozygotic (MZ) twins arise from division of one fertilized ovum into two separate embryos. The timing of this division has important implications.

Division within the first 72 hours after conception results in a **diamniotic, dichorionic (di/di)** monozygotic twin pregnancy. As neither the inner cell mass nor the outer layer of blastocyst (destined to become chorion) has formed, each embryo will have a separate amnion and chorion. This occurs in about 30% of MZ twins and has the lowest mortality rate—about 9%.

Division 4–8 days after fertilization results in a **diamniotic, monochorionic (di/mono)** twin pregnancy. As the amnion is not yet differentiated, separate amniotic sacs but shared chorion will result. This is the most frequent type of monozygotic twinning (68%), and in some series the mortality rate is as high as 25% due to complications of vascular anastomoses within the placentas.

Division 8–13 days after fertilization results in **monoamniotic, monochorionic (mono/ mono)** twins. These MZ twins occur least often (2% or less) but have the highest mortality rate— up to 50%.

Division at 2 weeks after fertilization, after the amniotic sac and embryonic disk are formed but division of the embryonic disk is incomplete, results in **conjoined** twins. The frequency of conjoined twins is not well established but is on the order of 1 in 60,000 births.

3. What mechanisms lead to fraternal twins?

Fraternal or dizygotic twins arise from the fertilization of two separate ova. **Superfecundation** refers to fertilization of different ova in the same menstrual cycle, at two separate episodes of intercourse. **Superfetation** occurs when two ova are fertilized during separate menstrual cycles, i.e., the second ovulation occurred after the first pregnancy was established; this is rare.

4. How does examination of the placenta help to establish zygosity?

Twins of the opposite sex (barring genetic abnormalities) are always dizygotic; placental examination reveals zygosity in cases of like-sex twins. Determination is based on the chorion/amnion status described in question 2. **Histologic evaluation of the membranes** as they join the body of the placenta at the so-called "T-section" (transverse section) may be needed to establish the presence of one or two chorions. Demonstration of **vascular anastomoses** by injection of milk or dye through the vessels may reveal communications between the placentas and also indicates MZ twinning. In indeterminate situations, zygosity can be established by blood types and chromosomal or DNA polymorphisms.

5. How does ultrasound help to establish zygosity?
    If fetal gender can be identified on ultrasound, twins of opposite sex are almost always dizygotic. If the separating membrane between the twins measures > 2 mm in thickness, the pregnancy is probably dichorionic.

6. What characteristics of multiple gestations distinguish them from singleton pregnancies?
    Preterm delivery: close to 50% are premature (born before 37 weeks). Prematurity is the most common cause of neonatal morbidity and mortality in multiple gestations. Overall, twins account for about 10% of all premature infants. The mean length of gestation in twins is 35 weeks and in triplets is 33 weeks.
    Intrauterine growth restriction (IUGR): up to two-thirds of twins. Although twin growth is similar to singleton gestations up to 30–32 weeks, after that point, a falloff in the growth rate can be expected. Growth restriction may occur in one or both fetuses. Asymmetric or discordant growth is identified in 10–25% of twin pregnancies and carries a higher perinatal mortality. IUGR in multiple gestations may be caused by placental insufficiency, velamentous cord insertion, and twin–twin transfusion as well as all intrinsic fetal conditions affecting a singleton pregnancy. IUGR is more common in MZ twins.
    Perinatal mortality: averaging 5 times higher than singletons. The risk is higher for MZ twins and twins displaying discordant growth. The largest single cause of perinatal death, however, is prematurity. Twins are responsible for 25% of preterm perinatal deaths and 10% of all perinatal mortality. In addition to prematurity, etiologies include congenital malformations, twin–twin transfusion syndrome, uteroplacental insufficiency, and birth trauma or hypoxia.
    Spontaneous abortion: at least twice as often as singleton pregnancies. With increasing use of ultrasound, early abortion or resorption of one twin—the "vanishing twin syndrome"—has been observed to occur more frequently than recognized clinically. It is estimated that only 50% of twins diagnosed by ultrasound in the early first trimester continue as such until delivery.
    Congenital malformations: twice as frequent, increased risk confined to MZ sets.
    Pregnancy-induced hypertension: 3–5 times more often in multiple gestations with increasing frequency correlated with higher order gestations; apt to occur earlier in pregnancy and to be more severe as compared with singleton pregnancies. It occurs with equal frequency in MZ and DZ twin pregnancies.
    Anemia: due to iron deficiency because of increased fetal requirements. Rarely, megaloblastic anemia from folic acid deficiency occurs. Additionally, physiologic dilution from plasma volume expansion contributes.
    Polyhydramnios: in one or both sacs, to a greater or lesser degree in 5–8% of twin pregnancies overall. It tends to be more common in MZ sets, usually from the twin–twin transfusion syndrome.
    Fetal malpresentation at birth: one of the main factors leading to more frequent cesarean delivery of twins.
    Abruptio placentae: may occur with the sudden decompression of the uterus immediately after delivery of the first twin.
    Placenta previa: the placenta occupies a much larger area of the uterine cavity than in singleton pregnancies.

7. What are the risks from placental vascular anastomoses in a monochorial placenta?
    The twin–twin transfusion syndrome occurs when one placenta is fed by an artery from the first twin and drained by a vein that leads to the second twin. This syndrome develops in 15% of MZ sets and varies in severity. In its full-blown picture, the donor twin is hypoperfused, anemic,

undergrown, hypotensive, and develops oligohydramnios. The oligohydramnios may be so severe that the donor twin appears "stuck." On the other hand, the hyperperfused twin is polycythemic; has hypertension, cardiac hypertrophy and edema; and develops polyhydramnios. Moderate and severe twin–twin transfusion syndrome usually manifests before 28 weeks' gestation. The hallmark is a rapidly expanding uterus with polyhydramnios and discordant fetal growth. Perinatal mortality is high—70–80% if diagnosed before 28 weeks. If one fetus dies, significant problems may occur in the remaining twin, such as multicystic encephalomalacia and renal cortical necrosis. Current theory holds that such defects result from significant hypotension, as the living twin loses blood to the dead twin through placental vascular anastomoses, rather than embolic events. The placentas in twin–twin transfusion syndrome often reflect the difference in perfusion between two twins. The recipient placenta has a more plethoric appearance and is larger, whereas the donor placenta appears pale and somewhat smaller.

8. How are twin–twin transfusion syndromes managed?

Management begins with **ultrasound documentation** of discordant fetal growth (> 20% of the larger fetus's weight) and amniotic fluid volumes in monochorial twins. In the third trimester, pregnancies are followed by **serial ultrasounds and nonstress tests** for fetal well-being. **Daily fetal movement charts** should be kept by the patient, who may note decreased fetal movement in the donor twin due to the oligohydramnios. If fetal hydrops develops, delivery by **cesarean section** should be considered. Gestational age and the effect of the syndrome on the other twin influence the timing of delivery.

Polyhydramnios in the recipient twin may cause preterm labor due to distention of the uterus. **Therapeutic amniocentesis** to remove excessive amniotic fluid may help and often must be repeated at frequent intervals as the fluid rapidly reaccumulates. It is important to remove excessive fluid slowly, because rapid decompression may increase the risk of abruption.

Fetoscopic laser coagulation of the communicating placental vessels is a promising new technique to treat twin–twin transfusion syndrome. It is available only in a few centers. **Selective fetocide** of the smaller infant with umbilical cord occlusion is also under study.

9. What are the principles of prenatal care for twin pregnancies?

1. Early diagnosis is associated with an improved perinatal outcome.
2. Frequent antenatal visits, at least every 2 weeks from 20–36 weeks.
3. Diet: additional calories (+300 kcal/day) and protein (to 80 gm/day); 60–100 mg/day of iron supplementation; folic acid, 1 mg/day.
4. Extra bedrest.
5. Prevent, recognize, and aggressively treat preterm labor.
6. Follow fetal growth by serial ultrasound examinations to detect discordant growth and IUGR; manage accordingly.
7. Watch for and treat pregnancy-induced hypertension and preeclampsia.
8. Watch for and manage less common complications: polyhydramnios, twin–twin transfusion syndrome, intrauterine death.
9. Have parents make plans for two babies at home.

10. How can preterm delivery be prevented?

One must anticipate a higher incidence of preterm labor with twins because of increased uterine distention. Because of the well-known substantial morbidity and mortality from prematurity in multiple gestation, a major effort should be devoted to its prevention. The overall objective, in the absence of other problems, is to achieve 34 weeks' gestation, beyond which poor outcomes owing to prematurity are unusual. The critical period for these efforts is between 24 and 32 weeks.

Bed rest, hospitalization, prophylactic oral tocolytic drugs (beta-mimetics), routine weekly cervical examination, and prophylactic cerclage have been promoted as measures to prolong twin gestation. None of these is consistently effective in reducing the rate of preterm delivery in twins.

Results of programs for early detection of preterm labor through frequent contact with health care providers and education of the patient have been mixed. The use of home uterine activity monitoring to identify uterine contractions more recently has been advocated. However, this is an expensive intervention, and the results of studies of its efficacy in reducing preterm delivery are conflicting. Many believe that the improved outcomes with such monitoring are related more to the intensified contact with trained nurses than to monitoring itself.

11. How is the management of preterm labor different for multiple gestations?

Intervention is similar to a singleton pregnancy with additional consideration of the altered maternal physiologic characteristics of multiple pregnancy. Plasma volume with twins exceeds that of normal pregnancy (as much as 50–60% of the nonpregnant state vs. 45%), and cardiac output (heart rate and stroke volume) is increased over that of a singleton gestation. Such changes pose a special risk with intravenous fluids and beta-mimetic tocolytics. Pulmonary edema and other cardiac problems are seen more often with tocolysis of twin gestation, which dictates that tocolytic agents be used with caution. It may be best to use magnesium sulfate as the initial to-colytic drug. The use of nifedipine or indomethacin in patients who fail magnesium sulfate may be successful. Steroid therapy (betamethasone or dexamethasone) to accelerate fetal lung maturity should be administered to patients with documented preterm labor between 24–34 weeks' gestation.

12. How should parents of multiple gestations plan for the future?

The diagnosis of twins usually comes as a shock to most parents, especially the mother. Increasing physical discomfort causes difficulty in performing the usual household chores, caring for other children in the family, and continuing with employment. At home following delivery, the reality of caring for two babies at once, especially if they are premature and/or have other medical problems, is a real challenge. Parents may feel exhausted and overwhelmed. Prospective parents of multiple gestations should plan ahead, and arrange for additional help from family and friends in the home after delivery. Many communities have twin parent support groups. Information about such groups should be made available to the parents early in the pregnancy.

13. What happens if one twin dies in utero?

If death occurs **in the first trimester**, the dead fetus may be completely resorbed or may persist as a fetus papyraceous (small, flattened, dried-out fetus). If the patient did not have an ultrasound during this time, the twin gestation may not be identified.

If death occurs **in the second or third trimester** (incidence 2.2–6.8%), the surviving fetus may face significant morbidity and mortality. Prognostic factors include the etiology of the demise, type of zygosity and placentation, gestational age at the time of demise, and length of time between death of the first twin and delivery of the surviving twin. Monozygotic twins with monoamniotic/monochorionic or diamniotic/monochorionic placentation are at highest risk of complications.

Neonatal morbidity in the surviving MZ twin involves structural defects of the central nervous system, skin, and kidneys. Cerebral palsy, microcephaly, multicystic encephalomalacia, renal cortical necrosis, and aplasia cutis have been reported. Thromboplastin from the dead twin was thought to cross via placental anastomoses to the living twin and to cause infarction of various organs. Current theory holds that such defects result from significant, prolonged hypotension as the living twin loses blood to the dead twin through placental vascular anastomoses. Maternal morbidity from disseminated intravascular coagulation is rare and usually does not occur until 4 or more weeks after fetal death.

Early delivery does not prevent or decrease the risk of such complications, which are likely to have occurred at the time of demise. Delivery should be done for the usual obstetric indications. Vaginal delivery is appropriate unless there is an obstetric indication for cesarean section.

14. Do twins differ from singletons in developing pulmonary maturity? How should pulmonary maturity be assessed?

Overall, twins appear to develop pulmonary maturity 3–4 weeks earlier than singletons, and many achieve maturity by 32 weeks. Lecithin/sphingomyelin (L/S) ratios and the risk of hyaline membrane disease after birth are usually similar for both babies, but on occasion differences may be marked. Pulmonary function is frequently more mature in the smaller, growth-restricted twin of a discordant set and in the presenting twin during preterm labor. When assessment of pulmonary maturity is necessary, amniocentesis from one twin for an L/S ratio is adequate in most cases. In cases of discordant growth, the sac of the larger twin should be tapped. In preterm labor, the sac of the nonpresenting twin should be sampled.

15. How are twins managed in labor and delivery?

One must anticipate and recognize the increased potential for complications of labor and delivery in twins. Continuous electronic fetal monitoring of both twins, intravenous fluid access, surveillance of patient and fetuses by a trained obstetric nurse, presence of an obstetrician, and immediate availability of anesthesia are mandatory. In addition, pediatricians and/or other nursery personnel are needed for neonatal resuscitation. Complications to be anticipated include uterine dysfunction, pregnancy induced hypertension, fetal malpresentations, prolapse of the umbilical cord, abruptio placentae, fetal distress necessitating emergent delivery, and postpartum hemorrhage.

16. What are the most common presentations of twins at labor and delivery?

Vertex-vertex	39%	Vertex-transverse	8%
Vertex-breech	26%	Breech-transverse	4%
Breech-vertex	13%	Others	2%
Breech-breech	9%		

17. What are locked twins?

Although rare (1 in 817 twins), the phenomenon of locked twins occurs when the first fetus is breech and the second is vertex. The chin of the first (breech) fetus locks in the neck and chin of the second (vertex) fetus. This situation may occur in both single- and double-sac twins. Unless they spontaneously disengage, delivery must be accomplished by cesarean section.

18. How does fetal presentation affect labor and delivery of twins?

On admission the presentation of both twins is established by ultrasound examination. Generally, vertex-vertex twins are delivered vaginally, and sets in which twin A is nonvertex are delivered by cesarean section. The management of vertex-nonvertex twins is controversial.

19. How are vertex-vertex twins managed?

After delivery of the first twin, the cord is left clamped and no blood is taken; placental anastomoses may compromise the blood supply to the second twin. Until the second twin's head is well engaged, its amniotic sac is left intact if possible. Unless electronic fetal monitoring is nonreassuring or bleeding suggests an abruption, the uterus is allowed to resume labor for delivery of the second twin. Oxytocin may be needed to restart uterine contractions. Generally, the second twin delivers within 15–30 minutes of the first twin. With continuous electronic fetal monitoring, this interval may be prolonged as long as the fetal heart rate tracing remains reassuring. Delivery, as with twin A, may be expedited by vacuum extraction or low forceps.

20. What are the delivery options if the presentation is vertex-breech?

External cephalic version of the second (breech) twin to a vertex presentation under ultrasound guidance. Versions are successful in 46–73% of attempts, depending on gestational age and maternal habitus. Delivery then proceeds as in a singleton vertex delivery. The disadvantages are fetal distress secondary to the version or other factors and unsuccessful version. In such cases, the woman must undergo immediate cesarean section or breech extraction for delivery of the second twin.

Breech extraction of the second twin is advocated by many, and several reports attest to its safety. The prerequisites for breech extraction are the same as for singleton breech deliveries— i.e., adequate pelvis, estimated fetal weight of 2000–3800 gm, flexed or military head, a physician experienced in performing breech extraction, and the *immediate* availability of general anesthesia. Adequate anesthesia is mandatory for managing soft-tissue dystocia, nuchal arms, and other problems with delivery of the aftercoming head, which is the cause of most morbidity in vaginal breech delivery. Many practitioners do not attempt this form of delivery if the estimated fetal weight of twin B is significantly greater than that of twin A.

In light of the potential problems associated with either external cephalic version or breech extraction, it seems reasonable to offer **cesarean section** as an option to patients with a vertex-breech presentation.

21. What are the postpartum risks for twin pregnancies?

Because the uterus of a multiple gestation is overdistended, it frequently contracts inadequately after delivery. Postpartum hemorrhage from uterine atony must be anticipated and steps taken for its prevention.

22. What is the role of selective reduction in multiple gestations?

With assisted reproductive technologies, higher-order gestations occur more frequently. Both maternal and neonatal outcomes from pregnancies complicated by quadruplets or greater are believed to be significantly improved by reducing the pregnancy to a lower gestational number early in gestation. Usually performed late in the first trimester, selective reduction is generally undertaken by intracardiac/intrafetal injection of potassium chloride. For pregnancies with triplets, studies have been varied with regard to the overall benefits of selective reduction to twins. Although many advocate comparable perinatal outcomes in selectively reduced triplets compared with triplets managed with close surveillance, at least one study suggests selective reduction of triplet pregnancies may lower the loss rate in the second trimester.

BIBLIOGRAPHY

1. Adams DM, Chervenak FA: Intrapartum management of twin gestation. Clin Obstet Gynecol 33:52, 1990.
2. Benirschke K: Multiple gestation: Incidence, etiology, and inheritance. In Creasy RK, Resnik R (eds): Maternal-Fetal Medicine: Principles and Practice, 3rd ed. Philadelphia, W.B. Saunders, 1994, pp 575–588.
3. Benirschke K: The placenta in twin gestation. Clin Obstet Gynecol 33:18, 1990.
4. Burke MS: Single fetal demise in twin gestation. Clin Obstet Gynecol 33:69, 1990.
5. Chitkara U, Berkowitz RL: Multiple gestations. In Gabbe SG, Niebyl JR, Simpson JL (eds): Obstetrics: Normal and Problem Pregnancies, 2nd ed. New York, Churchill Livingstone, 1991, pp 881–921.
6. Cunningham G, MacDonald P, Gant N, et al (eds): Williams Obstetrics, 19th ed. Norwalk, CT, Appleton & Lange, 1993, pp 891–918.
7. Hollenbach KA, Hickok DE: Epidemiology and diagnosis of twin gestation. Clin Obstet Gynecol 33:3, 1990.
8. Iams JD, Johnson FF, Creasy RK: Prevention of preterm birth. Clin Obstet Gynecol 31:599, 1988.
9. MacLennan AH: Multiple gestation: Clinical characteristics and management. In Creasy RK, Resnik R (eds): Maternal-Fetal Medicine: Principles and Practice, 3rd ed. Philadelphia, W.B. Saunders, 1994, pp 589–601.
10. Nageotte MP: Prevention and treatment of preterm labor in twin gestation. Clin Obstet Gynecol 33:61, 1990.
11. Yeast JD: Maternal physiologic adaptation to twin gestation. Clin Obstet Gynecol 33:10, 1990.

60. Rh ISOIMMUNIZATION

Susan Berman, M.D., M.B.A.

1. What is isoimmunization? Why is it a concern during pregnancy?

Isoimmunization refers to the maternal development of antibodies to fetal red blood cell (RBC) antigens. During normal pregnancy a small number—and in some situations a large number—of fetal RBCs cross the placenta and enter the maternal circulation. When the fetal RBC antigens differ from those of the mother, a maternal immune response is generated. Although this response may be relatively small at first exposure, recurrent exposures elicit a larger and quicker response of IgG. This maternal IgG, directed at the fetal RBC antigen, is capable of traversing the placenta into the fetal circulation, causing hemolysis.

2. What is hemolytic disease of the newborn?

Most often secondary to isoimmunization to the Rh (rhesus) antigen, fetal RBCs that contain an antigen foreign to the mother (such as an RhD-positive fetus with an RhD-negative mother) become a site of binding for the maternal IgG. Once the maternal IgG binds to the RhD antigen on the fetal RBCs, these cells are destroyed. Depending on the severity of this hemolysis, the fetus may become anemic and hydropic, ultimately resulting in stillbirth.

3. Why does the severely anemic fetus become hydropic?

Severe fetal anemia results in extramedullary production of RBCs (primarily in the fetal liver and spleen). Extensive hepatic erythropoiesis distorts the portal venous circulation, leading to obstruction and finally to hepatomegaly, ascites, and placental edema. Hypoalbuminemia secondary to liver dysfunction also may contribute to this generalized edema.

4. In addition to anemia, what are the risks to the RhD-positive newborn whose mother is sensitized?

Marked hyperbilirubinemia, which, if untreated, may lead to central nervous system damage.

5. How many red blood cell (RBC) antigens are there?

More than 400 antigens have been identified on the red blood cell surface. However, only a few are clinically important as causes of hemolytic disease of the newborn. In addition to the Rh antigen, others include A, B, Kell(k), Duffy(Fy), Kidd(Jk), M,N,S, Lutheran(Lu), Diego(Di), and Xg.

6. What is the most common cause of hemolytic disease of the newborn?

Rh antigen isoimmunization.

7. How many antigens comprise the Rh system on the human red blood cell?

Five: CDE and c,e. Small d has not been identified. There are three closely linked loci within the Rh complex (D,C,E) with allelic forms (d,c,e). Some consider each antigen to be a separate gene. These three sites tend to be inherited intact with little crossover and rearrangement.

8. In which populations is RhD-negative trait most common? In which population is it rarely encountered?

Basque people are 95% RhD-negative, whereas approximately 15% of Caucasians are RhD-negative. Less than 5% of Asians and North American Indians are RhD-negative.

9. Define D^u.

D^u refers to the situation in which "D" is not detected by anti-D sera at a level that types the person as RhD-positive. This situation can occur by two mechanisms. First, the person may genetically contain the D sequence, but its expression is decreased (or masked) by the presence of C at the rhesus loci on the other chromosome. These genetic RhD-positive individuals are not at risk for isoimmunization. Less often, however, D^u is the result of genetic absence of a portion of the D antigen. Such women are at low risk for isoimmunization. RhoGAM should be given to the D^u mother unless the "environmental" (C allele) can be differentiated from the "genetic" variety.

10. What is the difference between a direct and indirect Coombs' test in the fetus?
A direct Coombs' test detects the presence of attached immunoglobulin in red blood cells; an indirect Coombs' test detects the presence of free immunoglobin in sera.

11. What is immunoglobulin prophylaxis for RhD-negative, nonsensitized mothers? Why is it helpful?
It is RhD immune globulin (RhoGAM) prepared from subjects previously sensitized to RhD. It absorbs the fetal RhD-positive antigen thus blocking formation of maternal Rh antibody at the time of exposure, usually at delivery. An alternative theory is that RhoGAM works at the cellular level of IgG production.

12. When should RhoGAM be given?
All previously unsensitized RhD-negative women who deliver an RhD-positive fetus should be given the immunoglobulin within 72 hours of delivery. In addition, RhD-negative unsensitized women should receive RhoGAM at 28 weeks, as well as following an abortion, ectopic pregnancy, amniocentesis, external version, or significant antepartum bleeding.

13. The standard dose (300 μg) of RhoGAM given after delivery provides coverage for how large of a fetomaternal hemorrhage?
30 ml of fetal whole blood or 15 ml of fetal packed red blood cells.

14. What percentage of women have evidence of fetomaternal hemorrhage after delivery? In what percentage is this bleeding considered excessive (> 5 ml of fetal blood)?
Seventy-five percent have evidence of fetomaternal hemorrhage. It is > 5 ml in < 1%.

15. In what circumstances may a woman at delivery have experienced fetomaternal hemorrhage of > 15 ml (30 ml of fetal whole blood)?

Placental abruption	Placenta previa associated with bleeding
Manual removal of the placenta	Multifetal gestations

16. Which test can be used to estimate the amount of fetomaternal hemorrhage?
Kleihauer-Betke test. A maternal blood sample can be treated with an acid dilution procedure, allowing identification and quantification of fetal red blood cells.

17. After a first pregnancy in a woman who is RhD-negative with an RhD-positive fetus and who does not receive RhoGAM, what is the risk that she will become sensitized?
Approximately 18%.

18. What is sensibilization?
Approximately one-half of women who are RhD-negative, do not receive RhoGAM after their first RhD-positive pregnancy, and become sensitized to the RhD antigen respond immediately with immunoglobin production to the RhD antigen. The other half mount a small, often undetectable response and may quickly mount an immune response with subsequent exposure to the antigen.

19. After evacuation of a molar gestation, do women who are RhD-negative need RhoGAM?
With complete molar gestations, there is theoretically no production of fetal red blood cells, the only cells that expresses Rh antigen. However, the distinction of a complete mole with no

fetal red blood cells is often not available at the time the decision for RhoGAM is needed. For this reason, many advocate RhoGAM even after evacuation of a complete mole.

20. How should pregnant women be followed to avoid fetal complications from Rh antibodies?

At their first prenatal visit, all pregnant women should be typed according to blood group, with serum screening for antibodies (indirect Coombs) to all RBC antigens associated with hemolytic disease of the newborn. For RhD-negative mothers without antibodies, antibody status should be reevaluated at least once during pregnancy, generally at 26–28 weeks. Some recommend reevaluation of antibody status each trimester. RhoGAM is administered to RhD-negative women at 26–28 weeks to prevent the small risk of sensitization in the third trimester.

For RhD-negative women with evidence of antibodies, serial antibody titers are obtained on a monthly basis. Further evaluation of the fetus is initiated when the antibody titers reach a critical level (≥ 1:16 in most laboratories). If there is a history of a previously affected sibling in utero, many initiate further testing of the fetus at 4–6 weeks before the gestational age at which the sibling was affected.

21. How is amniocentesis used in the management of Rh isoimmunization?

Amniocentesis can serve two purposes: (1) assessment of fetal Rh status by DNA-based molecular studies of the amniocytes and (2) measurement of bilirubin pigments in the amniotic fluid. Amniotic bilirubin reflects ongoing erythrocyte destruction. It can be quantitated by measuring the absorbance of amniotic fluid on a continuously recording spectrophotometer at the 450-nm wave length ($\Delta OD450$). The $\Delta OD450$ is determined by measuring the absorbance of amniotic fluid at 365nm and 535nm and drawing a straight line. The $\Delta OD450$ is then determined by subtracting the actual value from the expected 450-nm value. Liley defined three zones that relate the fetal health to the bilirubin level and the suggested course of action for each zone. For the premature fetus with evidence of significant hemolysis based on amniotic fluid bilirubin analysis, assessment of the fetal hematocrit by percutaneous umbilical blood sample (PUBS) is the next step.

22. What is the risk that after amniocentesis a RHD-negative mother will become sensitized if she does not receive RhoGAM?

Even with placental localization by ultrasound and avoidance of the transplacental passage of the needle, amniocentesis is associated with a 1–2% risk of fetomaternal hemorrhage of ≥ 1.0 ml fetal RBC. This risk is similar for amniocentesis performed in the second trimester for genetic indications and in the third trimester. Given these risks, RhoGAM should be administered to unsensitized Rh-negative women after amniocentesis. Of note, in the previously Rh-sensitized woman, even this small degree of fetomaternal hemorrhage can be associated with a marked increase in antibody titers.

23. What factors are considered in transfusing an anemic fetus?

In general, a fetal hematocrit below 25% warrants transfusion if gestational age is remote from term. To determine the amount of RBCs to transfuse, the gestational age and weight of the fetus, total vascular volume of both fetus and placenta, and desired final hematocrit are incorporated into the calculation. For transfusion, O-negative, CMV-negative, irradiated blood is used.

24. How are in utero fetal transfusions performed?

Either intravascularly or intraperitoneally. The technique is essentially similar, with ultrasound visualization of placement of a 20-gauge spinal needle within the amniotic sac and further advancement of the needle into either the umbilical vein (intravascular transfusion) or the peritoneal cavity of the fetus (intraperitoneal).

25. What are the advantages and disadvantages of intravascular transfusion?

The advantages of intravascular transfusion are the ability to obtain a fetal hematocrit before and after the procedure and direct placement of the transfused packed red blood cells into the fetal vascular system with more rapid correction of the fetal hematocrit. Disadvantages include technical constraints due either to vessel size at early gestational age or posterior placentation and dislodgment of the needle from the umbilical vein by fetal movement during the procedure.

26. What are the advantages and disadvantages of intraperitoneal transfusion?

The advantages are technically easier placement for earlier gestational fetuses and ability to transfuse a potentially greater amount of fetal packed red blood cells without dislodgment of needle by fetal movement. The major disadvantage is that the total amount of the transfusion is limited by constraints of peritoneal space, with overtransfusion resulting in increased abdominal pressure and compromised cardiac function in the fetus. In addition, there is decreased absorption of blood in the hydropic fetus.

27. Can a fetus still be transfused if it is hydropic?

Yes. If an intraperitoneal transfusion is needed, the ascitic fluid may be removed before transfusion.

28. What are the risks of fetal transfusion and the anticipated complications?

The risk of procedure-related mortality is 4–9%. In addition, significant morbidity may include fetal bradycardia, abruption, preterm labor, preterm rupture of membranes, and emergent delivery due to fetal distress.

29. When are fetuses who have required intrauterine transfusion delivered?

Once fetal lung maturity has been obtained, the risk of intrauterine transfusion outweighs the risk of delivering the infant with transfusions performed in the neonatal intensive care unit.

30. Why do the lungs in infants with Rh sensitization generally mature at a slightly later gestational age?

The cause is unknown but may be related to hydropic changes in the placenta with increased insulin production, an etiology similar to delayed fetal lung maturation in insulin-dependent diabetics.

31. Can the Rh type of a fetus be determined early in pregnancy?

For several of the Rh antigens it is now possible to determine the Rh antigen status of a fetus through DNA molecular probes with chorionic villus sampling or amniocentesis. This technique allows the opportunity to determine RhD-antigen status of a pregnancy early in gestation and may be considered by couples who have had prior pregnancies complicated by intrauterine transfusion or fetal demise. The expectation is that subsequent pregnancies would be similarly or more severely affected.

32. Because RhD immunoglobulin (RhoGAM) has prevented much of the isoimmunization problem, what remains?

The Kell antigen. Kell type is not determined before blood transfusion. Approximately 10% of people are Kell-positive, suggesting that the risk of sensitization to Kell after a blood transfusion is approximately 10%.

33. How does ABO sensitization differ from RhD sensitization?

Although successive pregnancies with fathers homozygous for RhD usually become more severe, ABO sensitizations are the opposite: the first pregnancy is usually the worst.

34. What are private antigens?

In rare instances, a fetus may have inherited a rare red blood cell surface antigen from the father. As the red blood cells of the mother in all likelihood do not contain this antigen, during her first pregnancy she may become sensitized to this "private" antigen. Subsequent pregnancies, depending on the antigen's ability to elicit an antibody response, are at variable risk for isoimmunization.

BIBLIOGRAPHY

1. American College of Obstetricians and Gynecologists: Management of Isoimmunization in Pregnancy. ACOG Educ Bull 227, 1996.
2. Bowman JM: Maternal blood group isoimmunization. In Creasy RK, Resnick R (eds): Maternal-Fetal Medicine: Principles and Practice, 3rd ed. Philadelphia, W.B. Saunders, 1994, pp 711–743.
3. Fisk NM, Bennet P, Warwick RM, et al: Clinical utility of fetal RhD typing in alloimmunized pregnancies by means of polymerase chain reaction on amniocytes or chorionic villi. Am J Obstet Gynecol 171:50–54, 1994.
4. Harman CR, Bowman JM, Manning FA, Menticoglou SM: Intrauterine transfusion—intraperitoneal versus intravascular approach: A case-control comparison. Am J Obstet Gynecol 162:1053–1059, 1990.
5. Queenan JT, Tomai TP, Ural SH, King JC: Deviation in amniotic fluid optical density at a wavelength of 450 nm in Rh-immunized pregnancies from 14 to 40 weeks' gestation: A proposal for clinical management. Am J Obstet Gynecol 168:1370–1376, 1993.

61. PRENATAL DIAGNOSIS

Marsha Wheeler, M.D.

1. Who should be offered prenatal diagnosis?

Couples at risk for having a fetus with any of the following:

Chromosome abnormality	Abnormal maternal serum screening test
Genetic disease	Abnormal sonographic exam
Neural tube defect	Teratogen exposure

2. List risk factors for having an infant with a chromosomal abnormality.

Maternal age of 35 years or older

Previous child with a chromosomal abnormality

Chromosome abnormality in either parent, including balanced translocation, aneuploidy, or mosaicism

Chromosome abnormality in a close family member

Abnormal fetus on sonographic exam

Abnormal serum screening test such as alpha-fetoprotein (AFP), double test, or triple test

3. Why are women over 35 at risk for having infants with chromosomal abnormalities?

Increased maternal age poses increased risk for a fetus with nondisjunction. Nondisjunction is an error in meiosis that results in a gamete with one chromosome too few or too many. Fertilization of the gamete with one extra chromosome results in a conception with 47 chromosomes. Aneuploidy occurs when the chromosome number is not an exact multiple of 23. The most common aneuploidies are trisomy 21 (Down syndrome), trisomy 13, and trisomy 18. Nondisjunction may involve the sex chromosomes; therefore, abnormalities such as 47,XXY, 47,XYY, and 47,XXX also increase with increasing maternal age.

4. If a parent is a translocation carrier, what is the risk of an unbalanced offspring?

An unbalanced offspring has an abnormal amount of chromosomal material. All people have two copies of chromosomes except for the sex chromosomes. The offspring of a translocation carrier may have three copies of one chromosome and only one copy of another. Translocation may involve whole chromosomes or portions of chromosomes. The specific risk of having an abnormal child varies according to the type of translocation. In most cases, however, if the carrier is the mother, the risk is 10–12%; if the father is the carrier, the risk is 2–3%.

5. How should a couple with a previous child with spina bifida be screened?

If the couple appears to have a child with an isolated neural tube defect, the risk for recurrence with that couple is around 3% for each pregnancy. Because serum screening misses 10–20% of abnormalities, amniocentesis for amniotic fluid AFP and possibly acetylcholinesterase is recommended. The couple's family and medical histories should be reviewed. The medical records of the previous child should be examined to see if a specific diagnosis was made. Sometimes a neural tube defect is part of a syndrome, or it may be due to a chromosomal abnormality. In some cases the recurrence risk may be increased, often as high as 25%.

6. If a family history identifies a couple at risk for a specific inherited disease, how should the couple be counseled?

Medical records of the affected family members should be obtained to determine the specific diagnosis. Then the specific inherited disease must be investigated to see if prenatal diagnosis is available. The couple can be counseled according to what tests are available. For example, carrier testing for Tay-Sachs disease is available, and if both members of the couple are carriers, prenatal diagnosis is available. The metabolic defect can be determined from cultured amniocytes and chorionic villi. In this case amniocentesis or chorionic villus sampling may be offered.

7. What DNA techniques are used in prenatal diagnosis?

If the specific, most common mutations are known for a disease, mutations can be looked for in fetal cells such as amniocytes or chorionic villus. When multiple different mutations in a known gene are responsible for a specific disease, such as Duchenne muscular dystrophy, or if the gene has not been identified, linkage to DNA markers can be used. DNA markers are located near the gene on the chromosome. In such cases, the couple is given a probability rate that the fetus is affected. This area of prenatal diagnosis is rapidly growing, and information about specific diseases changes daily.

8. What techniques are used to make prenatal diagnosis?

Ultrasound	Fetoscopy
Magnetic resonance imaging	Chorionic villus sampling
Maternal serum alpha fetoprotein	Radiographs
Amniocentesis	Percutaneous umbilical blood sampling
Ultrasound-guided tissue biopsy	Triple test

9. What is genetic amniocentesis?

Amniocentesis is a technique in which amniotic fluid is removed from around the fetus. The fluid or the cells suspended in the fluid can be used for specific metabolic tests, recombinant DNA technique, or obtaining a karyotype (chromosomes). Traditionally, amniocentesis has been done between 16 and 18 weeks. Now it can be done as early as 12 or 13 weeks. The risk of procedure-related loss is stated to be 1/200. The risk of loss after early amniocentesis remains undetermined. Studies suggest both similar and higher loss rates compared with standard amniocentesis. Amniotic fluid AFP is routinely assessed to screen for neural tube defects.

10. What is chorionic villus sampling (CVS)?

CVS is a procedure in which placental tissue is removed between 9½ and 12 weeks. The tissue can be obtained by either transabdominal or transcervical approach. The tissue can be used for recombinant DNA techniques, enzyme assays, or cytogenetic testing. The advantage of the procedure is earlier diagnosis, which may result in decreased medical risks associated with earlier termination. The disadvantages include a fetal loss rate of about 1% over baseline and maternal cell contamination, resulting in a need for further studies. An amniotic fluid AFP cannot be done simultaneously. As a result, an ultrasound and maternal serum AFP screening are recommended at 16–18 weeks.

11. What concern has been raised about birth defects among infants exposed to CVS?

Initial studies suggested a markedly higher rate of limb reduction abnormalities in infants exposed to CVS. Similar anomalies have been noted in animals secondary to ischemic damage as a result of vasoconstriction. Most recent evaluation of collaborative studies from around the world indicate the risk for limb reduction may be 3-fold higher after CVS (1/3000 vs. 1/9000). General recommendations include preprocedural counseling about limb reduction defects.

12. Define double test, triple test, and multiple marker screen.

These tests use biochemical markers in the maternal serum to calculate the risk for a birth defect. The most common abnormalities for which risk can be calculated are Down syndrome, neural tube defect, and trisomy 18.

13. What markers are used in the triple test?

Alpha fetoprotein (AFP)
Human chorionic gonadotropin (HCG)
Unconjugated estriol

14. How are the markers in the triple test interpreted?

AFP was the first fetal biochemical analog found to have altered serum concentration in the mother of a fetus with Down syndrome. AFP is produced by the fetal liver. The AFP level and maternal age can be used to calculate a risk for Down syndrome. About 20–25% of fetuses with Down syndrome can be detected; amniocentesis and chromosome studies are needed in 3–5% of screened pregnancies. The AFP is about 20% lower in the serum of mothers of a fetus with Down syndrome. HCG is produced by the placenta and is about twice as high in the serum of women with a fetus with Down syndrome. Unconjugated estriol is 25% lower than normal. It is produced by the fetal adrenal, fetal liver, and placenta. The three values are combined, and a specific risk for an individual pregnancy is given.

15. What risks are obtained from the triple test?

Risk for Down syndrome
Risk for neural tube defect
Risk for trisomy 18

16. What other information is included in the calculation of the triple test?

Maternal age	Gestational age
Race	Number of fetuses
Diabetes mellitus	

17. What are the advantages and disadvantages of percutaneous umbilical blood sampling for prenatal diagnosis (PUBS)?

Ultrasound-guided aspiration of a fetal blood sample can be obtained generally from 18 weeks' gestation onward. Access is optimized with an anterior placenta, and immobilization of the fetus is generally not needed. Advantages include access to the entire spectrum of diagnostic studies afforded by a peripheral blood sample, including karyotype in 48 hours and hematologic, immunologic, and acid/base assessment. Disadvantages include a 1–2% fetal loss rate.

18. What new prenatal diagnostic options are on the horizon?

Preimplantation diagnosis. Early in human gestation, when the vast majority of cells are destined for trophoblastic development, a single cell at the 8-cell stage or a dozen cells at the blastocyst stage can be removed without subsequent damage to the fetus. These cells provide sufficient DNA for PCR-directed molecular analyses of inherited diseases or fluorescent in situ hybridization for aneuploidy. Preimplantation biopsy for prenatal diagnosis involves participation in an in vitro fertilization program and is currently available for a limited number of genetic conditions.

Fetal cells in maternal circulations. Acquisition of fetal DNA without invasive studies has been an area of research for several decades. Currently attempts are underway to identify the most efficient means of isolating the few fetal cells from the overwhelming number of maternal cells. Once isolated, fetal cells provide information about the fetus through PCR and molecular studies as well as fluorescent in situ hybridization for aneuploidy.

BIBLIOGRAPHY

1. American College of Obstetricians and Gynecology: Genetic Technologies. ACOG Tech Bull 208, 1995.
2. Burton BK: Outcome of pregnancies with unexplained elevated or low levels of maternal serum alpha fetoprotein. Obstet Gynecol 72:709, 1988.
3. Campbell TL: Maternal serum alpha fetoprotein screening: Benefits, risks and costs. J Fam Pract 25:461, 1987.
4. Crandall BF: Risks associated with an elevated maternal serum alpha fetoprotein level. Am J Obstet Gynecol 165:581, 1991.
5. Haddow JE, Palomaki GE, Knight GJ, et al: Prenatal screening for Down's syndrome with use of maternal serum markers. N Engl J Med 327:588, 1992.
6. Hook EB, Cross PK, Schreinmachers DM: Chromosome abnormality rate at amniocentesis and in liveborn infants. JAMA 249:2034–2038, 1983.

62. GENETIC DISEASE AND THE FETUS

Louise Wilkins-Haug, M.D., Ph.D.

1. What percentage of children are born with birth defects? What causes them?

Two percent have major malformations (incompatible with life or requiring major surgery), 5% a minor malformation. The etiology often cannot be determined. Chromosomal anomalies, single gene mutations, multifactorial disorders and teratogenic exposures account for only 40% of major malformations.

2. How often do chromosomal abnormalities occur in newborns? What is the most common autosomal disorder? The most common sex-chromosome disorder?

0.5%. Trisomy 21 (Down syndrome) is the most common autosomal disorder (1 in 800 livebirths) and 47,XXY (Klinefelter syndrome) the most common sex-chromosome disorder (1 in 1000 livebirths).

3. When was Down syndrome first described?

1866. Langdon Down noted a similar facial appearance and body habitus among a subgroup of mentally deficient children. Trisomy for chromosome 21 and the Down syndrome phenotype were not associated until 1959.

4. Is the entire extra chromosome 21 required to produce the features of Down syndrome?

No. The genes producing the characteristic phenotype have been mapped to a small segment of #21 (band 21q22). Involvement of this band alone in an unbalanced translocation can result in features of Down syndrome.

5. What are three other autosomal disorders presenting with "classic" phenotypes in newborns?

Trisomy 18 (Edward syndrome)—1/3500 livebirths; small-for-gestation postdate pregnancies with a small placenta and a single umbilical artery; short sternum; overlapping clenched fingers and "rocker bottom" feet are noted skeletal anomalies; less than 10% live to 1 year of age.

Trisomy 13 (Patau syndrome)—1/5000 livebirths; growth-retarded newborns with a triad of facial clefts, ocular abnormalities, and polydactyly; less than 3% survive to 3 years of age.

5p- (cri du chat syndrome)—1/20,000 livebirths; high-pitched, monotonous cry; round facies and marked epicanthal folds; variable mental retardation correlated to the extent of deletion of chromosome 5.

6. What is a Robertsonian translocation? A reciprocal translocation?

Robertsonian—fusion between two acrocentric chromosomes (i.e., #13, 14, 15, 21, 22) at their centromeres, creating a composite chromosome; the carrier of this new chromosome is genetically balanced but at risk for chromosomally unbalanced gametes.

Reciprocal—breakage and exchange between segments of two different chromosomes; the balanced carrier has the correct number of chromosomes (46), but the rearrangement increases the risk for unbalanced gametes.

7. Why is the diagnosis of a sex-chromosome anomaly often missed in the newborn period?

Aneuploidy involving the X or Y chromosome is often not associated with intrauterine growth retardation or significant structural anomalies. These individuals often present during childhood with growth disturbances or during adolescence with poorly developed secondary sex characteristics.

8. Describe three common sex-chromosome syndromes.

45,X (Turner syndrome)—1/2500 livebirths; primary amenorrhea in a short female with a webbed neck, diffuse pigmented nevi, renal anomalies, and cardiac defects (aortic coarctation); mosaics can present with oligomenorrhea and some secondary sex characteristics. Advanced maternal age is not a feature of Turner syndrome. Monosomy X usually results from the loss of the paternal sex chromosome.

47,XXY (Klinefelter syndrome)—1/500 livebirths; normal pubic and axillary hair but scant facial hair; tall body habitus with female adipose distribution and breast development; a 20 times increase in breast carcinoma over 46,XY males.

47,XYY—1/800 livebirths; originally associated with tall, mentally deficient males incarcerated for antisocial crime; prospective studies showed only a slight increase in incarceration (1% vs. 0.1% for 46,XY males); slightly lower IQ, normal genitalia, and normal testosterone levels.

9. Can individuals with sex-chromosome anomalies reproduce?

Variable. Most 45,X females are infertile, although pregnancies have been reported and are associated with miscarriage, stillborns, and chromosomally abnormal offspring (30%). XXY males are commonly infertile due to hyalinization of their seminiferous tubules. XYY males are usually fertile with only a rare report of transmission of chromosome anomaly from father to son.

10. Which chromosomal abnormalities are associated with reproductive loss?

First-trimester miscarriage (40–60% aneuploidy)—50% involve autosomal trisomies (#16 most common), 25% with 45,X, 20% with triploidy, and 5% with unbalanced translocations.

Second-trimester miscarriage (10–30% aneuploidy)—trisomy 13, 18, and 21 and XO.

Stillborns (10% aneuploidy)—trisomy 18 most common whether or not obvious malformations present.

Habitual aborters—balanced structural rearrangements are found in 4.7% of couples with two or more spontaneous losses. This rate is lower if only couples with no liveborn are considered. Of note, if multiple miscarriages occur in conjunction with a stillbirth or prior abnormal liveborn, the frequency of balanced translocations increases to 16.7%.

Oligospermia—marked oligospermia is associated with an increased risk of balanced translocations (3–5%). Because affected men are candidates for intracytoplasmic sperm injection (ICSI), the risk of chromosomally abnormal conceptions is conceivably greater than in naturally occurring pregnancies.

Gestational trophoblast disease—complete moles are typically diploid (46,XX or XY) and are entirely of paternal origin with no maternally derived chromosomes; partial moles are generally triploid (69,XXX, 69,XYY), with the additional set of chromosomes also of paternal origin. Triploidy as a result of an additional set of maternal chromosomes generally presents with intrauterine growth retardation, malformations, and a small placenta.

11. What is FISH? What are its advantages and disadvantages?

Fluorescent in situ hybridization (FISH) provides identification of specific chromosomes or chromosomal segments with fluorescence-labeled probes. FISH can be performed in situ on a microscopic slide targeted to DNA in either interphase cells or metaphase chromosomes. The use of interphase cells is advantageous because neither time nor tissue viability is needed for cell culture. Rapid results are possible from various cells, including amniocytes. In addition, archived tissues can be studied retrospectively. Additionally, FISH analysis in selected settings detects structural alterations, such as deletions of chromosome 22, not visible in the metaphase chromosome. Disadvantages include an 80–93% sensitivity rate for available probes. FISH results provide information about only the specific chromosome studied and do not provide an analysis of the full karyotype, as generally obtained from cell culture.

With an understanding of its limitations and benefits, FISH has been used for rapid chromosomal assessment in the setting of fetal malformations, for retrospective analysis of archived tissues from stillbirths and for further qualification of structural chromosomal abnormalities.

12. What percentage of newborns have mendelian inheritance of a genetic disease?

1%. Autosomal dominant disease accounts for 70%, autosomal recessive disease for 20%, and sex-linked recessive disorders for 5%.

13. What are common examples of the various types of mendelian inheritance?

Autosomal dominant—Huntington's chorea, Marfan syndrome, neurofibromatosis, familial polyposis

Autosomal recessive—sickle cell disease, cystic fibrosis, phenylketonuria, Tay-Sachs disease

X-linked dominant—vitamin D–resistant rickets, hereditary hematuria

X-linked recessive—Duchenne's muscular dystrophy, hemophilia, color blindness

14. Why do autosomal recessive disorders often have an increased frequency among specific populations?

Gene flow within reproductively isolated populations forms the basis for the differences now seen between various racial and ethnic groups. As each group continues to segregate genes among themselves, mutations are passed silently through balanced carriers, and when expressed in a double dose, a recessive disorder is produced. The normal phenotype of the unsuspecting recessive carrier serves to mask the supply of mutant genes.

15. Specify the autosomal diseases with increased prevalence among the following ethnic/racial groups and indicate the carrier frequency.

Jewish (Askenazic)—Tay-Sachs disease (carrier 1 in 30)

Blacks—sickle cell disease (carrier 1 in 10)

Caucasians (Northern European)—cystic fibrosis (carrier 1 in 20)

Mediterranean—beta-thalassemia (carrier 1 in 25)

16. Autosomal dominant disorders (i.e., achondroplasia, Marfan syndrome, tuberous sclerosis) often appear in a newborn with "normal" parents. What are three explanations?

1. **New mutation**—the gene producing achondroplasia theoretically undergoes mutation in 1/20,000 gametes.

2. **Form fruste**—the parent has unrecognized mild or subclinical manifestations

3. **Nonpaternity**

17. What are the various approaches for molecular diagnosis of genetic disease in a fetus?

Indirect methods—Restriction fragment length polymorphisms (RFLPs) in noncoding DNA are base sequence variations that alter the action of specific restriction endonucleases. RFLPs occur approximately every 200 base pairs. The DNA fragments resulting after specific enzyme cleavage are thus altered in size, and gel mobility dependent on the RFLP results. Useful RFLPs are highly variable (polymorphic); thus, the chance that two individuals share the same variation at a specific restriction endonuclease site is extremely rare. For genetic diseases in which the DNA sequence has not been determined, RFLP analysis of affected individuals and other family members may provide an indirect method of tracking the abnormal gene through a family. As with genetic linkage analysis involving segregation of associated traits for tracking an inherited disease, RFLP analysis can be confounded by crossing over between the gene in question and the RFLP and the need for multiple informative members from a family.

Direct methods—Detection by direct analysis of the abnormal gene is the most straightforward but most difficult method. PCR can amplify a predetermined segment of DNA selected by knowledge of the unique starting and stopping sequences of the DNA under study. Disorders secondary to deletion of DNA (alpha-thalessemia, Duchenne and Becker muscular dystrophy, cystic fibrosis, and growth hormone deficiency) were first detected. If the abnormal amplified DNA is not altered in size (by deletion or insertion), recognition of a change in the DNA sequence requires additional steps. If the mutation has been sequenced, allele-specific probes can test the suspect DNA for hybridization to the normal and mutant alleles. In this fashion, direct DNA diagnosis for Tay-Sachs disease, alpha- and beta-thalassemia, and cystic fibrosis are possible.

Although direct DNA diagnosis requires knowledge of the mutated sequence, in some cases it has been obtained without knowledge of an associated abnormal protein or how the disease symptoms are produced. Known as positional cloning (or reverse genetics), the abnormal sequence is localized to a chromosome (through naturally occurring rearrangements or somatic cell hybrids of isolated human chromosomes), isolated through yeast artificial chromosomes (YACs) and directly sequenced. Candidate genes for Duchenne muscular dystrophy, cystic fibrosis, and myotonic dystrophy have been sequenced in this fashion.

18. What are the practical considerations of the numerous molecular mutations now identified for some Mendelian disorders?

The molecular genetics of cystic fibrosis (CF) emphasizes this concept. DNA sequencing of the abnormal protein associated with cystic fibrosis (CFTR) revealed over 140 mutations. Loss of three bases at position 508 (delta 508) is the most common mutation among the Caucasian population. However, 24% of CF mutations in a Caucasian population result from one of the other mutations in this gene. Furthermore, in this population, almost 10% of CF mutations remain uncharacterized.

Clinically, when DNA testing for a genetic disease is initiated within a family, heterogeneity at the molecular level needs to be considered. Whereas for some disorders only a small number of identified mutations account for the majority of disease states, for others, such as cystic fibrosis, the extensive number of identified mutations precludes testing for all known. When a family member of an affected individual or an at-risk fetus is tested, care should be taken that the mutation within the family is known and that the appropriate molecular studies are initiated.

19. What are characteristics of multifactorial inheritance?

Traits with an increased familial aggregation and recurrence without a mendelian pattern of gene transmission. The malformation often involves a single organ and has an increased propensity for one sex.

20. What in general terms is the risk of recurrence for multifactorial traits?

2–3% recurrence for a second affected child, 4–6% for a third affected child; a parent with a multifactorial trait has a 2–3% risk of an affected offspring; unaffected siblings have a 1–2% risk of an affected offspring. For traits that are more common in one of the sexes, an affected offspring of the less commonly affected sex carries a higher recurrence risk.

21. Cite four congenital anomalies inherited in multifactorial fashion.

Neural tube defects (anencephaly, encephalocele, spina bifida), hydrocephaly, cleft lip with or without cleft palate, cardiac anomalies.

22. Why is a careful examination necessary to exclude other minor malformations when a presumed multifactorial disorder has been identified?

Anomalies commonly inherited in a multifactorial fashion can also be components of genetic syndromes with different prognoses and recurrence rates.

23. Each of the multifactorial disorders in question 21 can also be seen as a component of a genetic syndrome. For each disorder, name an associated genetic syndrome and the new recurrence risk.

Neural tube defects—Meckel syndrome (encephalocele, polycystic kidneys, polydactyly); autosomal recessive

Hydrocephaly—aqueductal stenosis; X-linked recessive

Cleft lip—lip pit syndrome with lower paramedian lip pits; autosomal dominant

Cardiac anomalies—Noonan syndrome with pulmonic stenosis, skeletal anomalies, and hypogonadism; autosomal dominant

24. What is fragile X syndrome? How is it inherited?

Fragile X syndrome is the most common cause of familial mental retardation. Affected males are characterized by large ears and testes, prominent jaw, and moderate-to-severe mental retardation. Classically associated with an X chromosome fragile site induced by folic acid-deficient media, the gene (FMR-1) responsible for the phenotype was partially sequenced in 1991. Within the region, tandemly arranged arrays of trinucleotides [p(CGG)n] of variable length were detected.

In males, the largest trinucleotide fragments are associated with abnormal methylation and full fragile X phenotype. Females with the full mutation have a 50% frequency of mental retardation; the degree of phenotypic expression is confounded by X-inactivation. Smaller increases in the fragment length (premutations) are identified in normal transmitting males who only rarely were mentally retarded. In females, carriers of the premutation have a 3% incidence of mental retardation.

Although the X chromosome is involved, transmission of the syndrome deviates from accepted theories of X-linked inheritance. In general, inheritance through normal transmitting males results in stability of the fragment size. Their daughters would be carriers of a premutation; sons are not at risk because the son's X chromosome is from his mother. For women, however, transmission of the premutation often results in expansion to full mutation. Sons are at a 50% risk of fragile X syndrome, and some of the daughters who inherit the full mutation may be symptomatic as well.

25. What are some of the newer genetic theories that influence the expected Mendelian inheritance of genes?

Uniparental disomy (UPD)—both chromosomes of a pair originate from one parent. UPD may occur through gamete complementation (fertilization by gametes with loss and gain in the same chromosome pair), monosomic duplication, or an initially trisomic conceptus with rescue or loss of one of the trisomic set. The latter theory is supported by reports of UPD 15 in diploid individuals following trisomy 15 from chorionic villus sampling. Each of the two chromosomes can be genetically dissimilar (heterodisomy) or identical (isodisomy), depending on whether the nondisjunctional event occurs during the first or second meiotic divisions, respectively. Although rare, clinical implications include autosomal recessive diseases with only one parent a heterozygotic carrier, father-to-son transmission of X-linked disorders, expression of X-linked disorders in females, and mimicking of syndromes classically produced by deletion of chromosomal material. Prader-Willi syndrome, the most common dysmorphic form of obesity, occurs from loss of paternally derived chromosome 15 genes—either through chromosomal deletion or maternal

UPD for chromosome 15. In Angelman syndrome, characterized by dysmorphia, severe mental retardation, and paroxysms of laughter and seizures, loss of maternal chromosome 15 genes, through either chromosome deletion or paternal #15 UPD, is responsible. These areas of chromosome 15 contain imprinted genes—those genes for which, in addition to sufficient copy number, both a maternally and paternally derived copy are required.

Unstable DNA—Tandemly arranged repeat sequences in DNA expand in size and disease severity from one generation to the next. Present examples include fragile X syndrome, myotonic dystrophy, and Huntington's disease. Gender of the transmitting parent often influences the chances of expansion and disease.

Mitochondrial inheritance—Thirteen structural genes have been located in the circular DNA of the mitochondria. Cytoplasmic mitochondria segregate with the nucleus of an ovum, but not with the nucleus of a sperm, and are passed only from mother to offspring. Several diseases, including Leber hereditary optic neuropathy, Leigh's disease, and myoclonic epilepsy with ragged red fibers, have been mapped to the mitochondrial DNA.

26. Why are all fetuses not affected similarly when exposed to a teratogenic agent?
   The effect produced will be altered by the timing during gestation, the duration of exposure, and the genetic susceptibility of the fetus. Dizygotic twins inadvertently exposed for the same duration and at the same gestational time to the same teratogenic agent will show varying degrees of insult mediated by their different genotypes.

27. For each recognized teratogen below, describe the classically associated congenital anomalies.
   Coumadin—"Warfarin syndrome" with chondrodysplasia punctata, nasal hypoplasia, mental retardation; 10% of exposed fetuses
   Dilantin—cleft lip and palate, cardiac defects, facial dysmorphia, growth and mental retardation; 10–30% of exposed fetuses
   Isotretinoin (Accutane)—microtia/anotia, CNS defects, cardiac defects; 14% of exposed fetuses

28. Which birth defects are associated with increased maternal age? Increased paternal age?
   Increased maternal age is a risk factor for chromosomal anomalies, whereas increased paternal age has been associated with autosomal dominant mutations (achondroplasia, neurofibromatosis).

BIBLIOGRAPHY

1. Engel EM, DeLozier-Blanchet D: Uniparental disomy, isodisomy and imprinting: Probable effects in man and strategies for their detection. Am J Med Genet 40:432–439, 1991.
2. Little M, Van Heyningen V, Hstie N: Dads and disomy and disease. Nature 351:609–610, 1991.
3. Milunsky A: Genetic Disorders and the Fetus, 3rd ed. New York, Plenum Press, 1993.
4. Simpson JL, Golbus MS: Genetics and Obstetrics and Gynecology, 2nd ed. Philadelphia, W.B. Saunders, 1992.
5. Wilkins-Haug L: Medical genetics. In Ryan KJ, Berkowitz RS, Berbieri RL (eds): Kistner's Gynecology, 6th ed. St. Louis, Mosby, 1995.

63. OBSTETRIC ULTRASOUND

Mary E. Norton, M.D., and Carolyn M. Zelop, M.D.

1. What equipment is used for obstetric ultrasound?

Ultrasound (US) equipment uses sound waves delivered at a high frequency, usually > 20,000 cycles per second (Hz). Most diagnostic applications of US operate at frequencies of 2–10 million cycles per second (2–10 MHz). The best resolution is obtained with the highest-frequency US, although depth of visualization is compromised. Abdominal US transducers, either linear array with a rectangular image or sector scanners with a pie-shaped image, operate at 3.5–5 MHz. Greater resolution of structures in close proximity to the transducer can be obtained with vaginal scanners operating at 5–7.5 MHz.

2. Are there any side effects of obstetric ultrasound?

There have been no confirmed biologic effects on patients or instrument operators of diagnostic US. The greatest risk is false-positive or false-negative diagnoses.

3. Should all pregnant patients have an ultrasound exam?

Routine performance of obstetric US remains controversial in the United States, although it is performed throughout Europe. Opponents of routine US cite the failure of randomized clinical trials to demonstrate a clear benefit, the deleterious effects of false-positive or false-negative diagnoses, the lack of adequately trained personnel to perform the procedures, and cost. The benefits of routine US screening include detection of unsuspected anomalies, accurate determination of fetal age, and earlier diagnosis of placenta previa or multiple gestation.

4. What is involved in a first-trimester ultrasound exam?

A first-trimester exam should include demonstration of the location of the gestational sac, identification of the embryo, and measurement of the crown-rump length. Presence or absence of fetal cardiac activity should be documented, as well as fetal number. The uterus, cervix, and maternal adnexae should also be evaluated.

5. What is involved in a second- or third-trimester exam?

A second- or third-trimester exam should document the presence of fetal cardiac activity, fetal number and presentation. Additionally, the amniotic fluid volume should be assessed, as well as appearance of the placenta and its location, especially with reference to the cervical os (i.e., presence or absence of placenta previa). Gestational age should be assessed, and maternal uterus and adnexae examined. Fetal anatomic examination should include, but is not limited to, evaluation of the cerebral ventricles, 4-chamber view of the heart, spine, stomach, bladder, cord insertion, and kidneys.

6. What are the helpful landmarks of a normal early pregnancy?

When the mean sac diameter measures > 25 mm by transabdominal US, a living embryo should be identified in a viable pregnancy. This generally occurs by 7–8 weeks of gestation. By transvaginal US, fetal cardiac activity should be documented by 6.5 weeks, or when the mean sac diameter measures 18 mm. A normal gestational sac can be seen transvaginally when the level of human chorionic gonadotropin reaches 1,000 mIU/ml.

7. What is a blighted ovum?

A blighted ovum is a fertilized ovum in which development has stopped. The absence of a fetal pole in a gestational sac with a diameter of 3 cm or more is consistent with the diagnosis of blighted ovum.

8. What is the chance of spontaneous abortion in a patient with documented fetal cardiac activity in the first trimester?

In patients with documented fetal cardiac activity in the first trimester, < 5% will subsequently experience a fetal loss. This rate depends somewhat on maternal age and is slightly higher for women over the age of 35.

9. Which measurements are used for gestational dating?

In the first trimester, the fetal crown-rump length (CRL) is used to assess gestational age. In the second and third trimesters, the biparietal diameter (BPD) and femur length (FL) are the measurements used for pregnancy dating.

10. What is a quick assessment of fetal age based on crown-rump length (CRL) if tables are not handy?

CRL + 6.5 weeks = weeks of gestation.

11. What is the accuracy of ultrasound dating?

US dating of pregnancy becomes less accurate as pregnancy progresses. CRL in the first trimester is accurate within 3–5 days, whereas measurements in the second trimester are approximate within 2 weeks and in the third trimester within 3 weeks.

12. What structures identify the appropriate level to measure the BPD?

The BPD is measured in a transverse axial plane at the level of the falx cerebri, the thalamic nuclei, and the cavum septum pellucidi.

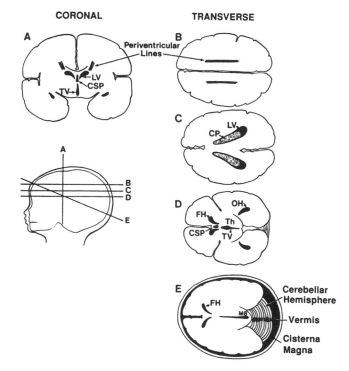

Normal ventricles. CP = choroid plexus; CSP = cavum septi pellucidi; FH = frontal horn; LV = lateral ventricle; MB = midbrain; OH = occipital horn; Th = thalamus; TV = third ventricle. (From Nyberg DA, Mahony BS, Pretorius DH: Diagnostic Ultrasound of Fetal Anomalies: Text and Atlas. St. Louis, Mosby, 1990, p 87, with permission.)

13. What structures identify the appropriate level to measure the abdominal circumference?

The abdominal circumference is measured in a transverse axial plane at a level including the left portal vein deep in the liver, and the fetal stomach.

14. What is the best time to obtain a single ultrasound exam in pregnancy?

At 18–20 weeks, one can judge placental position, estimate amniotic fluid volume, recognize early shortening of the cervix, and detect numerous fetal anomalies. Despite the somewhat improved accuracy of dating in the first trimester, these advantages make 18–20 weeks of gestation the ideal time to schedule a single US exam.

15. How accurate is fetal weight calculated by a third-trimester ultrasound exam?

When based on two or more fetal parameters using published regression formulas, an estimated fetal weight by US is predictive with 95% confidence that the true fetal weight is within a range of 7.5–10% above and below the estimated weight.

16. What is the amniotic fluid index?

The amniotic fluid index (AFI) is a quantitative technique to assess amniotic fluid volume. The maternal abdomen is divided into quadrants, using the umbilicus and linea nigra as reference points. The transducer head is maintained perpendicular to the floor, and the largest vertical pocket in each quadrant is measured. The sum of these four measurements (in cm) is the AFI.

17. What are the definitions of olio- and polyhydramnios?

The most common ways of determining amniotic fluid volume are by subjective assessment, measurement of the deepest vertical pocket, or using the AFI. Oligohydramnios is usually defined as a single vertical pocket of < 1 or 2 cm or an AFI < 5 cm. Polyhydramnios is usually considered a single vertical pocket > 8 cm or an AFI > 20 cm.

18. What are the components of a biophysical profile?

The biophysical profile (BPP) is a sonographic assessment of multiple fetal biophysical activities or components, including fetal body movements, fetal breathing movements, fetal tone, and amniotic fluid volume. The nonstress test (NST) is sometimes included as part of the BPP. Each component is scored as 0 when abnormal or 2 when normal; thus a normal score is 8 or 10, depending on whether the NST is included.

19. What is M-mode echocardiography?

M-mode echocardiography provides details about structural motion in the heart and accurate measurements of the dimensions of walls and cavities. It is used to document the presence of cardiac activity in early pregnancy, to evaluate ventricular cavity dimension and wall thickness as well as valve and wall motion, and to assess cardiac arrhythmias.

20. When is Doppler ultrasound useful?

Doppler ultrasonography demonstrates the direction and characteristics of blood flow and is used in evaluation of the fetal heart and great vessels as well as the uteroplacental and fetoplacental circulation. Doppler velocimetry can be used for further assessment of pregnancy complications such as intrauterine growth retardation, fetal hypoxemia or asphyxia, fetal cardiac anomalies, and cord malformations.

21. Can ultrasound detect Down syndrome or other chromosomal abnormalities?

US can detect many of the malformations associated with chromosomal abnormalities. Fetuses with trisomy 13 and 18 tend to have major malformations, most of which can be detected sonographically. In Down syndrome, many fetuses have either no major malformations or malformations that tend to be detected late in pregnancy, such as duodenal atresia. Thus only 30% of

Down syndrome fetuses are detected by routine US. Subtle biometric or morphologic abnormalities, such as shortened femurs, thickened nuchal folds, and renal pyelectasis, can be used to screen for and detect some cases of fetal Down syndrome.

22. What are the causes of an abnormal alpha-fetoprotein screen detected by ultrasound?
Maternal serum alpha-fetoprotein (MSAFP) was first noted to be elevated with open fetal neural tube defects. Elevated MSAFP also occurs with underestimation of gestational age, multiple gestation, fetal demise, cystic hygroma and other conditions associated with fetal edema, anterior abdominal wall defects, and other fetal anomalies associated with fetal skin defects. A low AFP can be associated with fetal chromosome abnormalities (e.g., Down syndrome, trisomy 18), dating errors, molar pregnancy, or fetal demise.

23. What ultrasound markers can be used to differentiate a mono- or dichorionic twin pregnancy?
Evaluation of chorionicity is an important component of the sonographic assessment of twins. Evidence of dichorionicity includes separate sacs in the first trimester, separate placentas, different genders, thick intertwin septa, or presence of a chorionic peak. A chorionic peak is a projecting zone of tissue extending from the chorionic surface of the placenta and tapering within the intertwin membrane.

24. What degree of discrepancy in estimated weight between twins implies a risk of morbidity?
A weight estimate discordance of 20% raises concern of significant birthweight disparity and risk of increased morbidity. Patients beyond viability with this degree of discordance should be monitored for fetal well-being.

25. What are the banana and lemon signs?
The banana and lemon signs are two sonographic signs of the Arnold-Chiari malformation seen in spina bifida. The frontal bones of the skull are scalloped, giving a lemonlike configuration. The cerebellum is flattened and centrally curved, obliterating the posterior fossa and giving the cerebellum a bananalike appearance.

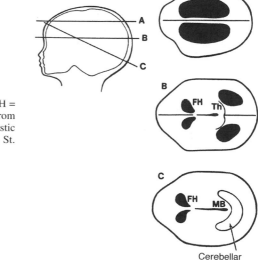

Cranial findings associated with spina bifida. FH = frontal horn; Th = thalamus; MB = midbrain. (From Nyberg DA, Mahony BS, Pretorius DH: Diagnostic Ultrasound of Fetal Anomalies: Text and Atlas. St. Louis, Mosby 1990, p 87, with permission.)

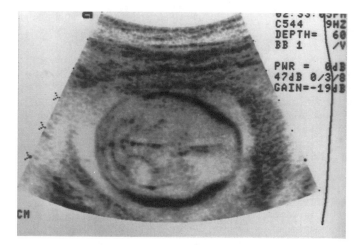

Ultrasound image demonstrating lemon and banana signs. (Courtesy M. Norton, Antenatal Diagnostic Center, Brigham and Women's Hospital.)

26. What is the difference between gastroschisis and omphalocele?

Gastroschisis and omphalocele are both anterior abdominal wall defects. Gastroschisis is a right paraumbilical defect through which small bowel (and occasionally other intraabdominal organs) eviscerates. The loops of bowel are not covered by a membrane. Omphalocele is an extrusion of the abdominal contents into the base of the umbilical cord. Thus, in omphalocele, the herniated mass is covered with parietal peritoneum, amnion, and Wharton's jelly. Gastroschisis is usually an isolated anomaly, whereas omphalocele is commonly associated with other malformations and/or chromosome abnormalities.

27. When does the normal physiologic herniation of the midgut resolve?

Before 12 weeks' gestation, the embryonic bowel is extraabdominal within the umbilical cord and should not be diagnosed as an abdominal wall defect. After this time, the bowel assumes its normal intraabdominal location.

28. What are the ultrasound features of hydrops fetalis?

Hydrops fetalis is a condition of excessive fluid accumulation within the fetus. It is characterized by varying degrees of ascites, pleural effusions, pericardial effusions, skin edema, placental edema, and polyhydramnios.

BIBLIOGRAPHY

1. American College of Obstetrics and Gynecology: Ultrasonography in Pregnancy. ACOG Tech Bull 187, 1993.
2. American Institute of Ultrasound in Medicine Bioeffects Committee: Bioeffects considerations for the safety of diagnostic ultrasound. J Ultrasound Med 7(Suppl 9):S1–38, 1988.
3. Callen PW: Ultrasonography in Obstetrics and Gynecology, 3rd ed. Philadelphia, W.B. Saunders, 1994.
4. Gabbe SG, Niebyl JR, Simpson JL: Obstetrics: Normal and Problem Pregnancies, 2nd ed. New York, Churchill Livingstone, 1991.
5. Simpson JL, Mills JL, Holmes LB, et al: Low fetal loss rates after ultrasound-proven viability in early pregnancy. JAMA 258:2555, 1987.

64. DISORDERS OF FETAL GROWTH

Thomas D. Shipp, M.D.

1. Is there a typical pattern of fetal growth throughout gestation?

Three phases of fetal growth occur during a normal gestation. The first 16 weeks of gestation are characterized by cellular hyperplasia. The second phase, which also lasts 16 weeks (gestational weeks 17–32), involves cellular hypertrophy in addition to continued cellular hyperplasia. The last phase, for the final 8 weeks of gestation, is primarily distinguished by cellular hypertrophy, with the greatest absolute increase in fetal weight.

2. How important are genetic and environmental factors in determining birth weight?

The intrauterine environment has the major role in determining birth weight by influencing 60% of the variance in fetal weight. Genetic factors account for 40% (20%, maternal; 20%, fetal) of the difference in fetal weight. Multiparous women deliver infants who weigh approximately 100 gm more than the infants of primiparas. Male neonates weigh approximately 200 gm more than females at term.

3. How good is ultrasound at predicting birth weight?

Ultrasound, when performed within 1 week of delivery by experienced operators, has been shown to give an estimated fetal weight within 10% of birth weight in 74% of cases and within 5% in 42% of cases.

4. What are average fetal weights at various points in gestation?

28 wk	1,000 gm
32 wk	2,000 gm
36-38 wk	3,000 gm

5. What is average weight gain per week in the fetus?

From 32–36 weeks, weight gain is an average of 210–245 gm (about ½ lb) per week, which decreases to 50–100 gm (about ¼ lb) at 38–40 weeks.

6. What is intrauterine growth restriction (IUGR)?

IUGR is a disorder of fetal growth in which the fetus does not meet its growth potential. Impaired growth places the fetus at risk for increased perinatal morbidity and mortality. It occurs in 3–7% of all deliveries.

7. Describe the two major classes of IUGR.

Symmetric IUGR, also known as type I, is characterized by globally impaired growth of the fetus. This type is usually diagnosed by the proportional lagging of the head, abdomen, and long bones of the fetus.

Asymmetric IUGR, or type II is also called "headsparing." It is characterized by disproportional growth of the fetus. The internal organs, as identified by the size of the abdomen, lag behind the size of the head and long bones.

Symmetric IUGR, seen in 25% of all cases, is thought to result from an insult early in gestation. Cellular hyperplasia is globally affected, leading to a proportionally small fetus. Asymmetric IUGR, the more common type, results from an insult later in gestation and affects cellular hypertrophy more significantly. This effect leads to decreased subcutaneous fat and smaller organ sizes with relatively small abdominal circumferences and appropriately developed head and long bones. Combinations of both types occur.

8. How often can the cause of IUGR be determined? Name the most common fetal and maternal causes of IUGR.

In 50% of all cases of IUGR, no cause is discovered. In those with known causes, the most common fetal factors are aneuploidy, genetic disorders, infection, major congenital malformations, and multiple gestations. The most common maternal factors are vascular disorders, inadequate nutrition, anemia, hypoxia, drugs, antiphospholipid antibody syndrome, and previous delivery of an infant with IUGR.

9. When used during pregnancy, what drugs are commonly associated with the development of IUGR?

IUGR has been associated with the use of tobacco and illicit drugs such as alcohol, cocaine, and narcotics. Medications used during pregnancy, such as anticonvulsants, alkylating agents, warfarin, aminopterin, and angiotension-converting enzyme inhibitors, also may lead to IUGR.

10. How is IUGR diagnosed?

The most commonly used definition of antenatal diagnosis is an estimated fetal weight < 10% for gestational age. An accurate assessment of gestational age is requisite for a reliable diagnosis of IUGR, because preterm delivery is also associated with low birth weight. Fetal growth must be assessed at 3–4-week intervals for reliable results, because lesser intervals lead to unacceptably high false appraisals of impaired fetal growth.

11. Is IUGR an associated finding in fetuses with structural malformations?

In a large study of fetuses with major congenital anomalies, 22.4% were found to have IUGR.

12. Are fetuses with IUGR at risk for major congenital anomalies?

Fetuses with IUGR have an approximately 8% risk for major congenital anomalies.

13. What is the risk for aneuploidy in fetuses with IUGR?

Without congenital anomalies, 2%; with congenital anomalies, 31%. A sonographically structurally normal fetus with early-onset, second-trimester fetal growth restriction, however, may have a risk of 25% for aneuploidy.

14. Of women who have previously delivered a growth-restricted neonate, what is the recurrence risk for growth restriction in subsequent pregnancies?

For the total obstetric population for whom a prior pregnancy resulted in a neonate with IUGR, the recurrence risk is 25%. For those in which growth restriction in the prior pregnancy led to delivery at < 34 weeks' gestation, the recurrence risk is 50%.

15. Can we prevent recurrent idiopathic IUGR?

Low-dose aspirin has been successfully used to decrease the risk of recurrence of IUGR.

16. What postnatal complications are associated with IUGR?

Intrapartum asphyxia	Meconium aspiration
Neonatal hypoglycemia and hypocalcemia	Neurodevelopmental delays

17. When a pregnancy is diagnosed with IUGR, what evaluation should be performed?

A search for factors known to lead to IUGR should be aggressively made, including a thorough search for associated major congenital anomalies. Continuing ultrasound evaluation of fetal growth is essential. Diagnostic studies to consider include karyotype and maternal viral and antiphospholipid studies, depending on gestational age and severity of growth restriction.

18. When a pregnancy is diagnosed with IUGR, what treatment should be given?

Correctable maternal factors should be corrected (e.g., anemia, drug use, hypoxia). Fetal well-being should be serially assessed. Amniotic fluid volume is an important part of this assessment.

Oligohydramnios is frequently seen with IUGR and may be a sign of fetal compromise. Nonstress tests and oxytocin challenge tests have long been used for following IUGR pregnancies. The biophysical profile is highly effective in assessing fetal well-being in IUGR pregnancies. Doppler evaluation of the umbilical artery also may be helpful in following the IUGR fetus, because abnormal blood flow velocity waveforms have been associated with uteroplacental compromise. Delivery should occur if there is evidence of fetal compromise or if fetal pulmonary maturity is documented.

19. What is macrosomia?

The most common definition is a birth weight > 4000 gm or birth weight > 90% for gestational age.

20. What factors are known to lead to higher neonatal weights?

Postdate pregnancies	Male fetus
Maternal diabetes	Maternal birth weight
Increased prepregnancy weight	Previous delivery of macrosomic infant
Excessive maternal weight gain	Genetic overgrowth syndromes
Multiparity	(Beckwith-Wiedemann)

21. What percentage of macrosomic neonates are born to women with identifiable risk factors?

Fewer than 40% of macrosomic infants are born to mothers with risk factors for macrosomia.

22. How accurate is ultrasound in predicting macrosomia?

The accuracy for ultrasound prediction of the large-for-gestational-age fetus ranges from 47–64%. At 4500 gm, the accuracy decreases to 22%. One-third of fetuses estimated to be > 4000 gm are < 4000 gm at birth; conversely, 10% of those thought to be < 4000 gm deliver at > 4000 gm. Given the current inaccuracies of ultrasound in the prediction of macrosomia, clinical decisions should incorporate more information than sonographically determined estimated fetal weight.

23. What are the risks of macrosomia?

Shoulder dystocia	Childhood and adolescent
Birth trauma	obesity

24. What are the risk factors for shoulder dystocia?

Diabetes, increasing birth weight, and possibly labor abnormalities are risk factors for shoulder dystocia. In diabetes, the risk has been shown to be 23.1% for infants with a birth weight from 4000–4499 gm and 50% for infants with a birth weight ≥ 4500 gm. In nondiabetic parturients, the incidence is 10% with birth weight of 4000–4499 gm and 22.6% for birth weight ≥ 4500 gm. The incidence of shoulder dystocia in all vaginal deliveries is < 2%.

25. What birth trauma has been attributed to macrosomia?

Birth injuries are greater with vaginally delivered than cesarean-delivered neonates. The most common potentially serious injury to the neonate is brachial plexus injury. Fractures, especially to the clavicle and humerus, usually are well tolerated by the neonate.

26. What is the risk for brachial plexus injury in an obstetric population?

Brachial plexus palsies occur in approximately 1:526 births. Overall, approximately 5% of brachial plexus injuries are persistent (1:10,520 births).

27. Why are diabetics at increased risk for birth trauma?

Neonates of diabetics have an increased shoulder/chest-to-head ratio compared with neonates of similar weights born to nondiabetic mothers. Therefore, even at normal weights, the fetuses of diabetics are at a greater risk for shoulder dystocia compared with fetuses of nondiabetics.

28. Can neonatal birth injuries be prevented?

The inaccuracies of antenatal ultrasound for predicting macrosomia limit its usefulness in keeping the risk for birth injuries low. Most (> 80%) cases of shoulder dystocia follow spontaneous vaginal deliveries, and a minority of birth injuries occur with cesarean delivery. Documented shoulder dystocia occurs in only 50% of neonates who have sustained a brachial plexus injury.

BIBLIOGRAPHY

1. Acker DB, Sachs BP, Friedman EA: Risk Factors for shoulder dystocia. Obstet Gynecol 66:762–768, 1985.
2. American College of Obstetricians and Gynecologists: Fetal Macrosomia. Washington, D.C. American College of Obstetricians and Gynecologists, 1991.
3. Creasy RK, Resnik R: Intrauterine growth restriction. In Creasy RK, Resnik R (eds): Maternal-Fetal Medicine: Principles & Practice. 3rd ed. Philadelphia, W.B. Saunders, 1994.
4. Nicolaides KH, Snijders RJM, Gosden CM, et al: Ultrasonographically detectable markers of fetal chromosomal abnormalities. Lancet 340:704–707, 1992.
5. Nimrod CA: The biology of normal and deviant fetal growth. In Reece EA, Hobbins JC, Mahoney MJ, Petrie RH (eds): Medicine of the Fetus and Mother. Philadelphia, J.B. Lippincott, 1992.
6. Pollack RN, Divon MY: Intrauterine growth retardation: Definition, classification, and etiology. Clin Obstet Gynecol 35:99–107, 1992.
7. Visser GHA, Huisman A, Saathof PWF, Sinnige HAM: Early fetal growth retardation: Obstetric background and recurrence rate. Obstet Gynecol 67:40–43, 1986.

65. DISORDERS OF AMNIOTIC FLUID VOLUME

Craig Stark, M.D.

AMNIOTIC FLUID DYNAMICS

1. What functions does amniotic fluid serve?

Amniotic fluid serves as a protective cushion preventing fetal damage to the mother who has suffered trauma. It allows the fetus to move freely and plays an important role in fetal lung development. Amniotic fluid also helps to maintain a steady temperature state and contains antibacterial agents which help to protect the fetus from bacteria that may enter the amniotic cavity.

2. What factors regulate amniotic fluid volume throughout pregnancy?

In the first trimester of pregnancy, amniotic fluid is an ultrafiltrate of maternal serum with little embryonic contribution to total volume. With advancing gestation, transudation of fetal plasma across the skin becomes a significant contributor to the total volume. As the pregnancy enters the second trimester, fetal urination and swallowing begin to become the major players in amniotic fluid volume and its regulation. Other less important sources of amniotic fluid include transudation across the fetal surface of the placenta and umbilical cord and the fetal gastrointestinal and respiratory tracts.

3. How does amniotic fluid volume vary throughout pregnancy?

There is a progressive increase in amniotic fluid volume throughout pregnancy. Amniotic fluid volume peaks at 750–800 cc by the 34th week and remains relatively stable until 41–42 weeks, when it often begins to drop rapidly. Despite a wide variation in volumes at different gestational ages, mean volumes have been calculated to be 55–60 cc at 12 weeks, 150–200 cc at 16 weeks, 250–500 cc at 20 weeks, 1000 cc at 33–34 weeks, 850 cc at term, and 550 cc at 41–42 weeks.

4. How do abnormal amounts of (both high and low) amniotic fluid affect perinatal outcome?

Both perinatal morbidity and mortality are increased in pregnancies with abnormal amniotic fluid volumes. The more fluid levels appear to deviate from normal, the more likely that perinatal outcome will be adversely affected.

OLIGOHYDRAMNIOS

5. Define oligohydramnios.

Oligohydramnios is the presence of abnormally low amounts of amniotic fluid. Because the normal amount of amniotic fluid varies with gestational age, definition based on a quantitative determination is neither possible nor practical.

6. What clinical clues point to the possibility of oligohydramnios complicating a pregnancy?
- Fundal height at least 3 cm less than estimated gestational age
- Easily palpated fetal parts on maternal exam
- Ultrasound exam in which the fetus appears to be crowded and visualization of anatomy is difficult

7. What ultrasonographic methods are used to diagnose oligohydramnios?

The most common method to assess amniotic fluid volume (AFV) and pathologic deviations from normal involves the use of ultrasound. Simple visual assessment of AFV and whether it is abnormally low or high is an accurate method of diagnosis in experienced hands. When an abnormality in AFV is suspected, most clinicians attempt to make a semiquantitative estimate of amniotic fluid. One method involves measuring the largest vertical pocket of amniotic fluid that is free of fetal parts or umbilical cord. Oligohydramnios is said to exist when the largest pocket visualized is not larger than either 1 or 2 cm in depth. The most common method of measuring AFV is to divide the uterine cavity into four quadrants, measure the largest isolated pocket in each quadrant, and add all four numbers to get an amniotic fluid index (AFI). AFI values < 5 are considered diagnostic of oligohydramnios. No one measurement has been accepted as the lower limit of normal by a majority of clinicians. In recent years, the AI has become more widely adopted as a method of estimating AFV.

8. How does the timing of the onset of oligohydramnios affect perinatal outcome?

Oligohydramnios diagnosed early in pregnancy (i.e., the second trimester) is often associated with severe congenital anomalies with a poor prognosis at best. Fetal demise is not uncommon even when no obvious etiology is noted. When diagnosed in the third trimester, oligohydramnios is more often associated with intrauterine growth retardation.

9. For what other reasons is oligohydramnios associated with an increase in perinatal morbidity and mortality?

In addition to the reasons mentioned above, oligohydramnios can be the result of chromosomal aneuploidies, preterm premature rupture of membranes, and postmaturity (dysmaturity).

10. What congenital anomalies are often associated with oligohydramnios?

Most common are urinary tract anomalies involving both kidneys, such as bilateral renal agenesis, dysplastic multicystic kidneys, and infantile polycystic kidney disease. When only one kidney is abnormal or missing, amniotic fluid volume is generally unaffected. Complete obstruction of the urinary tract outlet may also produce oligohydramnios. In males, the presence of posterior urethral valves is the most common anomaly associated with oligohydramnios.

11. What role does diagnostic ultrasound play in delineating the etiology of oligohydramnios?

Amniotic fluid is an excellent transmitter of sound waves. Decreased amniotic fluid volume can make it extremely difficult, if not impossible, to visualize clearly intraabdominal fetal structures such as the fetal kidneys. Hypertrophied adrenal glands have been confused with kidneys.

Recent studies utilizing color flow Doppler techniques to visualize fetal renal arteries have proved helpful in clarifying the presence or absence of the kidneys. Some have suggested intraamniotic placement of sterile normal saline in an effort to enhance ultrasonic visualization of the fetus. Visualization of a fluid-filled bladder essentially rules out bilateral renal agenesis. A large bladder in the presence of oligohydramnios is usually consistent with urethral obstruction. Filling and emptying of the fetal bladder should lead one to look for other nonrenal causes of oligohydramnios.

12. What is the relationship between oligohydramnios and intrauterine growth retardation?
Asymmetric growth retardation is generally related to uteroplacental insufficiency. In this setting, decreased amniotic fluid is attributed to shunting of blood away from the fetal kidneys and a secondary decrease in urinary output. Symmetric growth retardation coupled with oligohydramnios has been associated with an increased incidence of fetal trisomies and triploidies. Affected women should receive genetic counseling and be offered prenatal diagnostic testing. Chorionic villus sampling, fetal blood sampling, and aspiration of the fetal bladder have provided adequate tissue for karyotype analysis.

13. Why is congenital pulmonary hypoplasia commonly seen in pregnancies with the onset of oligohydramnios in the second trimester?
Although it is somewhat unclear, it appears that normal fetal lung development depends on filling of the pulmonary tree with amniotic fluid. Loss of this distending force at critical times in pulmonary development is associated with varying degrees of pulmonary hypoplasia. Generally, however, the degree of pulmonary hypoplasia is severe and a common cause of early neonatal death. The earlier in gestation and the more prolonged the duration of oligohydramnios, the more significant the hypoplastic process tends to be. In one study in which oligohydramnios was related to preterm premature rupture of membranes, a 26% incidence of lethal pulmonary hypoplasia was reported when the oligohydramnios was first noted before 26 weeks and was present for > 5 weeks.

14. Can an accurate diagnosis of pulmonary hypoplasia be made prenatally?
Although many attempts have been made to diagnose the severely affected fetus in utero, no clinically applicable test exists today. Comparisons of both thoracic to abdominal circumference and thoracic to cardiac circumference have been studied but have not been found to be accurate enough to use for clinical decision making. The presence or absence of fetal breathing motion also has not proved to be an accurate predictor of postnatal pulmonary function.

15. What signs of oligohydramnios are seen on antepartum testing?
Often when patients with oligohydramnios undergo antipartum testing, variable decelerations are noted. This finding is believed to result from cord compression due to the loss of the cushioning effect of adequate amniotic fluid.

POLYHYDRAMNIOS

16. What is hydramnios? Polyhydramnios?
Both terms are synonymous with abnormally excessive amounts of amniotic fluid. Because amniotic fluid volume changes with gestational age, the amount considered to be pathologically increased also changes.

17. What ultrasound criteria are used to make the diagnosis of polyhydramnios?
As with oligohydramnios, the diagnosis can be made either on qualitative or semiquantitative criteria. The first clue that often leads to the diagnosis is that one finds it easy to see the fetus clearly and to delineate the fetal anatomy. However, often with severe polyhydramnios, the fetus is lying so posteriorly that it is difficult to visualize the whole fetus. A vertical pocket of amniotic fluid > 9 cm is considered diagnostic of mild polyhydramnios; 11–13 cm suggests moderate polyhydramnios; and pockets > 13 cm suggest a severe problem. An amniotic fluid index (AFI) > 20 also is used to confirm the diagnosis.

18. What are the different clinical presentations of polyhydramnios?

Acute polyhydramnios is characterized by a rapid accumulation of excessive amounts of amniotic fluid and is generally diagnosed in the later stages of the second and early portions of the third trimester. Delivery often follows shortly after diagnosis; extreme prematurity is a common problem. Chronic polyhydramnios is a more gradual accumulation of amniotic fluid with an onset in the mid-to-late third trimester. Prematurity is not as significant a problem.

19. What is the differential diagnosis for polyhydramnios?

In approximately one-third of cases no apparent cause can be found. Possible associations include diabetes (both gestational and previously diagnosed disease), congenital malformations, both immune and nonimmune hydrops, and multiple gestations. In some series, approximately 10% of cases demonstrate a chromosomal abnormality when karyotyping is performed.

20. Which organ systems are most often anomalous in polyhydramniotic pregnancies?

The central nervous system (CNS) and the gastrointestinal (GI) system are the most common sites of anomalies. Cardiovascular anomalies, including arrhythmias, are also occasionally seen. Finally, musculoskeletal and genitourinary tract anomalies have been reported.

21. What specific anomalies are associated with polyhydramnios?

As many as one-third of pregnancies with polyhydramnios are associated with a congenital anomaly. Anencephaly is one of the most common CNS anomalies associated with polyhydramnios. Facial clefts and neck masses, which may interfere with the normal swallowing process, and atretic lesions of the GI tract have also been frequently noted. The skeletal dysplasias, including thanatophoric dwarfism and achondroplasia, are occasionally noted.

22. What obstetric complications most frequently complicate polyhydramniotic pregnancies?

As in all pregnancies in which an overdistended uterus is present, preterm labor, premature rupture of the membranes, and preterm delivery are frequent. Severe cases may involve compromise of maternal respiration and urinary tract obstruction.

23. What therapeutic options are available for polyhydramnios?

Rarely, correction of the underlying cause of the polyhydramnios is possible. An example is conversion of fetal supraventricular tachycardia to a normal sinus rhythm with a subsequent return of amniotic fluid levels to normal. Resolution of congenital parvovirus is another example. Generally, however, the cause is either unknown or results from a congenital anomaly not amenable to in utero therapy. Efforts are then directed to decreasing fluid levels in hopes of preventing preterm rupture of membranes and preterm labor and delivery. Frequent therapeutic amniocentesis is advocated by many, with the patient undergoing the procedure once to several times a week. Maternal administration of indocin has also been shown to decrease amniotic fluid levels. Often there is a rapid return to previous excessive levels when the medicine is discontinued. Long-term indocin therapy has been associated with both fetal and neonatal morbidity, and many limit therapy to 48-hour courses.

BIBLIOGRAPHY

1. Brace RA: Amniotic fluid dynamics. In Creasy R, Resnick R (eds): Maternal Fetal Medicine: Principles and Practice, 2nd ed. Philadelphia, W.B. Saunders, 1989.
2. Devoe LD, Ware DJ: Oligohydramnios: Definition and diagnosis. Contemporary Obstet Gynecol. Sept: 31–40, 1994.
3. Harrison M, Golbus M, Filly R (eds): The Unborn Patient: Prenatal Diagnosis and Treatment, 2nd ed. Philadelphia, W.B. Saunders, 1990, pp 139–140.
4. Neyberg DA, Mahony BS, Pretoria DH: Diagnostic Ultrasound of Fetal Abnormalities: Text and Atlas. Chicago, Yearbook, 1990.
5. Queenan JT: Polyhydramnios and oligohydramnios. Contemp Obstet Gynecol. Dec:60–81, 1991.
6. Stoll CG, Alembik Y, Dott B: Study of 156 cases of polyhydramnios and congenital malformations in a series of 118,265 consecutive births. Am J Obstet Gynecol 165:586–590, 1991.

66. POSTDATE PREGNANCY

Martin E. Nowick, M.D.

1. What is the definition of postdate pregnancy?
Postdate pregnancy is defined as a gestation that has entered in its 42nd week (287 days) from the last menstrual period. Without intervention, approximately 10% of pregnancies proceed past 42 weeks.

2. Does postdate pregnancy have clinical significance?
Yes. There is an increased incidence of fetal demise—as high as 3–5% by completion of the 43rd week.

3. Is postdate pregnancy a new entity?
Postdate pregnancy and its risks were described as early as 1902 by Ballantyne. The entity gained clinical significance in the late 1960s.

4. What information is evaluated in diagnosing a postdate pregnancy?
- The patient's accurate recording of the first day of her last normal menstrual period
- Early examination and recording of uterine size by an experienced clinician
- Auscultation of fetal heart tones by fetoscope at 18–20 weeks
- Regular and precise recording of uterine growth supplemented by evidence of cessation of growth
- Ultrasound evidence of placental insufficiency, such as decreased amniotic fluid, placenta calcification, absent fetal breathing movements, decreased fetal tone
- A nonreactive nonstress test or a nonstress test with late component decelerations
- Amniotic fluid index of < 7.1 with the deepest pocket < 2.7 cm
- Doppler flow studies showing decreased umbilical artery end-diastolic flow or middle cerebral artery to umbilical artery flow ratio < 1.05

5. Is it true that postdate pregnancy is a recognized cause of placental insufficiency?
Yes. It is the evidence of deterioration of the fetal environment that prompts action.

6. What causes postdate pregnancy?
The cause of the majority of cases is unknown. Rare associates include anencephaly, fetal adrenal hypoplasia, placental sulfatase deficiency, and extrauterine pregnancy. The majority of cases occur in perfectly healthy and normal gestations.

7. How does the typical patient present?
Many patients are primigravidas. The patient may have noticed a decrease in the quality and frequency of fetal movements. Vaginal exam usually reveals an uneffaced, undilated cervix. The fetus is usually in vertex presentation, often with an occiput posterior position. The vertex may or may not be engaged and well applied to the cervix. Ultrasound may show evidence of a large fetus and/or decreased amniotic fluid.

8. What is done after the diagnosis of postdate pregnancy has been made?
The obstetrician may continue to observe the patient with serial fetal surveillance, including nonstress testing and biophysical profiles. Many centers now use frequent Doppler flow ultrasound studies, especially in a pregnancy with 42 completed weeks. Observation is acceptable only with reassurance of fetal well-being and in anticipation that the patient will go into spontaneous labor and deliver within a few days.

9. What if labor does not begin spontaneously?

This is usually the case. Sooner or later, in a certain number of patients, the obstetrician is forced into action.

10. What should be undertaken before labor is initiated?

This is the golden opportunity to formulate a plan that is fully discussed before implementation. The obstetrician has a conference with the patient and her husband. The data are presented, and the use of prostaglandin gel or suppositories and intravenous pitocin for labor induction is discussed. The possibility of cesarean section should be considered for fetal distress or if the labor does not progress normally.

11. Does the mother sign a consent form?

A consent form is an excellent idea. The conference is the time to answer questions in a relaxed environment. The consent for induction of labor and possible cesarean section should be obtained when the woman is not under the stress of labor and has accepted the obstetrician's recommendations.

12. Once the consent is signed, how is labor initiated?

The patient is admitted to the hospital labor service. Prostaglandin gel or suppository is introduced into the vagina every 4–6 hours for a total of 3 doses. The cervix usually effaces and slightly dilates, often with contractions beginning. Once the cervix begins to dilate, an amniotomy is performed. If labor does not progress, intravenous pitocin is started. It is a good idea at this point to place a scalp electrode and intrauterine pressure monitor. From this point, labor generally progresses in a normal fashion.

13. Is it safer simply to wait for the patient to go into labor?

The decision for action is based on a deteriorating fetal environment. The question is not whether the mother is at risk but to what degree the fetus is at risk. About 1–2% of infants suffer extreme morbidity from procrastination. A recent study of 10,000 births reported 14 deaths among 702 patients who had passed 42 completed weeks.

14. What if the patient's cervix is already dilated?

Prostaglandin should be omitted, because its purpose is effacement in preparation for dilation. In such patients amniotomy and carefully administered intravenous pitocin usually cause an active labor.

15. Do patients with postdate pregnancy have a higher cesarean section rate?

Yes. But postdate pregnancies represent only 5–10% of the obstetric population and thus contribute a minute fraction to the overall 15–20% primary cesarean section rate. The incidence of fetal macrosomia is 10% at 38–40 weeks, 20% at 40–41 weeks, and 42% at 43 weeks of gestation.

16. Is a cesarean section ever done with no trial of labor?

Yes. If fetal macrosomia is suspected (in excess of 4,000 gm) or the patient had a previous difficult labor with a large child and a history of shoulder dystocia.

17. What are the clinical secrets?

Be sure to use serial fetal surveillance to ensure the proper diagnosis of deteriorating fetal environment. Explain clearly to the patient that her baby is at risk and obtain proper consent in advance of initiating induction of labor. Always admit the patient to a medical facility that is capable of handling unforeseen complications. Careful planning reduces the fetal morbidity and mortality that may arise from postdate pregnancy.

BIBLIOGRAPHY

1. Charles D, Glover DD (eds): Current Therapy in Obstetrics. Toronto, B.C. Decker, 1988.
2. Creasy RK, Resnik R (eds): Maternal-Fetal Medicine: Principles and Practice, 2nd ed. Philadelphia, W.B. Saunders, 1989.
3. Jimerrez JM, Tyson JG, Reisch JS: Clinical measures of gestation age in normal pregnancies. Obstet Gynecol 61:438–443, 1983.
4. Pitkin RM, Scott JR, Phelan JP (eds): Postdatism. Clin Obstet Gynecol 32:219–303, 1989.
5. Devine PA, Bracero LA, Lysikiewicz AJ, et al: Middle cerebral to umbilical artery Doppler ratio in post date pregnancies. Obstet Gynecol 84:856–860, 1984.
6. Hasib Ahemed AI, Versi A: Prolonged pregnancy. Curr Opin Obstet Gynecol 5:669–674, 1993.
7. Vottn RA, Gibilis LA: Active management of prolonged pregnancy. Am J Obstet Gynecol 168:557-562, 1993.
8. Fischer RL, McDonnel M, Biaculli DW, et al: Amniotic fluid volume estimation in the postdate pregnancy: A comparison of techniques. Obstet Gynecol 81:698–703, 1993.
9. Chervenak, JL: Macrosomia in the postdate pregnancy. Clin Obstet Gynecol 35:151–155, 1992.

67. ANTEPARTUM FETAL SURVEILLANCE

Kent Heyborne, M.D.

1. Describe in general terms the tests used for antepartum fetal surveillance.

Fetal movement record (FMR)—quantification by the mother of the number of fetal movements perceived within a given time frame.

Nonstress test (NST)—external fetal cardiac monitoring allows evaluation of the fetal heart rate, including baseline, response to fetal movement, and variability.

Contraception stress test (CST)—External fetal cardiac and uterine contraction monitoring allows evaluation of the heart rate in response to contractions.

Biophysical profile (BPP)—combined analysis of NST and several ultrasound parameters provides more comprehensive evaluation of the fetus.

Doppler flow studies—Doppler ultrasound evaluation of fetal blood flow velocity obtained at various uterine and fetal vessels.

2. Which patients should receive antepartum fetal surveillance?

Any patient with an increased chance of fetal compromise is a candidate. Examples include present pregnancy complications (hypertension, diabetes, preeclampsia, or growth retardation) or previous in utero demise. Surveillance usually is initiated with FMR and NST.

3. What advantages does a maternally recorded FMR offer as a means of antepartum surveillance?

The FMR is essentially free, simple, and noninvasive; it involves the patient actively in the assessment of her fetus. Fetal movement is typically recorded daily. A daily total below a set threshold (10–15 total movements) or any drastic change in fetal activity perceived by the mother prompts further evaluation, such as NST.

4. How is NST performed and interpreted?

The fetal heart rate is recorded with an external monitor for 20–40 minutes. Three components of the heart rate are assessed. To achieve a reactive NST, there must be a normal baseline (120–160 bpm), heart rate variability of 6–10 bpm, and 2–4 heart rate accelerations by at least 15 bpm for at least 15 seconds associated with fetal movement. Because of central nervous system immaturity, the NST is often nonreactive before 30–32 weeks.

5. Define FAST and describe its role during NST.

Many NSTs are nonreactive by the criteria described previously, perhaps owing to a fetal sleep cycle. Fetal acoustic stimulation testing (FAST) causes the fetus to wake up and potentially enter a more active state. FAST can be performed with an artificial larynx or an electric toothbrush held briefly to the maternal abdomen. FAST has been shown to shorten the amount of time necessary to obtain an NST and to decrease the number of falsely nonreactive NSTs.

6. In which patients have falsely reactive NSTs been most commonly observed (i.e., reactive NSTs within 1 week of fetal death in utero)? What implications does this have for fetal surveillance?

Falsely reactive NSTs occur most commonly in association with insulin-dependent diabetes, postdate pregnancies, and preeclampsia with IUGR. For this reason, twice-weekly NST monitoring has been advocated in such situations.

7. How should a nonreactive nonstress test be evaluated?

A BPP or CST should be performed.

8. How is the CST performed and interpreted?

Uterine contractions and fetal heart rate are monitored with the patient in a left lateral recumbent position. Uterine contractions may be spontaneous or induced with maternal nipple stimulation or intravenous oxytocin. Three moderate contractions in 10 minutes must be achieved for an adequate CST. The CST is interpreted as follows:

Positive CST—declerations of fetal heart rate after more than half of the uterine contractions.

Negative CST—no late decelerations noted.

Equivocal CST—decelerations with uterine hyperstimulation, isolated late deceleration, or technical problems such as inability to achieve adequate contractions.

Many physicians also include reactive or nonreactive in their report, using the same criteria as described previously for nonstress tests (i.e., reactive negative CST). At least 50% of patients with a positive CST can deliver vaginally.

9. How do NSTs, CSTs, and BPPs compare in terms of false-positive rates?

Each of these three tests has approximately a 50% false-positive rate. More recent studies suggest, however, that well-performed biophysical profiles may have as low as a 20% false-positive rate.

10. How do the three tests compare in terms of false-negative rates?

The NST has the highest false-negative rate at 1.4 per 1000 tests. CST and biophysical appear to be relatively comparable at 0.4 per 1000 and 0.6 per 1000, respectively.

11. BPP involves more comprehensive evaluation of the fetus than simply heart rate. What four ultrasound components of BPP are evaluated in addition to NST?

Fetal breathing movement, fetal body and extremity movement, fetal tone, and amniotic fluid volume. Some physicians use placental grade as a fifth component. A standard scoring system is available with points given in each category; the overall score is then interpreted as an indicator of fetal well-being.

12. What are the putative advantages of BPP over NST?

BPP can potentially diagnose disorders of amniotic fluid volume and fetal anomalies. It also appears to have a higher specificity than NST; fewer healthy infants are subjected to further surveillance and intervention.

13. What is a modified BPP? What are its advantages?

A modified BPP consists of NST and evaluation of amniotic fluid volume. It is quicker than a complete BPP and appears to have the same sensitivity for detecting fetal compromise.

14. How is the Doppler principle applied to antepartum surveillance?

The Doppler shift phenomenon is used to approximate velocity of flow in various vessels (uterine artery, umbilical artery). Increased ratios of systolic-to-diastolic velocity (S/D ratio) correlate with high resistance in distal vascular beds (i.e., spiral arteries, placenta). High umbilical artery S/D ratios correlate histologically with abnormal placental vasculature and clinically with adverse perinatal outcome (IUGR and preeclampsia).

15. What is the significance of absent diastolic flow?

Although decreased diastolic flow and increased diastolic systolic ratios remain controversial as to their predictive abilities for fetal compromise, the finding of absent diastolic and, in severe cases, reversal of diastolic flow in general are harbingers of fetal distress.

16. Do abnormal Doppler flow analyses in the setting of a fetus with growth retardation always reflect uteroplacental etiology of the fetal compromise?

No. Abnormal Doppler flow is also seen with increased frequency among karyotypically abnormal infants.

17. Describe the attributes of the perfect antepartum test. Do any of the tests described above meet this description?

The ideal test should be cheap, quick, simple to interpret, and noninvasive. It should have few false-positive or false-negative results. It should be able to identify the fetus at risk before serious compromise has occurred. Unfortunately, none of the current tests fulfills these criteria. Using several tests in combination may partially overcome some of the shortcomings.

BIBLIOGRAPHY

1. American College of Obstetricians and Gynecologists: Antepartum fetal surveillance. ACOG Tech Bull 188, 1994.
2. Clark SL, Sabey P, Jolley K: Nonstress testing with acoustic stimulation and amniotic fluid volume assessment: 5973 tests without unexpected fetal death. Am J Obstet Gynecol 160:694, 1989.
3. Devore L, Castillo R, Sherline D: The nonstress test as a diagnostic test: A critical reappraisal. Am J Obstet Gynecol 152:1047–1053, 1985.
4. Schulman H: The clinical implications of Doppler ultrasound analysis of the uterine and umbilical arteries. Am J Obstet Gynecol 156:889–893, 1987.
5. Vintzileos AM: Antepartum Fetal Surveillance. Clin Obstet Gynecol 38:1–143, 1995.

68. FETAL DEMISE

Louise Wilkins-Haug, M.D., Ph.D.

1. What is the commonly accepted definition of fetal demise? How often does it occur?

According to the American College of Obstetricians and Gynecologists, fetal demise is death of a gestation in utero past 20 weeks' gestation. This definition is followed by the majority of states. However, several states as well as various countries use definitions as diverse as all products of conception and only gestations of greater than 28 weeks. In the United States, the overall fetal death rate is 7.5/1000, representing approximately 50% of the total perinatal mortality rate.

2. What maternal variables influence the fetal death rate?

Maternal age: Extremes of maternal age are associated with an approximate 2% fetal demise; women under 15 years of age have a stillbirth rate of 19/1000 births, and for women older than 40 years, a rate of 22/1000 births has been reported.

Race: Although comparable proportionate decreases in the fetal death rate have occurred over the past decades in both white and black populations, the starting and end points differ. From 1945–1988, in the white population fetal death rates decreased from 21 to 6/1000 births, whereas in the black population the decrease was from 42 to 11/1000 births.

Maternal weight: Prepregnant weight outside the ideal for the individual's height, either significantly underweight or obese, increases the risk for fetal demise. Additionally, for extremes of prepregnant weight, risk of fetal demise is tied to weight gain during pregnancy.

3. How is third-trimester demise recognized? How is it confirmed?

Most often, the mother reports absent fetal movement. With prolonged demise, the mother may lose weight, no longer feel pregnant, and experience breast regression. Demise can be confirmed by ultrasound with visualization of lack of cardiac activity by two proficient examiners observing for a minimum of three minutes.

4. How can the diagnosis be made if ultrasound is not available?

Absence of heart tones by auscultation does not confirm fetal demise. Especially with a fetoscope, heart tones can be present but obscured by maternal obesity, anterior placenta, or polyhydramnios. Radiographic examination has classically been used for confirmation of fetal death by using the following parameters:

Spalding's sign—overlapping of the fetal skull bones, although this may also appear in fetuses with oligohydramnios or with molding of normal labor.

Halo sign—extravasation of fluid between the fetal cranium and subcutaneous fat; may be mimicked by fetal hydrops.

Exaggerated curvature of the fetal spine.

Intravascular gas—from decomposition of the fetal blood, considered an irrefutable sign, although it may take up to 10 days to appear and is not present in 100% of cases.

5. How often can the cause of fetal demise be determined?

Despite extensive evaluation, a specific cause is determined in only approximately 40% of cases. Approximately one-half of the etiologies are maternal, and one-half are intrinsic to the fetus. Although variable over time as well as by population and with some overlap between categories, approximate groupings of etiology include:

Percentage of All Demises	
Maternal disease	10–35%
Hypertension	5–25%
Other medical	5–10%
Fetal—intrinsic	25%
Sporadic malformation	7%
Cytogenetic	6%
Multifactorial	3%
Mendelian	1%
Fetal-maternal hemorrhage	3–5%
Isoimmunization	3–10%
Cord/placental abnormalities	10–20%
Infections	5–10%

6. How often does syphilis cause fetal demise?

In the early part of this century, 40% of fetal demise was due to syphilis. In recent decades, syphilis has rarely been identified. However, the recent increase in syphilis argues for continued surveillance of this treatable disorder.

7. Once a fetal demise is recognized, from a medical standpoint, does labor need to be induced immediately?

No. 75–90% of demises deliver without intervention within the next two weeks. Exception to expectant management should be made in cases of rupture of membranes, because delay in delivery increases the risk of maternal infection. Whether the mother should deliver immediately or await spontaneous labor is an individual choice. However, the risks of prolonged induction, including side effects of induction agents, possible infection, and maternal morbidity, should be seriously considered.

8. What are the concerns if delivery is not immediate?

If not delivered by 4 weeks, 25% of women develop mild coagulopathy. This results when thromboplastic substances from the demise are carried into the maternal circulation and initiate disseminated coagulopathy.

9. What is the most clinically helpful parameter to follow for detecting a coagulopathy?

Fibrinogen. A gradual decrease can be noted at 4 weeks, with an anticipated decrease of 20–85 mg/dl/week thereafter. Fibrinogen levels in pregnancy are generally around 450 mg/dl; clinically significant coagulopathy is usually not apparent until levels fall below 100 mg/dl.

10. How can induction of labor be accomplished with a fetal demise?

Prostaglandins: Vaginal suppositories, 20 mg of prostaglandin E_2 (PGE$_2$), have been approved by the Food and Drug Administration for labor induction up to 28 weeks' gestation. Side effects include nausea and vomiting, diarrhea, tachycardia, and fever. PGE$_2$ is relatively contraindicated in asthmatics; women with cardiac, renal, or hepatic disease; diabetics; and women with a previously scarred uterus. Prostaglandins have also been used via intravenous (IV PGE), intraamniotic (F_2 alpha), and intramuscular (15 methyl PGF$_2$ alpha) routes. With any route, preinduction placement of osmotic dilators in the cervix (laminaria) may decrease the amount of prostaglandin used.

Amnioinfusion: Intraamniotic placement of a hypertonic solution, usually sodium chloride, glucose, or urea induces contractions. This method is seldom used because maternal deaths have been attributed to amnioinfusion.

Oxytocin: Oxytocin (pitocin) is often used for third-trimester demise after cervical ripening with low-dose prostaglandin vaginal suppositories or osmotic cervical dilators. Prolonged, higher doses of pitocin may be accompanied by maternal water intoxication. Intravenous fluid replacement should be an electrolyte-containing solution, input and output volumes should be carefully monitored, and intake should be restricted if necessary.

11. What should be considered if a patient with a third-trimester fetal demise fails to deliver despite prolonged pitocin augmentation?

Abdominal pregnancy

12. Which maternal laboratory studies should be considered for a fetal demise?

Blood type and antibody screen	Toxicology screen for maternal drug use
Kleihauer-Betke stain	Viral titers (rubella, parvovirus)
Venereal Disease Research Laboratory	Lupus anticoagulant, anticardiolipin antibody
test for syphilis	HgA1C

Studies obtained in the first trimester should be repeated because isoimmunization and infectious disease states have the potential for changing over the intervening months. For cost efficacy, some studies may be indicated only with collaborating evidence from evaluation of the fetal demise and placenta.

13. How is fetal-maternal hemorrhage (FMH) evaluated?

A small degree of fetal-maternal hemorrhage (< 0.1 ml) occurs in essentially all pregnancies at delivery. However, a large FMH during pregnancy can lead to fetal anemia and demise. A maternal Kleihauer-Betke stain, based on the different acid elution characteristics of fetal and adult hemoglobin, provides quantitative assessment of the volume of fetal blood within the maternal circulation. In most cases, for the evaluation of fetal demise, given the magnitude of fetal blood in the maternal circulation, a Kleihauer-Betke stain after delivery is as useful as one obtained before labor.

14. What studies should be done once the infant delivers?

Fetal examination, including measurements.

Placental examination with attention to number of cord vessels, infarcts, and size; placenta should be submitted for histology examination.

Autopsy of infant, which may include full-body radiographs and photographs.

Chromosomal analysis, especially in cases of noted malformations, maceration, or growth retardation.

Molecular genetic studies in selected instances; suspected viral infection and some inherited disorders can be investigated with DNA technology

15. If the parents decline full autopsy, what additional options should be discussed?

Unfortunately, in some situations when the parents decline an autopsy, no further evaluation is initiated. Although the parents may be opposed to internal examination of the infant, several options should be offered:

Limited autopsy—especially in situations in which ultrasound has suggested congenital malformation, internal autopsy can be limited to that specific area.

Radiologic studies—radiographs and other radiologic modalities provide valuable information.

Gross examination including photographs—visual examination by a pathologist or dysmorphologist should be offered, even if full autopsy is declined.

Placental pathology—often provides information suggesting possible maternal causes, placental abnormalities, or fetal conditions, such as infection.

Chromosomal studies—most efficacious when fetal autopsy has identified a malformation; however, they are an option when autopsy has been declined, especially in the setting of maceration, which may obscure recognizable facial dysmorphology.

16. What are sources for chromosomal analysis?

With a recent fetal demise, cardiac puncture for 10 ml heparinized blood can be obtained. Alternatively, skin biopsy can be sent in sterile saline. With macerated demises, culture failure rate as high as 90% has been reported. For such cases, internal tissue (diaphragm or lung), fascia lata, or a chorionic plate biopsy may provide a more successful culture rate. Some advocate amniocentesis at identification of demise to increase the chances of successful karyotype. Additionally, fetal tissue or placental cell suspension without culture and evaluated by fluorescent in situ hybridization (FISH) provides information limited to specific chromosomes (usually 13,18,21,X and Y). In some instances, FISH provides limited retrospective evaluation of paraffin-embedded archival materials in instances in which a full karyotype was not obtained.

17. Which physical findings should be noted and documented when the stillborn infant is examined by the obstetrician?

Overall appearance—maceration, meconium-staining, and skin lesions.

Posterior surface—integrity of the skull, neck, and spine.

Anterior surface—presence of orbits and integrity of the palate should be included in the general description of the face. Abdominal wall should be described for defects as well as scaphoid appearance (diaphragmatic hernia) or possible masses. Genital sex should be assigned.

Extremities—symmetry and proportions, digits on all four extremities, and abnormal palmer creases.

18. What support services should be available to couples after fetal demise?

After fetal demise, couples often experience classic grief reactions (shock, guilt, anger, disorientation, and reorganization). After the first month, literature about perinatal death and community support groups may help to alleviate feelings of isolation. Arrangements should be made, generally at 6–8 weeks, for a follow-up appointment in which available records and studies are reviewed, possible recurrence risks and interventions discussed, and additional support for adjustment to the grief reaction assessed.

19. What is the recurrence risk for fetal demise?

Without an identifiable cause, stillbirth rarely recurs. Estimates in the range of 1/300 are provided by at least one study. In a subsequent pregnancy, many advocate antepartum surveillance, usually with nonstress testing, although the timing of initiation of surveillance is variable. If recurrent maternal risk factors are present, such as diabetes and hypertension, the risk of recurrent still birth has been estimated at 10%.

BIBLIOGRAPHY

1. American College of Obstetricians and Gynecologists: Diagnosis and Management of Fetal Death. ACOG Technical Bulletin 176, 1993.
2. Brady K, Duff P, Harlass FE, Reid S: The role of amniotic fluid cytogenetic analysis in the evaluation of recent fetal death. Am J Perinatol 8:68–70, 1991.
3. National Center for Health Statistics: Vital statistics of the United States, 1988, Vol II, Mortality, Part A. DHHS Pub No. 91-1101. Washington, DC, U.S. Government Printing Office, 1991.
4. Owen J, Stedman CM, Tucker TL: Comparison of predelivery versus postdelivery Kleihauer-Betke stains in cases of fetal death. Am J Obstet Gynecol 161:663–666, 1989.
5. Pauli RM, Reiser CA: Wisconsin Stillbirth Service Program. II: Analysis of diagnoses and diagnostic categories in the first 1000 referrals. Am J Med Genet 50:135–153, 1994.
6. Samueloff A, Xenakis EM, Berkus MD, et al: Recurrent stillbirth. Significance and characteristics. J Reprod Med 38:883–886, 1993.
7. Vance JC, Najman JM, Thearle MJ, et al: Psychological changes in parents eight months after the loss of an infant from stillbirth, neonatal death or sudden infant death syndrome—a longitudinal study. Pediatrics 96:933–938, 1995.
8. Weeks JW, Asrat T, Morgon MA, et al: Antepartum surveillance for a history of stillbirth: when to begin? Am J Obstet Gynecol 172:486–492, 1995.

VII. The Placenta

69. PATHOPHYSIOLOGY OF THE PLACENTA

Debra Klaisle, M.D.

1. How and when does placental development begin?

Implantation of the blastocyst occurs 6–7 days after fertilization. Enlargement of trophoblasts helps to anchor the blastocyst to the endometrial lining. Close interdigitation between the microvillae and the lumens of the endometrial epithelial surface allows junctional complexes to be formed. The reactions that then allow the embryo to be completely interstitial within the endometrial layer are poorly understood. Immunologic, biochemical, and phagocytic processes have all been proposed. The developing placenta is thus composed of two parts: (1) the chorion frondosum (chorionic plate), which is the fetal contribution arising from extraembryonic mesoderm, and (2) the decidua basalis, which is the maternal contribution from the endometrial surface (see figure below).

2. What are decidual changes? How are they anatomically related to the developing embryo?

Transformation of fibroblast-like cells into plump glycogen and lipoid-rich cells characterizes the decidual reaction. This occurs as a response to ovarian steroids (estrogen and progesterone) and is seen in pregnancy and to a lesser degree in the nonpregnant uterus during the later half of the menstrual cycle (see figure below).

Decidua basalis—the decidual reaction that occurs between the blastocyst and the myometrium

Decidua capsularis—the decidual reaction occurring over the blastocyst closest to the endometrial cavity, destined to be compressed to a remnant layer overlying the membranes

Decidua vera (parietalis)—reaction changes in the endometrium opposite the site of implantation

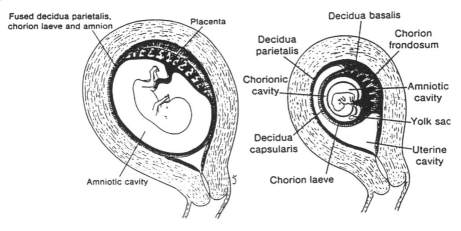

The developing placenta. (From Langman J: Medical Embryology, 4th ed. Baltimore, Williams & Wilkins, 1981, p 86, with permission.)

3. At what gestational age do the developing embryo, gestational sac, and placenta fill the endometrial cavity?

By the end of the third month (12 weeks), the endometrial cavity is obliterated as the membranes from the enlarging embryo fuse with the decidua vera opposite the implantation site. Until this time, the gestational sac is a distinct entity within the endometrial cavity. An incompletely filled endometrial cavity can sometimes be visualized on first-trimester ultrasound.

4. What is the origin of the fetal membranes?

Amnion—single cell layer of fetal ectodermal origin without vasculature; surrounds the developing embryo and with embryo enlargement meets the chorionic membrane at about 12 weeks' gestation.

Chorion—layer consisting of remnants of the decidua capsularis, hyalinized villi, and chorion laeve; stretches and thins during gestation.

5. What is the role of the placenta as an endocrine gland?

The chorionic villi are the functional endocrine units of the placenta. A central core with abundant capillaries is surrounded by an inner layer (cytotrophoblast) and an outer layer (syncytiotrophoblast). The cytotrophoblast primarily produces neuropeptides, whereas the syncytiotrophoblast is responsible for producing the protein hormones (hCG, hPL) and the sex steroids (estrogen, progesterone).

6. What part does the placenta play in estrogen and progesterone synthesis?

After the seventh week of gestation, most progesterone is produced by the syncytiotrophoblast from maternally derived cholesterol precursors. Progesterone production is exclusively a maternal-placental interaction, with no contribution from the fetus.

In contrast, production of placental estrogen involves an intricate pathway, requiring maternal, placental, and fetal contributions. The placenta lacks 17-hydroxylase activity and thus cannot produce estrogen directly by the common pathway from cholesterol. To compensate, the fetal adrenal gland plays a major role by converting pregnenolone to dehydroepiandrosterone sulfate (DHEA-S). DHEA-S is then transported to the placenta where sulfatase converts it to DHEA. The placenta converts DHEA to androgens, which are aromatized to estrone and estradiol. Further conversion to estriol is accomplished by the maternal liver, as the placenta lacks 17-hydroxylase. However, most estriol is produced by fetal contributions of DHEA-S to the placenta and then can be converted directly to estriol. Estriol production thus reflects both fetal and placental contributions.

7. What other hormones are produced by the placental endocrine unit?

Human chorionic gonadotropin (hCG)—produced by the syncytiotrophoblast; functions to maintain the corpus luteum in early pregnancy; detected as early as 9 days after conception; peaks at 8–10 weeks.

Human placental lactogen (hPL)—also produced by the syncytiotrophoblast; its concentration in maternal blood is directly related to placental mass; actions include promotion of lipolysis and an anti-insulin action that serves to direct nutrients to the fetus.

Human chorionic thyrotropin (hCT)—functional role is unknown, although increased amounts are thought by some investigators to account for the higher incidence of thyrotoxicosis associated with gestational trophoblastic disease.

8. What other endocrine unit is created during placental development?

Decidua-fetal membranes—the source of production of relaxin, prolactin, and prostaglandin.

9. What is relaxin?

Relaxin is produced by the corpus luteum as well as the decidua. Its importance is unclear but it may play a role in cervical ripening, inhibition of uterine contractions, and rupture of membranes.

10. What is the role of prolactin during pregnancy?

During pregnancy prolactin is produced by the maternal pituitary, the fetal pituitary, and the decidualized endometrium. Rising during the first trimester, it peaks at 10 times normal by term. Fetal prolactin has been linked to lung maturation. The highest prolactin levels are measured in the amniotic fluid, and here it may play a role in regulating osmotic exchanges.

11. What are some placental transport mechanisms?

Most forms of transport can be identified in the placenta and include active transport and diffusion. Without a specialized mechanism of transport, permeability is determined by size and lipid solubility. Molecules with a molecular weight less than 5,000 and with high lipid solubility cross with ease.

12. What features of a placenta should be evaluated following its delivery?

Of immediate consequence is whether or not the placenta has delivered intact. Either missing cotyledons on the maternal surface or vessels that run to edge with a sheared-off appearance suggest a fragmented placenta. If an accessory lobe (succenturiate lobe) or placental fragment remains in the uterus, postpartum hemorrhage or infection may result. Inspection of the maternal surface may suggest abruption as evidenced by an old clot that has depressed the underlying placenta.

The membranes are inspected for color and consistency, with attention to meconium staining or signs of infection. The length of the umbilical cord is noted. Short cords of less than 30 cm may result in traction during labor and delivery, leading to avulsion of the cord, abruption, or inversion of the uterus. Long chords are more likely to prolapse, become twisted around the fetus, or tie in true knots.

13. What is amnion nodosum?

Amnion nodosum consists of small elevations on the fetal membranes, measuring in millimeters. It is associated with oligohydramnios and results from fetal cells that are not washed off by the normal fluctuations of amniotic fluid. Amnion nodosum should not be confused with a similar appearing lesion, squamous metaplasia, which occurs in mature placentas and is not easily removed.

14. What is a battledore placenta?

The term refers to the insertion of the umbilical cord at the margin of the placenta. It has no clinical significance unless the cord is avulsed during delivery.

15. What is a velamentous placenta?

It is an abnormality in which the cord has a membranous insertion. In a small number of cases (2%), it may be associated with significant fetal hemorrhage, especially if the membrane carrying the vessels is positioned across the internal os (vasa previa).

16. Why is a circumvallate placenta important?

A circumvallate placenta is recognized by a white, slightly raised circumferential edge to the fetal surface. In effect, it results in placental villi around the border of the placenta that are not covered by the chorionic plate. It is associated with premature labor and hemorrhage.

17. What is Nitabuch's layer? With what abnormality is its absence associated?

Nitabuch's layer is a zone of fibrinoid degeneration between the invading trophoblast and the decidua basalis. Its absence is associated with an abnormally adherent placenta (accreta).

18. How many umbilical vessels are there normally? Does deviation from the normal number have any significance?

Normally there are three umbilical vessels: two arteries and one vein. One umbilical artery is found in approximately 1% of all singleton births and in 7% of twin gestations. It is seen more commonly in diabetic mothers and is associated with low birthweight infants. Congenital malformations are seen in 25–50% of infants with one umbilical artery. In decreasing order of frequency, the following organ systems are affected: genitourinary, cardiovascular, orofacial (cleft palate), and musculoskeletal.

19. Name the three types of fetal membranes that are seen with twin placentas.
Dichorionic, diamniotic (di, di)
Monochorionic, diamniotic (mono, di)
Monochorionic, monoamniotic (mono, mono)

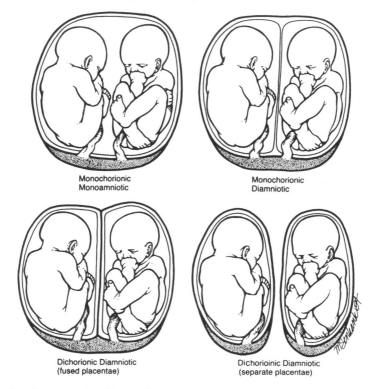

Placentation in twin pregnancies. (From Gabbe SG, Niebyl JR, Simpson JL (eds): Obstetrics: Normal & Problem Pregnancies. New York, Churchill Livingstone, 1986, p 741, with permission.)

20. Dizygotic twins (two ova, fraternal twins) are always associated with which type of fetal membranes? Monozygotic twins?
Di, di. Monozygotic (identical) twins are associated with all three types of membranes, depending on when during gestation the twinning event occurred. In other words, if the membranes are di, di, the pregnancy is probably dizygotic (97% chance) with only a 3% chance it is a monozygotic pregnancy. If the membranes are mono, di, or mono, mono, then they have to be from a monozygotic pregnancy.

21. What tumors have been found in the placenta?
Chorioangioma, a benign proliferation of fetal vessels, has been reported measuring up to 7–8 cm and is associated with hydramnios, fetal cardiomegaly, and death. Malignant melanoma is the most common metastatic tumor to the placenta.

22. What is villitis? What are some of its common causes?
Villitis, inflammation of the villi, occurs with a frequency of 1–9%. In most placentas with villitis, no etiologic agent is identified and the baby shows no signs of infection. Viruses, including cytomegalovirus, rubella, herpes, vaccinia, and varicella, are seen in association with villitis. The only bacterial cause is *Listeria monocytogenes*, which often produces microabscesses.

23. What are the causes of placentomegaly?
Pathologically, an enlarged placenta is one weighing more than 600 gm. Ultrasound diagnosis is less specific but is suggested by placental thickness greater than 5 cm. Associations include maternal diabetes, maternal anemia, blood group incompatibility, Rh sensitization, syphilis, fetal lung malformations, twin-twin transfusion, congenital neoplasms (neuroblastoma, chorioangioma), and alpha-thalassemia.

BIBLIOGRAPHY

1. Bernirschke K: The placenta: Normal development. In Creasy R, Resnik R (eds): Maternal-Fetal Medicine: Principles and Practice, 2nd ed. Philadelphia, W.B. Saunders, 1989.
2. Russell P: Inflammatory lesions of the human placenta. II. Villitis of unknown etiology in perspective. Am J Diag Gynecol Obstet 1:339, 1979.
3. Salazar H, Kanbour AI: Amnion nodosum: Ultrastructure and histopathogenesis. Arch Pathol 98:39, 1974.
4. Sieracki JC, Panke TW, Horvat BL, et al: Chorioangiomas. Obstet Gynecol 46:155, 1975.
5. Simon JA, Buster JE: Placental endocrinology and diagnosis of pregnancy. In Gabbe S, Niebyl J, Simpson J (eds): Obstetrics: Normal and Problem Pregnancies. New York, Churchill Livingstone, 1986.
6. Yen SSC: Endocrinology of pregnancy. In Creasy R, Resnik R (eds): Maternal-Fetal Medicine: Principles and Practice, 2nd ed. Philadelphia, W.B. Saunders, 1989.

70. ABNORMAL PLACENTATION

Michael W. Trierweiler, M.D.

1. How is placenta previa defined?
Complete—implantation of the placenta across the cervical os
Partial—placenta covers part of internal os
Marginal—placenta just reaches the edges of the internal os

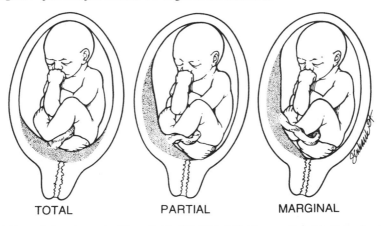

TOTAL   PARTIAL   MARGINAL

Three variations of placenta previa. (From Gabbe SG, Niebyl JR, Simpson JL (eds): Obstetrics: Normal & Problem Pregnancies. New York, Churchill Livingstone, 1986, p 495, with permission.)

2. How often does previa occur in term gestations? In second-trimester pregnancies?

1 in 200 deliveries at term. Earlier in gestation, complete previa is noted in about 5% of second-trimester pregnancies, with 90% resolving by term. Asymptomatic partial or marginal previas are noted in as many as 45% of second-trimester pregnancies, with over 95% resolving before delivery.

3. What are predisposing factors for previa implantation?

Advanced maternal age, increased parity, and previous uterine surgery (whether vertical or low transverse incision).

4. What role does cigarette smoking play in the risk of placenta previa?

Several studies have shown an increased risk of placenta previa among women who smoke. In general, the risk is two-fold greater if the mother is a smoker. Reports of the relationship between risk and quantity and duration of smoking vary. One hypothesized mechanism is the relative carbon monoxide hypoxemia associated with smokers, which may result in compensatory placental hypertrophy with increased surface area more likely to cover the cervical os.

5. What are the maternal complications of placenta previa?
- Life-threatening maternal hemorrhage
- Cesarean delivery
- Increased risk of placenta accreta
- Increased risk of postpartum hemorrhage

6. What is the significance of a history of prior cesarean section delivery when evaluating a patient with placenta previa?

The risk of placenta accreta increases above that for placenta previa alone. Without prior uterine surgery, the risk of accreta at the time of delivery with placenta previa is 1–5%, increasing to 25% if there has been one previous cesarean section and to as high as 45% when there have been two or more previous uterine surgeries.

7. How does placenta previa usually present?

Classically, there is painless, bright red, vaginal bleeding in the third trimester. However, as many as 20% are associated with uterine contractions that are often premature. Abnormal lie, either transverse or breech, and fundal height slightly greater than dates are commonly noted. One-fourth present with the first bleeding episode prior to 30 weeks, whereas half present with bleeding prior to labor during the 34–40 week gestation period.

8. How is placenta previa diagnosed?

Presentation of vaginal bleeding during the third trimester is a contraindication to a pelvic exam until the diagnosis of previa is excluded. Ultrasound visualization of the placenta usually supplies the needed information. However, a false-positive rate of 10% has been reported, with the false impression of previa usually created by an overdistended bladder, a myometrial contraction, or an extraamniotic clot. A false-negative rate of 7% has been noted and is most often attributed to missing a lateral previa that is obscured by the fetal head. Transperineal and, in some centers, transvaginal ultrasound may be helpful, especially late in the third trimester when the cervix is difficult to visualize by transabdominal ultrasound.

9. How is placenta previa remote from term managed?

Maternal hemodynamic instability or fetal distress mandates immediate cesarean section delivery, even for the preterm pregnancy. If the bleeding ceases, as is often the case with the first episode, and the mother and fetus are stable, then expectant management can be undertaken. Maternal blood studies should include serial hematocrit, blood type to assess the need for supplemental RhoGAM, and cross and type for two units of packed red blood cells. Many advocate transfusion to maintain the maternal hematocrit greater than 30.

Expectant management involves bed rest in hospital until rebleeding necessitates delivery or fetal maturity is confirmed by amniocentesis and delivery is undertaken electively. Some advocate the use of steroids for fetal lung maturation in the patient with previa remote from term who is having intermittent bleeding and threatened delivery.

Aggressive expectant management in placenta previa remote from term has been advocated by some centers. Such an approach includes the use of tocolysis. Although retrospective analysis has shown significant prolongation of pregnancy without increase in maternal or fetal complications, this approach remains to be evaluated in a prospective study.

10. What is the role of a "double setup"?

A double setup refers to a pelvic examination for suspected placenta previa that is performed when immediate operative delivery of the infant is possible. Under ideal circumstances, two teams of obstetricians are present; one performs the amniotomy and digital examination and the other is scrubbed and gowned in preparation for cesarean section delivery if excessive vaginal bleeding occurs. A double setup is used less commonly today because improvements in ultrasound resolution have resulted in fewer instances of equivocal diagnoses of marginal previa as opposed to low-lying placenta.

11. How can localization of the placenta facilitate choice of uterine incision when operative delivery is performed for placenta previa?

An anterior placenta previa is best managed with a low vertical or classic uterine incision, so as not to incise the placenta directly. With posterior or lateral localization of the previa, often a low transverse incision may be used if the segment is sufficiently developed.

12. What is the risk of recurrence for placenta previa?

In one large study that had a baseline incidence of 0.3% for placenta previa at delivery, recurrence was 2.4%, an 8-fold increase over the general population.

13. What is placenta accreta?

Attachment of the placenta directly to the uterine muscle without intervening decidua; histologic diagnosis requires specifically the absence of the decidua basalis.

14. How does accreta differ from placenta increta and percreta?

Increta—placental penetration into the myometrium
Percreta—placental penetration through the uterine wall to the serosa

15. What are predisposing factors for abnormal placental adherence?

Placenta previa	Uterine scars	Submucosal leiomyomas
Prior cesarean section	Chronic endometritis	Intrauterine synechiae

Uteroplacental relationships found in abnormal placentation. (From Gabbe SG, Niebyl JR, Simpson JL (eds): Obstetrics: Normal & Problem Pregnancies. New York, Churchill Livingstone, 1986, p 498, with permission.)

NORMAL decidua

INCRETA—17%

ACCRETA—78%

PERCRETA—5%

16. What are the complications of abnormal placental adherence?

Uterine rupture, uterine inversion during placental removal, and hysterectomy for incompletely removed placenta with maternal bleeding.

17. What is the relationship between maternal serum alpha feto-protein (MSAFP) and abnormal placentation?

Second-trimester elevations of MSAFP in women with ultrasound evidence of placenta previa are associated with an increased risk of placenta accreta, percreta, and increta. As MSAFP is governed by both fetal production and placental transference, abnormally deep invasion of the placenta results in elevations of MSAFP even in the second trimester.

18. What is placenta membranacea?

Placenta membranacea is a rare abnormality of placental development in which the chorion remains covered with villae instead of differentiation into chorion laeve and frondosum. If often presents clinically with vaginal bleeding. Ultrasound usually suggests a diffuse placenta occupying anterior and posterior uterine walls as well as previa location. The risk of postpartum hemorrhage and abnormal placental invasion requiring hysterectomy is high.

BIBLIOGRAPHY

1. Besinger RE, Moniak CW, Paskiewicz LS, et al: The effect of tocolytic use in the management of symptomatic placenta previa. Am J Obstet Gynecol 172:1770–1775, 1995.
2. Handler AS, Mason ED, Rosenberg DL, Davis FG: The relationship between exposure during pregnancy to cigarette smoking and cocaine use and placenta previa. Am J Obstet Gynecol 170:884–889, 1994.
3. Hertzberg BS, Bowie JD, Caroll BA, et al: Diagnosis of placenta previa during the third trimester: Role of transperineal sonography. Am J Roentgenol 159:83–87, 1992.
4. Monica G, Lilja C: Placenta previa, maternal smoking and recurrence risk. Acta Obstet Gynecol Scand 74:341–345, 1995.
5. Williams MA, Mittendorf R, Lieberman E, et al: Cigarette smoking during pregnancy in relation to placenta previa. Am J Obstet Gynecol 165:28–32, 1991.
6. Zelop C, Nadel A, Frigoletto FD, et al: Placenta accreta/percreta/increta: A cause of elevated maternal serum alpha fetoprotein.

71. PLACENTAL ABRUPTION

Scott M. Barton, M.D.

1. What is placental abruption? What is its incidence?

Placental abruption is premature separation of the placenta before delivery of the fetus, secondary to bleeding into the decidua basalis. If vaginal bleeding is associated with abruption, it is termed an external hemorrhage (90%). If abruption occurs without vaginal bleeding, the hemorrhage is said to be concealed (10%). The incidence varies with the population studied but averages about 0.83% (1/120 deliveries).

2. What factors are associated with placental abruption as possible causes?

Maternal hypertension is seen in 50% of severe abruptions and is thought to be a risk factor. In one-half of such cases, the hypertension is chronic, whereas in the other half it is pregnancy-related. Advanced parity and maternal age are thought to increase the likelihood of abruption, but age is believed merely to reflect the effect of parity. Smoking is thought to contribute to placental abruption by causing decidual necrosis. More recently, abruptions have been seen with cocaine use, perhaps because of its hypertensive effects. Trauma, short umbilical cords, sudden decompression of the uterus (either by loss of fluid or after delivery of a first twin), uterine anomalies, and myomas are sometimes associated with abruption. Folic acid deficiency as a cause of placental abruption is not well documented, and inferior vena cava compression, which increases the pressure in the intervillous space, has not been proved in humans.

3. Do pregnancies complicated by preterm premature rupture of the membranes (PPROM) have an increased risk of abruption?

In a recent study, expectant management of PPROM is associated with a 5-fold higher rate of abruption, regardless of the gestational age at rupture of membranes or latency period to delivery. Of note, vaginal bleeding before PPROM occurred significantly more often in pregnancies (15%) that subsequently had abruption.

4. How does placental abruption present?

The clinical presentation of placental abruption varies, but the classic symptoms and signs are vaginal bleeding, abdominal pain, uterine contractions, and uterine tenderness. Furthermore, evidence of maternal hypovolemia or fetal distress is sometimes present. A differential diagnosis may include placenta previa, preterm labor, chorioamnionitis, vasa previa, and uterine rupture.

5. Is the bleeding that occurs with an abruption maternal or fetal in origin?

Generally, most blood lost with an abruption comes from the mother. However, it may be either maternal or fetal in origin. Furthermore, it is common to underestimate actual blood loss on the basis of observation alone.

6. Is ultrasound helpful in the diagnosis of abruption?

Ultrasound may show detachment of the placenta with retroplacental collection of blood in a minority of cases only; therefore, normal findings on ultrasound do not exclude the possibility of abruption. However, ultrasound is useful in excluding placenta previa, another important cause of obstetric hemorrhage.

7. What laboratory studies are helpful in the diagnosis and management of abruption?

Laboratory studies have limited utility in the **diagnosis** of abruption. Various studies, such as Kleihauer-Betke stain, D-dimer (a measure of fibrinolytic activity) and CA-125 have been proposed. Each, however, is limited by relatively poor sensitivity as well as the time required to obtain results.

Laboratory studies indicated for the **management** of abruption, however, often include maternal hematocrit, blood type, Kleihauer-Betke stain for determination of quantity of RhoGAM for Rh-negative mothers, and, in severe abruption, assessment for disseminated intravascular coagulation.

8. What are potential complications of placental abruption?

Complications may be maternal or fetal. Potential maternal complications are hemorrhagic shock, disseminated intravascular coagulation (DIC), and ischemic necrosis of distal organs. DIC is thought to be due to entry of thromboplastins into the circulation from the site of placental injury, which initiates widespread activation of the clotting cascade. Ischemic necrosis of distal organs usually involves the kidneys, liver, adrenal glands, or pituitary. Ischemic necrosis of the kidney may take the form of acute tubular necrosis (ATN) or bilateral cortical necrosis. Both ATN and bilateral cortical necrosis are characterized by oliguria or anuria. However, bilateral cortical necrosis results in death from uremia within 1–2 weeks unless dialysis is instituted, whereas ATN usually resolves spontaneously. Fetal complications include hypoxia, anemia, growth retardation, increased incidence of anomalies (especially of the central nervous system), and death. Death of the fetus occurs in 4 of 1,000 abruptions and accounts for 15% of all perinatal deaths. The major causes of perinatal death in abruption are anoxia, prematurity, and exsanguination. It is believed that early and more liberal use of abdominal delivery has lowered the perinatal mortality rate associated with abruption.

9. For low-birth-weight (LBW) infants (< 2500 gm), do outcomes differ for infants delivered after abruption compared to other LBW infants?

For infants under 2500 gm, neonatal and infant outcome appears to depend on severity of the abruption. Compared with infants delivered for other indications, preterm infants delivered due to a severe abruption have lower APGAR scores and higher rates of intraventricular hemorrhage. Follow-up at 2 years of age shows a similar significant increase in cerebral palsy. This difference remains even after correction for possible confounders of abruption and infant outcome, such as social class, level of education, gestational age, and birthweight.

10. How should placental abruptions be managed?

On presentation of significant abruption, initial measures include administration of intravenous fluids and supplemental oxygen. Type and crossmatch, usually for 4 units of packed red blood cells, should be obtained. Placement of an indwelling urinary catheter allows close monitoring of urinary output. Finally, electronic fetal monitoring is recommended for continuous assessment of fetal well-being.

Hemorrhagic shock requires vigorous blood and volume replacement with packed red blood cells and crystalloid. Goals of blood and volume replacement are to maintain the hematocrit at or above 30% and the urinary output $\geq$ 30 ml/hr. Platelet count, fibrinogen level, and serum potassium level should be checked after each 4–6 units of packed red blood cells administered. Invasive central monitoring (either central venous pressure or pulmonary capillary wedge pressure) is sometimes advisable.

The patient should be tested for **DIC** every 4 hours until delivery. Quantification of fibrin split products (FSPs) is the most sensitive lab test. However, once elevated, FSPs are not helpful in guiding therapy, and repeat testing is not necessary. Although normal results do not exclude DIC, fibrinogen levels and platelet counts are more indicative of the ongoing process and are more useful in terms of management. The ultimate therapy for DIC is delivery, which results in spontaneous resolution. Blood and volume replacement is all that is usually necessary until delivery. If a cesarean section needs to be performed and the platelet count is < 50,000 or the fibrinogen level is < 100 mg/100 ml, these components should be replaced individually. Fibrinogen may be replaced with fresh frozen plasma (FFP) or cryoprecipitate. Heparin should not be used unless there is evidence of microvascular plugging (such as gangrene), which is rare.

11. When should a pregnancy complicated by abruption be delivered?

The method and timing of delivery depend on the gestational age of the fetus and the severity of abruption. If the pregnancy is at term and abruption is mild, vaginal delivery may be attempted. This may include cautious augmentation of labor with oxytocin, if needed. Amniotomy is generally considered to be advantageous because it may decrease extravasation of blood into the myometrium and entry of thromboplastic substances into the circulation. On the other hand, when the fetus is immature, mild abruptions may be managed expectantly and a trial of tocolysis considered. If distress occurs in a potentially viable fetus and vaginal delivery is not imminent, cesarean section should be performed immediately. Furthermore, severe maternal hemorrhage may necessitate immediate abdominal delivery. Finally, when a fetal demise has occurred, but the maternal condition is stable, vaginal delivery should be attempted.

12. What is the risk of recurrence with placental abruption?

It is estimated that 5.5%–16.6% of subsequent pregnancies will again be complicated by placental abruption. This risk increases to 25% during a third pregnancy if there have been two consecutive abruptions previously. Despite the significant risk of recurrence, it is impossible to predict which pregnancies will be affected and at what gestational age the abruption will occur. Therefore, a history of placental abruption with a prior pregnancy qualifies a present pregnancy as high risk.

BIBLIOGRAPHY

1. Combs CA, Nyberg DA, Mack LA, et al: Expectant management after sonographic diagnosis of placental abruption. Am J Perinatol 9:170–174, 1992.
2. Creasy RK, Resnik R (eds): Maternal-Fetal Medicine: Principles and Practice, 3rd ed. Philadelphia, W.B. Saunders, 1994.
3. Cunningham FG, MacDonald PC, Gant NF, et al (eds): Williams Obstetrics, 19th ed. Norwalk, CT, Appleton & Lange, 1993.
4. Major CA, de Veciana M, Lewis DF, Morgan MA: Preterm premature rupture of membranes and abruptio placentae: Is there an association between these pregnancy complications? Am J Obstet Gynecol 172:672–676, 1995.
5. Scott JR, Disaia PJ, Hammond CB, Spellacy WN (eds): Danforth's Obstetrics and Gynecology, 7th ed. Philadelphia, J.B. Lippincott, 1994.
6. Spinillo A, Fazzi E, Stronati M, et al: Severity of abruptio placentae and neurodevelopmental outcome in low birth weight infants. Early Hum Devel 35:45–54, 1993.

VIII. Labor and Delivery

72. CERVICAL CERCLAGE

Errol R. Norwitz, M.D., Ph.D.

1. Who is a candidate for cervical cerclage?

Only women with proven cervical incompetence are candidates for cervical cerclage. The presence of uterine contractions and an advanced cervical examination before 30 weeks of gestation suggest a diagnosis of premature labor, not cervical incompetence. However, because a dilated cervix may in turn precipitate contractions, it is often difficult to distinguish between these two diagnoses by history alone. Placement of a cerclage in women who do not have a history of cervical incompetence (such as women with a history of intrauterine diethylstilbestrol [DES]-exposure or cervical cone biopsy) remains contentious and is not well supported in the literature.

2. What is cervical incompetence?

Cervical incompetence has been defined as the inability to support a pregnancy to term due to a functional or structural defect of the cervix and implies an intrinsic abnormality of the cervix. Cervical incompetence is characterized by acute, painless dilatation of the cervix, usually in the mid-trimester, culminating in prolapse and/or rupture of the fetal membranes with resultant preterm and often previable delivery.

3. What causes cervical incompetence?

The pathophysiology of cervical incompetence is not clear. Embryologically, the body and cervix of the uterus are derived from fusion and recanalization of the paramesonephric (müllerian) ducts, a process that is complete by the fifth month of pregnancy. Histologically, the cervix consists of fibrous connective tissue, muscular tissue, and blood vessels. Muscular connective tissue constitutes on average 15% of the cervical stroma, but it is not uniformly distributed throughout the cervix. The isthmus (upper third) of the cervix continues approximately 30% muscular tissue, whereas the middle third contains around 18% and the lower third only 7%. Conversely, the fibrous connective tissue component of the cervical stroma increases as one moves from the external os to the uterine corpus. This tissue is believed to confer tensile strength to the cervix. During the fourth and fifth months of pregnancy, the isthmus thins out to become part of the lower segment of the uterus. The junction of the isthmus and middle third of the cervix ("cervicoisthmic junction") therefore serves as the physiologic internal cervical sphincter during the remainder of the pregnancy. Defects in this region may result in premature dilatation of the cervix and recurrent pregnancy loss.

4. How common is cervical incompetence?

The incidence of cervical incompetence is estimated at 0.05–1% of all pregnancies. It is reported to be responsible for approximately 15% of habitual immature deliveries from 16–28 weeks' gestation.

5. Is there a reliable diagnostic test for cervical incompetence?

No. Cervical incompetence is a diagnosis made primarily on the basis of history. Clinical and ultrasound evaluation of the cervix are less important. A number of tests have been developed in an attempt to diagnose cervical incompetence before pregnancy—for example, the ability to pass a no. 16 Foley catheter or no. 8 cervical dilator (positive Hegar test) through the cervix or an abnormally wide uterocervical canal (≥ 8 mm at the level of the internal os) on hysterosalpingography. But these tests are of little clinical value. Recent studies have shown that cervical length of ≥ 2.5 cm at 24 weeks of gestation on transvaginal ultrasound is predictive of preterm delivery, but this does not make a diagnosis of cervical incompetence.

6. Will cervical incompetence always recur in subsequent pregnancies?

No. In women with documented cervical incompetence, the probability of recurrence in a subsequent pregnancy is around 15–30%. Even in women who have had two consecutive midtrimester pregnancy losses, the chance of carrying the next pregnancy to term without intervention is in the range of 70%.

7. What are the risk factors for cervical incompetence?

Risk factors for cervical incompetence can be either congenital or acquired. Congenital factors include congenital cervical hypoplasia and intrauterine DES-exposure. Exposure of the developing uterus to DES in utero results in a cervix with a higher muscular/connective tissue ratio compared with unexposed controls. This "muscular cervix" is intrinsically weak (i.e., it has less tensile strength and is more elastic). Acquired risk factors for cervical incompetence include previous trauma to the cervix (such as cervical conization or amputation, obstetric laceration, or forceful dilatation).

8. Do abortions predispose to cervical incompetence?

Data from European studies suggest that a single late second-trimester abortion or two or more elective first-trimester pregnancy terminations may increase the risk of cervical incompetence and premature delivery in subsequent pregnancies, but studies in the U. S. failed to confirm these findings.

9. When is the best time in gestation to place a cerclage?

Elective (prophylactic) cerclage at 13–16 weeks of gestation in patients with a history of cervical incompetence is now well established, and reported fetal salvage rates suggest a viable delivery in 75% or more of cases. In contrast, the efficacy of emergent cerclage (i.e., after the cervix has already effaced and dilated), which is usually placed at 18–23 weeks' gestation, is less well established. Indeed, it is unclear whether emergent cerclage has any benefit over no cerclage.

10. Is it ever too late to place a cerclage?

Given the questionable efficacy of emergent cerclage, most clinicians do not place a cerclage after the limit of fetal viability has been reached (currently 24 weeks' gestation). At this point, the risk of placing the suture outweighs the potential benefit.

11. What are the contraindications to cervical cerclage?

Cervical cerclage should not be placed in the setting of ruptured membranes, intrauterine infection, unexplained vaginal bleeding (abruption), intrauterine fetal demise (IUFD), major fetal anomaly incompatible with life, intrauterine growth restriction (IUGR), life-threatening maternal condition, or uterine contractions and/or active labor. An ultrasound is recommended before cerclage placement to confirm a viable intrauterine pregnancy and to exclude gross anatomic defects such as anencephaly. Evidence of fetal membranes that bulge through the cervical os is a relative contraindication to cerclage placement; the literature suggests a high incidence of rupture of membranes in this setting. The presence of bacteria on Gram stain or a positive culture from preoperative amniocentesis is associated with a failure rate in excess of 90%. However, unless there is clinical evidence of chorioamnionitis, preoperative amniocentesis is not routinely performed.

12. Is placenta previa a contraindication to cervical cerclage?

No. In fact, cervical cerclage has been proposed as a treatment for placenta previa. A randomized trial of McDonald cerclage in 25 patients with bleeding at 24–30 weeks and sonographic evidence of placenta previa resulted in later deliveries (35 vs. 32 weeks), larger birth weight (2709 vs. 1812 gm), fewer hospital admissions, and fewer neonatal complications in the group randomized to cerclage compared with controls. Currently no other data support these findings.

13. What are the alternatives to cervical cerclage? How successful are they?

Over the years, numerous noninvasive modalities have been used to treat cervical incompetence, including prolonged bedrest, beta agonists, and progesterone, but none has been shown to be effective. Elective cervical cerclage has become the standard therapy for cervical incompetence and in a recent meta-analysis was shown to be more effective than bedrest alone.

14. What is the place of cerclage in multiple pregnancies?

Multiple pregnancies carry a high risk of preterm delivery; however, no evidence suggests that prophylactic cerclage is of any benefit in uncomplicated twin pregnancies. There are no data on higher-order multiple gestations.

15. Should all DES-exposed women get a cerclage?

This question remains controversial. The majority of clinicians believe that a history of DES-exposure alone—without history of prior pregnancy losses—is not an indication for cerclage. However, a small, nonrandomized, prospective trial suggested that placement of a prophylactic cerclage may increase gestational age at delivery and improve perinatal outcome. As a result, some clinicians have suggested that elective cervical cerclage at 13–16 weeks' gestation be offered to all women known to be DES-exposed.

16. What is the difference between a Shirodkar cerclage and a McDonald cerclage?

Both Shirodkar and McDonald cerclages are placed transvaginally. The Shirodkar cerclage involves a single suture around the cervix at the level of the internal os after making an incision in the vaginal mucosa above the cervix and reflecting the bladder and a similar incision below the cervix, with reflection of the rectum. The sutures is then secured and the mucosal incisions closed. In his original description in 1955, Shirodkar used a $4\frac{1}{2} \times \frac{1}{4}$ strip of fascia from the patient's thigh.

In 1957, McDonald published his modification of the transvaginal cerclage, which involved a simple pursestring suture around the cervix with absorbable suture material. The suture is placed as high as possible without dissection of the bladder or rectum. If necessary, a second or even a third suture can be placed. Since the 1950s, transvaginal cervical cerclage has been the mainstay for the management of cervical incompetence. Current techniques suggest using permanent suture material such as a no. 1 polypropylene (Proline), no. 2 nylon (Ethibond), or a 5-mm Mersilene band. Confirmation of fetal viability both before and immediately after the procedure (either by auscultation of the fetal heart or by ultrasound) is advised.

17. Which is better—a Shirodkar or a McDonald cerclage?

Although they have not been tested head-to-head in a prospective, randomized, controlled clinical trial, it is probably fair to say that they are equally efficacious. Careful patient selection and the experience of the surgeon are far more important determinants of success than the choice of suture technique. However, under certain circumstances, one or other technique may be preferable. For example, if the cervix is very short or lacerated, a Shirodkar cerclage may be technically easier to place.

18. What is a Wurm procedure?

A Wurm procedure is a modification of the McDonald cerclage in which interrupted sutures (usually no. 0 Nylon or polypropylene) are placed between the anterior and posterior lips of the cervix. Usually five or six sutures are required to close the cervix.

19. Is there any alternative to transvaginal cerclage?

Transabdominal cerclage (TAC) was first performed in 1965 by Benson and Durfee. The perinatal salvage rate in this series was reported as 11% (5 viable infants out of 45 pregnancies) before and 82% (11/13) after TAC placement. A number of investigators have since used this procedure in carefully selected patients with cervical incompetence, and similar results have been reported. No evidence suggests that TAC is superior to transvaginal cerclage (either Shirodkar or McDonald), and placement of a TAC is a far more morbid procedure, requiring laparotomy and subsequent delivery by cesarean section. Transabdominal cerclage should therefore be reserved for patients with documented cervical incompetence in whom a prophylactic cerclage is indicated, but who have either failed previous transvaginal cerclages or in whom a transvaginal cerclage is technically impossible to place. Indications for TAC placement include one or more unsuccessful transvaginal cerclages; congenitally short or absent cervix; acquired short or absent cervix; marked scarring, lacerations, or defects of the cervix (trauma, previous cerclages); cervicovaginal fistula; and/or subacute cervicitis.

20. Are prophylactic antibiotics and tocolysis necessary?

There is no consensus in the literature about the use of prophylactic antibiotics, prophylactic tocolysis, or the choice of anesthesia for cervical cerclage. Such decisions should be individualized. Regional anesthesia is generally preferred because patients awakening from general anesthesia often cough and retch, which may put additional strain on both the cerclage and fetal membranes. Prophylactic tocolysis (indomethacin, ritodrine, magnesium sulfate or terbutaline) may be used for 2–3 days to inhibit the transient uterine contractions associated with placement of the suture, but no evidence suggests that this improves perinatal outcome. In the setting of emergent cerclage, prophylactic antibiotics are recommended because of the risk of chorioamnionitis. The use of antibiotics for elective cerclage, however, is at the discretion of the surgeon. If antibiotics are to be given to prevent ascending infection, broad-spectrum agents that cover both anaerobes and aerobes are recommended, such as third-generation cephalosporin, ampicillin and sulbactam (Unasyn), or a combination of ampicillin, gentamicin, and clindamycin.

21. Can a cerclage be placed before conception?

Because the presence of a vaginal cerclage is a contraindication to coitus, there are no studies looking at transvaginal cerclage placement before conception. However, there are a number of reports of TAC placement before conception. In such patients the combined perinatal salvage rate before TAC placement was 8% (10/133) compared with 78% (25/32) after TAC placement. TAC placed before conception may induce cervical stenosis and thereby interfere with fertility, but this risk remains theoretical. Of interest, dilatation of the cervix and uterine curettage were carried out successfully and without difficulty in all patients with first-trimester pregnancy losses without removal of the cerclage, and a number of these patients subsequently carried pregnancies to term with the same cerclage in place. No cases of attempted dilatation and curettage for late second-trimester pregnancy losses are described.

22. Do you abandon the procedure if you find membranes prolapsing through the external os?

No. A number of techniques have been described to help reduce the fetal membranes before placement of the suture, including placing the patient in steep Trendelenburg position, placing a 30-ml Foley catheter through the cervix, filling the bladder, and/or performing therapeutic transabdominal amniocentesis. Intravenous nitroglycerin also has been used to relax the uterus and allow the membranes to recede.

23. Should the suture be secured anteriorly or posteriorly?

Once again, there is no consensus on this issue. Securing the suture anteriorly may make it easier to visualize during pregnancy and easier to remove, but it also has been shown to increase the incidence of bladder discomfort.

24. What are the complications of cervical cerclage?

Complications associated with cervical cerclage are increased with increasing gestational age and cervical dilatation. Short-term complications (i.e., ≤ 48 hours) occur in 3–20% of cases, including excessive blood loss (occasionally requiring blood transfusion), premature rupture of the fetal membranes (PROM), abortion, and complications from the anesthesia. Premature rupture of the membranes is the most common cause of suture failure. Long-term complications from cervical cerclage include cervical lacerations (3–4%), chorioamnionitis (4%), and cervical stenosis (1%) as well as rare complications (such as IUGR, fetal demise, placental abruption, thrombophlebitis, migration of the suture, bladder discomfort, and abdominal pain). The use of cervical cerclage is also associated with increased intervention during pregnancy, including higher rates of admission to hospital, administration of oral tocolytics, induction of labor, and cesarean delivery. Puerperal infection occurs in approximately 6% of patients with cerclages, twice as common as the incidence in gestational age-matched controls with no cerclages.

25. How should pregnant patients with cerclages be followed?

Weekly cervical checks should be carried out at least for the first month to assess the integrity of the suture. Patients should be made aware of the increased risk of PROM and preterm labor and should be on a strict regimen of pelvic rest for the remainder of the pregnancy (i.e., avoiding coitus or placement of any object in the vagina). A protocol of modified bedrest (i.e., ≥ 8 hours of rest during the day) is usually recommended until around 34 weeks' gestation, especially following emergent cerclage placement. All patients with cerclages are instructed to report any symptoms of pelvic or back pressure, increased vaginal discharge, or pelvic aching and cramping. Fetal growth should be monitored sonographically every 3–4 weeks throughout the remainder of the pregnancy, given the association with IUGR. The reason for this association is unclear, but it may be related to impairment of blood supply to the lower segment of the uterus.

26. Does the presence of a cerclage increase the risk of PROM in the third trimester?

No. Studies to date show no association between the presence of a cerclage (either McDonald or Shirodkar) and PROM remote from placement.

27. Should the cerclage be removed if the membranes rupture?

There is currently no consensus regarding the management of cervical cerclage in the setting of PROM. If there is evidence of amnionitis, the cerclage should be removed immediately. In the absence of infection, there is no clear benefit either way. The risk of prematurity (assuming you believe that cerclages work) must be weighed against the risk of ascending infection. Recent studies suggest that neonatal and maternal morbidities do not change with expectant management of PROM. However, there are no conclusive data to show that expectant management (including tocolysis, corticosteroid therapy, and antibiotics) improves neonatal outcome.

28. When should the cerclage be removed if the pregnancy progresses uneventfully to term?

Most clinicians recommend removal of the cerclage at around 37–38 weeks to prevent laboring against an intact cerclage with possible laceration of the cervix or uterine rupture. The cerclage may be removed in the office. However, it may require a return visit to the operating room and anesthesia. This is especially true of Shirodkar cerclages, in which the knot may retract and be buried below the vaginal mucosa. Removal of a TAC transvaginally through a posterior colpotomy, although technically feasible, has proved more difficult than was originally reported and often results in excessive blood loss. It is therefore not widely recommended. Patients with a TAC require delivery by elective cesarean section at 37–38 weeks' gestation after confirmation of lung maturity. If the couple desires future fertility, the TAC is usually left in place at the time of cesarean section.

BIBLIOGRAPHY

1. Arias F: Cervical cerclage for the temporary treatment of patients with placenta previa. Obstet Gynecol 71:545–548, 1988.
2. Benson RC, Durfee RB: Transabdominal cervicouterine cerclage during pregnancy for the treatment of cervical incompetency. Obstet Gynecol 25:145–155, 1965.
3. Danforth DN: The fibrous nature of the human cervix, and its relation to the isthmic segment in gravid and nongravid uteri. Am J Obstet Gynecol 53:541–560, 1947.
4. Dor J, Shalev J, Mashiach S, et al: Elective cervical suture of twin pregnancies diagnosed ultrasonically in the first trimester following induced ovulation. Gynecol Obstet Invest 13:55-60, 1982.
5. Harlap S, Shiono PH, Ramcharan S, et al: Prospective study of spontaneous fetal losses after induced abortion. N Engl J Med 301:677–681, 1979.
6. Iams JD, Goldenberg RL, Meis PJ, et al: The length of the cervix and the risk of spontaneous premature delivery. N Engl J Med 334:567–572, 1996.
7. Ludmir J, Landon MB, Gabbe S, et al: Management of the diethylstilbestrol-exposed pregnant patient: a prospective study. Am J Obstet Gynecol 157:665-669, 1987.
8. McDonald IA: Suture of the cervix for inevitable miscarriage. J Obstet Gynecol Br Emp 64:346–350, 1957.
9. Medical Research Council/Royal College of Obstetricians and Gynecologists Multicentre Randomized Trial of Cervical Cerclage. MRC/RCOG working party on cervical cerclage. Br J Obstet Gynecol 100:516–523, 1993.
10. Norwitz ER, Goldstein DP: Transabdominal cervicoisthmic cerclage: Learning to tie the knot. J Gynecol Tech 2:49–54, 1996.
11. Romero R, Gonzales R, Sepulvade W, et al: Infection and labor. VIII: Microbial invasion of the amniotic cavity in patients with suspected cervical incompetence: prevalence and clinical significance. Am J Obstet Gynecol 167:1086–1091, 1992.
12. Shirodkar VN: A new method of operative treatment for habitual abortion in the second trimester of pregnancy. Antiseptic 52:299, 1955.
13. Wong GP, Farquharson DF, Dansereau J: Emergency cervical cerclage: A retrospective review of 51 cases. Am J Perinatol 10:341–347, 1993.

73. PRETERM LABOR

Kim Cox, M.D.

1. How is preterm labor defined?

Preterm labor is strictly defined as frequent uterine contractions with or without pain in the face of progressive cervical dilatation or effacement, occurring after the second trimester up to 37 weeks' gestation.

2. What are the common symptoms of preterm labor? How are they evaluated?

- Regular uterine contractions with or without pain more frequently than every 15 minutes for greater than 1 hour's duration
- Pelvic pressure
- Dull, constant back pain
- Change in vaginal discharge
- Intermittent abdominal cramping

These symptoms may be evaluated with ambulatory external tocodynamometry.

3. What causes preterm labor?

In the majority of cases, preterm labor is idiopathic. Because approximately 50% of patients who complain of premature contraction resolve these without treatment or cervical change, the diagnosis, causes, and incidence of true preterm labor are difficult to assess accurately. Dehydration, urinary tract infection, systemic infection, vaginitis, or cervicitis may contribute or predispose to preterm labor.

4. What are the risk factors for preterm labor?

Previous induced abortion (two or more first-trimester or one second-trimester abortion)
Low socioeconomic status
Smoking
Previous preterm delivery
Hemorrhage
Congenital anomalies
Chorioamnionitis
Preterm premature rupture of membranes
Abruption
Fetal demise
Placenta previa
Poor nutritional status
Uterine anomalies
Advanced maternal age
Maternal age less than 20
Previous cervical surgery
Diethylstilbestrol (DES) exposure
Urinary tract infection
Vaginitis
Polyhydramnios
Serious systemic infection
Multiple gestation
High-frequency, low-amplitude contractions

5. How frequently does preterm labor occur?

Preterm labor complicates 5–10% of all pregnancies; this incidence varies with the population studied.

6. What are the consequences of preterm labor?

Prematurity is the major consequence, resulting in risk of neonatal morbidity and death; this mostly occurs from pulmonary immaturity, resulting in increased intraventricular hemorrhage, neonatal respiratory distress syndrome, persistent pulmonary hypertension, and bronchopulmonary dysplasia. Premature neonates are also at higher risk for sepsis, necrotizing enterocolitis, and apneic and bradycardic episodes. The majority of neonatal mortality occurs prior to 28 weeks.

7. How is preterm labor treated?

Elimination of risk factors, bed rest, and parenteral and oral tocolytics have been used. Tocolytics are routinely used at less than 34 weeks' gestation, if there are no contraindications to treatment. Treatment is individualized from 34–37 weeks. Therefore, gestational age must be carefully documented prior to initiating tocolytic therapy. Antibiotics have been controversial in preventing preterm labor.

8. What are relative contraindications to tocolysis?

Severe hemorrhage
Abruption
Severe preeclampsia
Eclampsia
Intrauterine fetal death
Chorioamnionitis
Pulmonary hypertension
Maternal hyperthyroidism
Known intolerance to tocolytics
Fetal maturity
Lethal fetal anomaly
Severe intrauterine growth retardation (IUGR)

9. What are parenteral agents for treating preterm labor?

Intravenous beta agonists (ritodrine and terbutaline) have been used to treat premature labor. Ritodrine is used in doses of 50–350 µg/min; terbutaline is used in doses of 10–50 µg/min. Both are begun at a low rate and increased in an incremental fashion every 10 minutes to achieve tocolysis. Intravenous magnesium sulfate is usually given in a 4–6 gm bolus over 20 minutes and then continued at 2–4 gm/hour as titrated to contractions. Infusions of magnesium sulfate and beta agonists are usually continued for up to 24 hours once tocolysis is achieved. Terbutaline has also been used subcutaneously in doses of 0.25 mg every 3–4 hours.

10. What are the oral tocolytic agents?

Terbutaline, 5 mg every 4–6 hours, has been used as has ritodrine, 10–20 mg every 4–6 hours. Ritodrine is the only FDA-approved tocolytic. Oral magnesium preparations have also been used with some reported success. Each of these has side effects that may limit their tolerance.

Calcium channel blockers such as nifedipine and verapamil have been used with some success and are tolerated well by patients. In animal studies, fetal deaths have been reported with calcium channel blocker infusions; these have not been confirmed in preliminary human studies.

Prostaglandin synthetase inhibitors such as indomethacin and ibuprofen have been used in standard doses, especially in early gestation between 28 and 32 weeks. They are effective tocolytics. Their use appears to be complicated by oligohydramnios and possible premature closure of the ductus arteriosus; the maternal side effects are those well known of nonsteroidal antiinflammatory drugs in the nonpregnant population. For these reasons, calcium channel blockers and prostaglandin synthetase inhibitors have been used mostly as second-line tocolytics, usually in a controlled fashion.

11. Is tocolysis effective?

Clinical studies have been mixed in showing an actual effectiveness in prolonging gestation more than 48 hours. The efficacy of maintenance oral tocolytic therapy is likewise being questioned.

12. What are the postulated mechanisms of action of the various tocolytics?

Beta-adrenergic agonists (terbutaline, ritodrine) activate beta-adrenergic receptors and thus increase adenylate cyclase, with a concomitant increase in intracellular cyclic adenosine monophosphate (AMP). Cyclic AMP reduces intracellular calcium and the sensitivity of the myosin-actin contractile unit to calcium.

Magnesium sulfate has an unclear mechanism of action; according to one theory, it competes for calcium entry into muscle cells or calcium storage in muscle cell endoretriculum.

Calcium channel blockers (*nifedipine*) interfere with influx of calcium into cells through voltage mediated channels.

Prostaglandin synthetase inhibitors (*indomethacin*) prevent formation of prostaglandins from arachidonic acid.

13. What are the side effects of the usual tocolytics?

Use of beta agonists may be complicated by hypotension, pulmonary edema, cardiac arrhythmias, chest pain, tachycardia, myocardial ischemia, hyperglycemia, glucose intolerance, and hypokalemia. Twin gestations are at greater risk of pulmonary edema secondary to tocolysis.

Magnesium sulfate infusions may be complicated by hypotension, flushing, lethargy, hyporeflexia, pulmonary edema, and respiratory and cardiac depression and arrest. Neonatal suppression may also occur.

14. How should patients on tocolytics be followed?

For patients on beta agonists, it is necessary initially to evaluate the hematocrit, electrolytes, especially potassium, and glucose. Each patient should be examined for a history of cardiac ischemia, valvular lesions, congestive heart failure, and arrhythmias, or for previous intolerance to these medications. Along with routine physical exam, a careful cardiac and pulmonary exam should be performed.

These patients should be followed with serial electrolytes, glucose, and physical exam for pulmonary edema every 6–24 hours or as symptoms require. Oral and parenteral fluids should be limited to not more than 100–125 cc/hr to decrease the risk of pulmonary edema. For complaints of chest pain, an electrocardiogram, and cardiac enzymes if indicated, should be done, and the infusion should be stopped.

Patients on magnesium sulfate should be followed with serial blood pressure evaluations and examined for deep tendon reflexes, alertness, and urine output. Fluid intake should be strictly limited in these patients also. Serial magnesium and calcium levels may be followed to assess adequacy of infusion: 5–8 mg/dl is considered therapeutic; cardiac and respiratory depression may occur at greater than 10 mg/dl. Magnesium sulfate is renally excreted; therefore, renal function and adequate urine output must be assured.

If evidence of cardiac or respiratory depression occurs, one ampule of 10% calcium gluconate may be given to competitively inhibit the elevated magnesium concentration, along with stopping the infusion.

15. What are key points in the initial evaluation and treatment of the patient with possible preterm labor?

1. Baseline history for pregnancy complications, gestational age, history of preterm premature rupture of the membranes (PROM), any infectious symptoms (especially cystitis, pyelonephritis, or chorioamnionitis), and hydration, and cardiac history and risk factors for preterm labor.

2. Baseline physical exam with special attention to any fever, cardiac and respiratory exam, estimated fetal weight, uterine tenderness, any evidence of PROM, and cervical change. External monitoring of the fetus and contractions for confirmation of contractions, possible abruption, and baseline fetal heart rate.

3. Baseline laboratory studies include a complete blood count (CBC) for leukocytosis and hematocrit, urinalysis to assess degree of hydration and infection, cervical cultures for group B streptococcus, and ultrasound for any question regarding gestational age or rupture of membranes. If tocolysis is contemplated, levels of electrolytes, glucose, calcium, and magnesium may also be measured. Isotonic intravenous fluids are begun (normal saline or lactated Ringer's) in 500-cc bolus over 30 minutes; the patient is put at bed rest to assess for contractions and cervical change.

16. What role does fibronectin play in the assessment of labor?

The appearance of fetal fibronectin in cervical samples correlates to a certain extent with the onset of labor in both term and preterm pregnancies. A fetal fibronectin assay has been proposed by some as an alternative scoring system to assess success of induction of term and postterm pregnancy.

As a predictor of preterm delivery, fetal fibronectin has been evaluated in several populations. As a screening tool in low-risk and some high-risk populations, the efficacy of fibronectin assays is limited. Although sensitivity is low, negative predictive values (NPV), indicating true absence of preterm delivery in the absence of fibronectin, are high. The frequency with which the assays need to be repeated remains unclear.

Among pregnancies complicated by premature contractions, some have advocated incorporating fetal fibronectin assays in management. Again, the negative predictive values are high—76–83% for delivery before 37 weeks. In one study, a high NPV (99%) was noted for delivery within 7 days. In the same populations with premature contractions, positive predictive values for a preterm delivery ranged from 60–80%.

17. Does home uterine activity monitoring (HUAM) decrease preterm deliveries?

Controversial. During the 1990s there have been strong advocates as well as opponents of this new technology. Initial studies that supported the ability of HUAM to decrease preterm labor and preterm birth and to improve neonatal outcomes were criticized for methodologic flaws. In addition, increased nursing contact with the patients in the group receiving twice-a-day HUAM have played a role in their more favorable outcomes. More recent attempts to evaluate this question have reached varying conclusions. A metaanalysis of randomized studies in 1995 found statistically significant decreases in preterm labor with dilation > 2 cm and preterm birth in singleton pregnancies. These findings were not present in twin gestations. Additionally, no significant differences could be detected in infant referrals to the intensive care unit or mean birth weights between the monitored and unmonitored groups. The 1995 Collaborative Home Uterine Monitoring Study (CHUMS) failed to find significant differences in gestational ages at delivery or neonatal outcomes in over 1000 patients at high risk for preterm labor who were randomized to monitoring vs. sham monitoring devices.

18. What are general guidelines for survival of the preterm infant?

Viability of a preterm gestation depends on several factors. Certainly immediate accessibility of neonatal support and the absence of congenital malformations are associated with better outcomes. Although gestational age is sometimes used a a predictor of neonatal viability, birth weight is felt by some to be a more sensitive predictor. Generally infants weighing 1,000–1,500 gm have > 90% survival. Below 1,000 gm, survival decreases 10–15% for each decrement of 100 gm. Below 500 gm survival is rare but has been documented. For comparison, viability by gestational age is provided in the table below.

How Do Survival Rates Correlate with Gestational Age at Delivery?

GESTATION (WKS)	SURVIVAL (%)
22	0
23	15
24	31–56
25	55–80
26	63–75
27	77
28	87

Data compiled from three recent series: Allen, 1993[1]; Whyte, 1993[14]; and Synnes, 1994.[13]

19. What are the short- and long-term complications of the extremely premature infant (≤ 27 weeks)?

Neonatal complications include intraventricular hemorrhage (IVH), bronchopulmonary dysplasia (BPD), sepsis, and necrotizing enterocolitis (NEC). At these early gestational ages, respiratory complications predominate, with BPD in two-thirds of infants. IVH occurs in approximately 20%, sepsis in 10–20%, and NEC in < 10%. Long-term outcome is compromised by cerebral palsy, blindness, and deafness. Two-thirds of 23-week-gestation survivors are considered impaired. This rate decreases to one-third for survivors of delivery at 24 and 25 weeks' gestation. By 26–27 weeks, developmental disability among survivors occurs in 10–20%.

20. What are the complications in preterm infants delivered at 28–32 weeks?

Both short-term and long-term complications decrease from 28–32 weeks. Developmental disability occurs in approximately 10% of survivors in the 28–30-week range, with retinal scarring in 2–3% and blindness in < 1%. Respiratory complications compromise approximately 50% of these neonates.

21. What are the general risks of hyaline membrane disease (HMD) at various gestational ages?

Gestational age	*Percent HMD*
26–28 weeks	60–80%
28–30 weeks	30–60%
30–32 weeks	20–30%
32–34 weeks	10–15%

22. How can fetal lung maturity be assessed during preterm labor?

Various tests have been developed to analyze the components of fetal lung maturation. The ratio of lethicin to sphingomyelin or the appearance of phosphatidyglycerol are commonly employed as markers of fetal lung maturation. The various tests are listed in the table at the top of the next page.

Assessment of Fetal Pulmonary Maturity*

TEST	PRINCIPLE	MATURE LEVEL
L/S ratio	Quantity of surfactant lecithin compared to sphingomyelin	≥ 2.0
Lung profile	Includes determination of PG and PI, which improve surfactant function in mature, saccular alveoli	> 50% acetone precipitated lecithin; 15–20% PI; 2–10% PG
Lecithin concentration	Direct measure of primary phospholipid in surfactant	≥ 3.5 mg/100 ml lecithin; ≥ 1 mg/100 ml phosphorus
Saturated lecithin	Measurement after oxidation with osmium tetroxide	≥ 500 mg/dl
Microviscosimeter	Fluorescence depolarization used to determine phospholipid content	P < .310–.336
"Shake test"	Generation of stable foam by pulmonary surfactant in presence of ethanol	Complete ring of bubbles 15 minutes after shaking at 1:2 dilution
Foam stability index (FSI)	Quantitative measure of foam stability of surfactant and ethanol	≥ 0.48
Optical density	Evaluates turbidity changes dependent on total phospholipid concentration	At 650 nm, ≥ 0.15

* From Main DM, Main EK: Ob-Gyn: A Pocket Reference. Chicago, Year Book Medical Publishers, 1984, p 46, with permission. Adapted from Gabbe SG: Recent advances in the assessment of fetal maturity. J Reprod Med 23:227, 1979 (an excellent review article). For saturated lecithin, see Torday J, Carson L, Lawson EE: Saturated phosphatidylcholine in amniotic fluid and prediction of respiratory distress syndrome. N Engl J Med 301:1013, 1979. For FSI, see Sher G, Statland BE, Freer DE: Clinical evaluation of the quantitative foam stability index test. Obstet Gynecol 55:617, 1980.

23. In the classic studies of steroid use in preterm gestations, how was the incidence of HMD altered?

The original findings of Liggins and Howie in 1972 have since been repeated in several studies and serve as a landmark contribution to the decreased mortality of premature neonates. Two doses of IM betamethasone 24 hours apart, with delivery 24 hours after the last dose and before 7 days from the first dose, were associated with a marked decrease in HMD. The findings were most significant for gestations 30–34 weeks, with decreased effect for gestations of 27–30 weeks.

24. When does it appear that infants receive the greatest respiratory benefit from maternal betamethasone treatment?

Overall decrease in hyaline membrane disease (HMD) is greatest in infants delivered between 1 and 7 days after maternal treatment. However, benefits are still derived if an infant is delivered within 24 hours of treatment (30% reduction in HMD) or at more than 7 days after treatment (40% reduction).

Currently, the gestational age at which infants benefit by reduction in HMD is not restricted to those at 30–34 weeks' gestation. Because few infants over 34 weeks develop HMD, benefits are difficult to ascertain; however, benefits to infants under 30 weeks appear equal to those in the 30–34 week range.

25. What other fetal benefits have been attributed to maternal steroid therapy?

Reduction in intraventricular hemorrhage by 60% and decrease in necrotizing enterocolitis by 65%.

26. What fetal/neonatal and maternal complications have been ascribed to steroid administration?

No significant short-term fetal/neonatal complications have been definitely identified. Although an increased rate of neonatal infection has been suggested when steroids are administered in the presence of premature rupture of membranes, current estimates are imprecise. Twelve-year follow-ups of children treated in utero have shown no demonstrable effects on growth and development of the central nervous system. These studies have helped to alleviate initial concerns in animals for impaired myelination with third-trimester in utero steroid exposure.

Maternal complications include glucose intolerance with increased insulin requirements and the potential for increased pulmonary edema when steroids are used in conjunction with tocolytics. For increased pulmonary edema, the role of tocolysis vs. the combination of tocolysis and steroids has been difficult to assess. A concern for possible increase in postpartum maternal infection remains unresolved.

27. What role does surfactant administration play in outcomes of premature infants?

Administered neonatally, synthetic surfactant has been shown to reduce neonatal morbidity and mortality. Initially used as a rescue treatment in markedly premature infants (< 1000 gm), studies have also supported its efficacy as a prophylactic measure in extremely premature infants and as a rescue treatment in larger infants (< 2000 gm). Debate continues about the greater efficacy of synthetic (Exosurf) vs. modified bovine surfactant extract (Survanta). Enhanced beneficial effects of maternal steroid administration (dexamethasone) and subsequent rescue surfactant use have been reported, although animal studies remain inconclusive.

BIBLIOGRAPHY

1. Allen MC, Donohue PK, Dusman AE: The limit of viability—neonatal outcome in infants born 22 to 25 weeks gestation. N Engl J Med 320:1597–1601, 1993.
2. Bartnicki J, Casal D, Kreaden US, et al: Fetal fibronectin in vaginal specimens predicts preterm delivery and very-low-birth-weight infants. Am J Obstet Gynecol 174:971–974, 1996.
3. Blanch G, Olah KS, Walkinshaw S: The presence of fetal fibronectin in the cervicovaginal secretions of women at term—its role in the assessment of women before labor induction and in the investigation of the physiologic mechanisms of labor. Am J Obstet Gynecol 174(1 Pt 1):262–266, 1996.
4. Collaborative Home Uterine Monitoring Study (CHUMS) Study: A multicenter randomized controlled trial of home uterine monitoring: Active versus sham device. Am J Obstet Gynecol 173:1120–1127, 1995.
5. Colton T, Kayne HL, Zhang Y, Heeren T: A metaanalysis of home uterine activity monitoring. Am J Obstet Gynecol 173:1499–1505, 1995.
6. Ekman G, Granstrom L, Malmstrom A, et al: Cervical fetal fibronectin correlates to cervical ripening. Acta Obstet Gynecol Scand 74:698–701, 1995.
7. Hellemans P, Gerris J, Verdonk P: Fetal fibronectin detection for prediction of preterm birth in low risk women. Br J Obstet Gynaecol 102:207–212, 1995.
8. Iams JD, Casal D, McGregor JA, et al: Fetal fibronectin improves the accuracy of diagnosis of preterm labor. Am J Obstet Gynecol 173:141–145, 1995.
9. Kari MA, Hallman M, Eronen M, et al: Prenatal dexamethasone treatment in conjunction with rescue therapy of human surfactant: A randomized placebo-controlled multicenter study. Pediatrics 93:730–736, 1994.
10. Lockwood CJ, Wein R, Lapinski R, et al: The presence of cervical and vaginal fetal fibronectin predicts preterm delivery in an inner-city obstetric population. Am J Obstet Gynecol 169:798–804, 1993.
11. Nageotte MP, Casal D, Senyei AE: Fetal fibronectin in patients at increased risk for premature birth. Am J Obstet Gynecol 170(1 Pt 1):20–25, 1994.
12. NIH Consensus Developmental Panel: The effect of corticosteroids for fetal maturation on perinatal outcomes. JAMA 273:413, 1995.
13. Synnes AR, Ling EW, Whitfield MF, et al: Perinatal outcome of a large cohort of extremely low gestational age infants (twenty-three to twenty-eight complete weeks gestation). J Pediatr 125:952–960, 1994.
14. Whyte HE, Fitzhardinge PM, Shennan AT, et al: Extreme immaturity: Outcome of 568 pregnancies of 23–26 weeks gestation. Obstet Gynecol 82:1–7, 1993.

74. PRETERM PREMATURE RUPTURE OF MEMBRANES

Jean C. Ryan, M.D., and Vanessa A. Barss, M.D.

1. How is premature rupture of membranes (PROM) defined?
Rupture of membranes before the onset of labor.

2. How is preterm rupture of membranes defined?
Rupture of membranes before the onset of labor in a gestation < 37 weeks.

3. What is prolonged rupture of membranes?
Ruptured membranes for > 24 hours before delivery.

4. What is the latency period?
The interval between rupture of membranes and the onset of labor.

5. What is the incidence of premature rupture of membranes?
PROM occurs in 10–15% of all pregnancies, including 10% of term pregnancies. Preterm PROM complicates 2–4% of preterm pregnancies.

6. What is the major complication of preterm PROM?
Premature delivery. Preterm PROM is associated with 30–40% of preterm births and 10% of all perinatal mortality.

7. What causes preterm PROM?
Preterm PROM probably occurs because of weakness of the chorioamnion. Physical stress, bacteria, and macrophages produce proteases, elastases, phospholipases, cytokines, and eicosanoids that produce uterine irritability, cervical ripening, and membrane weakness and rupture.

8. List the risk factors for preterm PROM.
- History of premature PROM (most common risk factor)
- Cervicovaginitis: sexually transmitted diseases, including gonorrhea, trichomonas, bacterial vaginosis, group B streptococci, possibly chlamydia
- Incompetent cervix
- Cigarette smoking
- Amniocentesis
- Prior cervical surgery
- Vaginal bleeding in the first or second trimester
- Hydramnios
- Connective tissue disease such as Ehlers-Danlos syndrome

9. What is the recurrence rate for preterm PROM?
20–30%, compared with a 4% incidence if the prior pregnancy was an uncomplicated term pregnancy.

10. Which characteristics are no longer believed to be risk factors for premature PROM?

Coitus	Maternal exercise
Cervical exams	Vitamin or mineral deficiencies
Changes in barometric pressure	Parity
Male fetal sex	

11. How soon does labor follow PROM?
- 80–90% of term patients are in labor within 24–48 hours of membrane rupture.
- 50% of preterm patients are in labor within 24–48 hours.
- 70% of preterm patients are in labor within 7 days.

In some, but not all, studies there is an inverse relationship between gestational age at PROM and latency period, with very early preterm PROM having a longer latency.

12. What is the major neonatal complication of preterm delivery in patients with preterm PROM?

Hyaline membrane disease occurs in 10–40% of deliveries and is responsible for 30–70% of neonatal deaths.

13. What is the second most common complication of preterm PROM after preterm labor?

Infection occurs in 15–30% of patients, including choriamnionitis, fetal infection, and endometritis. Neonatal sepsis accounts for 3–20% of neonatal deaths.

14. What organisms have been cultured from infected amniotic fluid in patients with preterm PROM?

Infections are usually polymicrobial. Cultured organisms include *Ureaplasma* spp., *Mycoplasma* spp., group B streptococci, peptostreptococci, *Fusobacteria* spp., *Gardnerella vaginalis*, *Escherichia coli*, enterococci, *Bacteroides* spp., and others (more rarely).

15. List the other complications of preterm PROM.
- Cord prolapse, especially in nonvertex presentations
- Increased number of cesarean sections because of nonvertex presentations
- Fetal pulmonary hypoplasia and orthopedic deformations with severe, early, and prolonged oligohydramnios
- Placental abruption

16. How is PROM diagnosed?

History of fluid leaking through the vagina is the most common indicator. Urinary incontinence, excessive vaginal discharge, and mucous discharge are in the differential diagnosis.

17. What is the work-up for PROM?
- **Never** do a digital exam because even one digital exam can increase the chance of infection by carrying vaginal organisms into the cervix and uterus.
- Do a sterile speculum exam to look for pooling of amniotic fluid and to assess the cervix.
- Confirm the diagnosis by testing the fluid for pH using nitrazine paper. The pH of the vagina in pregnancy is 4.5–5.5. Nitrazine paper changes from yellow to blue at a pH above 6. Since the pH of amniotic fluid is about 7, the nitrazine paper turns blue if there is amniotic fluid in the vagina. False-positive nitrazine tests may occur from semen, blood or serum, trichomonas or bacterial vaginitis infections, or soap. False-negative tests occur in < 10% of cases.
- Do a fern test. A swab from the posterior vaginal fornix should be rolled on a slide and allowed to air dry for at least 10 minutes. Under the microscope a typical "fern" pattern will appear if amniotic fluid is present. False-positive tests have been attributed to fingerprints, talc, and semen.
- Ultrasound often shows decreased amniotic fluid volume.
- A definitive diagnosis can be made when the above tests are equivocal by injecting indigo carmine dye into the amniotic cavity under ultrasound guidance. A tampon is placed in the vagina, left for 2 hours, and then removed. If the membranes are ruptured, the tampon will turn blue from the colored amniotic fluid.

18. Are tocolytics useful to prolong pregnancy when preterm labor complicates preterm PROM?

This is a controversial subject. Most experts, however, believe tocolytics are not effective in prolonging pregnancy in the setting of PROM and are more effective for prolonging pregnancy in preterm labor with intact membranes.

19. Are corticosteroids to accelerate fetal lung maturation contraindicated in pregnancies complicated by preterm PROM?

No. They are indicated in pregnancies < 34 weeks to reduce the incidence and severity of hyaline membrane disease, intraventricular hemorrhage, and necrotizing enterocolitis in the event of preterm delivery. They do not increase the risk of chorioamnionitis or neonatal sepsis but may increase the risk for postpartum endometritis.

20. Can ruptured membranes seal again?

Resealing can happen but is rare. It is most common after a high leak, especially after genetic amniocentesis.

21. Do antibiotics prolong the latency period and prevent infection?

Probably not. This area is under investigation, but most studies do not show a better pregnancy or neonatal outcome if prophylactic antibiotics are given in preterm PROM.

22. What are the management options for patients with preterm PROM?

- Expectant management with delivery in presence of labor, infection, or nonreassuring fetal status
- Delivery when fetal lung maturity is documented, regardless of gestational age
- Delivery when the risks of prematurity are small compared with the risk of infection

23. What are the serious complications of chorioamnionitis?

1. 4-fold increase in neonatal mortality
2. 3-fold increase in neonatal morbidity from hyaline membrane disease, sepsis, and intraventricular hemorrhage

24. During what time of day is PROM most common?

Between 2 and 4 A.M.

25. How does the incidence of chorioamnionitis differ between term and preterm PROM?

1% at term, 15–30% preterm.

26. What is the outcome of preterm PROM before 26 weeks?

Most of the adverse neonatal outcome is due to prematurity; the longer the latency period and the greater the gestational age at delivery, the better the prognosis. Overall outcome: chorioamnionitis, 40%; neonatal survival, 46%; normal child at long-term follow-up, 60% of survivors.

27. At what gestational age do the complications of prematurity become so low that one might consider delivery to avoid potential problems from sepsis or cord prolapse?

34 weeks.

28. Other than confirming the diagnosis of PROM, what information is available from a sterile speculum exam?

1. Presence of cord prolapse or fetal part can be determined.
2. The dilatation and effacement of the cervix can be estimated.
3. Amniotic fluid can be aspirated from the vagina for lung maturity testing.
4. Cultures for gonorrhea, chlamydia, and group B streptococci can be obtained.

29. Why is PROM associated with a high prevalence of nonreassuring fetal tracings in labor?

Umbilical cord compression secondary to oligohydramnios.

30. What procedure may decrease the number and severity of variable decelerations on the fetal heart rate tracing?

Amnioinfusion with saline.

BIBLIOGRAPHY

1. Duff P (ed): Premature rupture of membranes. Clin Obstet Gynecol 34:685–793, 1991.
2. Ghidini A, Romero R: Premature rupture of membranes: When it occurs in the second trimester. Contemp OB/GYN August 1994, pp 685–793.
3. Garite TJ: Premature rupture of membranes. In Creasy RK, Resnik R (eds): Maternal-Fetal Medicine: Principles and Practice, 3rd ed. Philadelphia, W.B. Saunders, 1994, pp 625–637.

75. BREECH PRESENTATION

Robert Wester, M.D.

1. How often are infants in a breech lie at term? Does the incidence vary for preterm infants?

After 37 weeks, approximately 5–7% of infants present breech. This varies markedly from the mid-trimester (21–24 weeks) when 33% are noted to be breech, and from the early third trimester (29–32 weeks), during which a 14% incidence of breech presentation is common.

2. Which maternal and fetal characteristics increase the chances for a persistent breech lie?

Maternal—uterine anomalies (septum, unicornate uterus) and pelvic tumors (fibroids as well as adenexal masses)

Fetal—abnormalities of amniotic fluid (both polyhydramnios and oligohydramnios), fetal anomalies (especially anencephaly or hydrocephaly), and fetal neuromuscular disorders (myotonic dystrophy)

3. What is external version?

Converting the fetus from a breech to a vertex lie can be accomplished by applying pressure to the maternal abdominal wall to turn the infant in a somersault fashion. The success rate of version is higher when performed early in the third trimester. However, intervention before 37 weeks results in a higher reconversion rate (10%), manipulation of a significant percentage of breeches that would have converted to vertex spontaneously, and a risk of delivery of a preterm infant if complications are encountered.

Version after 37 weeks confines the procedure to infants with a minimal chance of spontaneous vertex positioning and has a success rate of about 50%. Maternal parity, placental location, dilation, station, and estimated fetal weight are the most predictive of successful version. Scoring systems to predict success are available incorporating these variables.

4. What are the potential complications of external version?

External version carries a risk to the fetus of morbidity and mortality. Fetal morbidity related to version is usually the result of abruption or cord entanglement and, on the average, is in the range of 3/1,000 versions. The use of general anesthesia during version has been associated with higher fetal mortality (reported to be in the 1–2% range by some authorities). Contraindications to attempted version include abruption, low-lying placenta, maternal hypertension, previous uterine incisions, multiple gestation, and evidence of uteroplacental insufficiency (nonreactive nonstress test). Rh-negative mothers should receive RhoGAM after an external version attempt.

5. How often will the fetus convert spontaneously to a vertex lie during the third trimester?

In early third trimester (29 weeks), as many as 75% of breech lies will spontaneously convert to vertex by the 38th week. With advancing gestation, however, fewer breeches spontaneously convert. Primiparous women, breeches with extended legs, and a prior delivery of a breech fetus all decrease the likelihood of spontaneous version.

At 37 weeks, spontaneous version is still a possibility, with rates as high as 18% reported. A "knee-chest" position for 15 minutes every 2 hours for 5 days has been reported by some authorities to increase the chance of spontaneous version in the late third trimester.

6. What are the three types of breech presentation?

Frank—flexed thighs, extended knees (50–75% of breeches)
Footling—one or both legs extended below the buttocks (20–24% of term breeches)
Complete—flexed thighs, flexed knees (5–10% of term breeches)

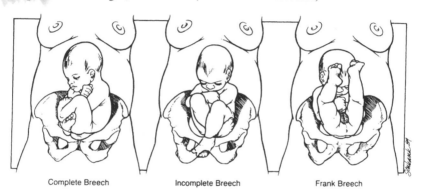

| Complete Breech | Incomplete Breech | Frank Breech |

Three possible breech presentations. (From Gabbe SG, Niebyl JR, Simpson JL (eds): Obstetrics: Normal & Problem Pregnancies. New York, Churchill Livingstone, 1986, p 465, with permission.)

7. How much higher is perinatal mortality with vaginal breech delivery compared with vaginal vertex delivery?

In some studies, perinatal mortality with vaginal breech delivery is 13 times higher than for vaginal vertex delivery. Morbidity is generally considered to be 5–7 times higher. This figure is heavily influenced by the gestational age at delivery and type of breech presentation.

8. What are the four main causes of increased perinatal mortality in breech presentations?

Multiple congenital anomalies, hypoxia, birth injury, and prematurity.

9. What is the incidence of congenital anomalies in cephalic presentations? Is it different in breech presentations?

In vertex presentations, approximately 2–3% of the infants will have congenital abnormalities. Among breech presentations, this rate is much higher (6–18%) and contributes significantly to the morbidity and mortality rate of a breech, whether delivery occurs by either a vaginal or abdominal route.

10. What is head entrapment?

In a breech presentation, the unmolded head of the fetus may be trapped above an incompletely dilated cervix and can impede delivery. Depending on fetal size, the more pliable abdomen and thorax of the breech fetus may descend through a cervix that does not allow passage of the unmolded head. Arrest of the fetal head occurs in approximately 88/1,000 vaginal breech deliveries and can result in significant morbidity and fetal mortality. Attempts to maintain flexion of the fetal head through external maternal suprapubic pressure and allowing spontaneous delivery of the body without traction help to reduce this risk.

11. What are Dührssen incisions (hysterostomatomy)?

If the incompletely dilated cervix cannot be slipped over the trapped head, radial incisions can be made in the cervix. Three incisions are placed at 2, 6, and 10 o'clock; if space permits, application of ring forceps to the cervical edge facilitates hemostasis. Maternal hemorrhage and extension into the lower uterine segment often result, relegating the application of Dührssen incisions to cases in which fetal morbidity or death is a strong possibility. For rapid delivery of a vertex infant with fetal distress, these incisions should not be substituted for emergent abdominal delivery, which carries a lower morbidity risk to the mother.

12. At what gestational age does fetal abdominal circumference equal head circumference?

At about 36 weeks. Prior to 36 weeks, head circumference is generally significantly larger than abdominal or thoracic measurements.

13. Should Piper forceps be routinely used for delivery of the aftercoming head in a vaginal breech delivery?

Yes. Advocated by most obstetricians, the Piper forceps requires skill in application. Their use facilitates the proper angle of traction for the aftercoming head, helping to maintain the flexed positioning of the head in the pelvic hollow.

14. What percentage of breeches have hyperextended heads during labor?

3–5% of breech presentations will have an angle between the fetal spine and jaw of greater than 105 degrees—a "star-gazing fetus." Hyperextension is associated with greater perinatal mortality and morbidity as well as with trisomy 21.

15. Why are membranes kept intact as long as possible in a woman in labor with breech presentation?

The pressure of the intact membranes may help to dilate the cervix as well as prevent cord prolapse and compression.

16. How often does cord prolapse occur with breech presentations?

The incidence of this potentially fatal complication varies with the type of breech presentation. Filling of the lower uterine segment with the frank breech presentation is associated with the lowest rate (0.5%), whereas complete breech has a 4–5% incidence of prolapse and footling breech carries the highest rate at 10%.

17. By performing cesarean section deliveries for all term breeches, neonatal outcome will be as good as in uncomplicated vaginal vertex deliveries. True or false?

False. Even when delivered through an abdominal incision, the breech delivery requires skill and inherently carries a greater risk of morbidity to the infant.

18. What is the Pinard maneuver? When is it useful?

Often at cesarean section and sometimes at vaginal delivery of a breech, a frank or complete breech does not deliver spontaneously. In these situations, breech decomposition with conversion to a footling breech may aid in extraction. This can be accomplished with the **Pinard maneuver**, which involves slipping two fingers along the inner surface of one thigh of the infant, applying gentle pressure away from the midline with resulting spontaneous flexion at the knee. The foot can then be grasped and the leg delivered below the buttocks. When completed on the opposite leg, this places both lower extremities below the buttocks and enables a breech extraction to be performed. Grasping of both feet in one of the operator's hands will allow gentle traction to be applied and the breech extracted to the level of the buttocks. At the level of the buttocks, the infant generally rotates to a spine anterior position and the operator's hands are repositioned with thumbs over the sacrum and fingers around the infant's hips. Care should be taken not to grasp the infant higher around the abdomen, as visceral damage is possible.

19. What is a nuchal arm? How can it be prevented?

Delivery of the breech proceeds with gentle traction until the scapulae appear. At this point the infant is rotated so that the biacromial diameter is anterior-posterior. At the level of the axilla, the shoulders are ready for delivery. Undue traction at this time can result in the arm(s) remaining extended above the head and wrapping around the infant's neck (**nuchal arm**) as rotation for delivery occurs. If the shoulders do not spontaneously deliver after the axilla, the operator should place two fingers along the infant's humerus and sweep the upper extremity across the infant's chest to effect delivery of each arm. The humerus should be splinted with the operator's fingers and not grasped, as grasping increases the chance of fracture. Nuchal arms can sometimes be freed by manually rotating the fetus in a fashion to bring the trapped arm down across the infant's face.

20. When is the Mauriceau maneuver used?

Often employed at cesarean section when Piper forceps are not applied to the aftercoming head, this maneuver will help maintain flexion of the head to facilitate delivery. The operator's hand is placed so that the index and fourth fingers are over the maxilla. If used in a vaginal delivery, the infant's body rests on the operator's hand and forearm. Gentle pressure will effect continued flexion of the infant's head for completion of delivery of the head. The operator's fingers should not be placed in the infant's mouth to facilitate traction, as this has been associated with jaw injury to the infant.

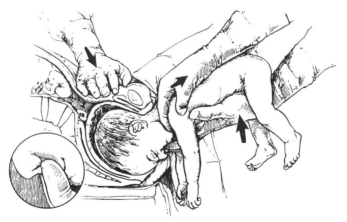

Delivery of aftercoming head using the Mauriceau maneuver. Note that as the fetal head is being delivered, flexion of the head is maintained by suprapubic pressure provided by an assistant and simultaneously by pressure on the maxilla (inset) by the operator as traction is applied. (From Cunningham FG, MacDonald PC, Gant NF (eds): Williams Obstetrics, 18th ed. Norwalk, CT, Appleton and Lange, 1989, p 398, with permission.)

21. What criteria should be considered if a vaginal breech delivery is to be undertaken?

Recommendations vary but general guidelines include:

1. Ultrasound examination to evaluate fetal anomalies, placental location, and extension of the fetal head, and to corroborate clinical estimation of fetal weight and type of breech

2. Inclusion of singleton, frank breech presentations with estimated weight between 2,500 and 3,800 gm

3. Adequate pelvimetry by x-ray: pelvic inlet with transverse diameter ≥ 11.5 cm and anteroposterior (AP) diameter ≥ 10.5 cm, and mid-pelvis with transverse diameter ≥ 10 cm and AP diameter ≥ 11.5 cm

4. Availability of an obstetrician experienced in breech delivery, an experienced assistant, anesthesia, and facilities for emergent cesarean delivery

5. No maternal or fetal indications for cesarean delivery (placenta previa, failure of progress in labor)

BIBLIOGRAPHY

1. Collea JV, Rabind SC, Weghorst GR, Quilligan EJ: The randomized management of term frank breech presentation: Vaginal vs. cesarean delivery. Am J Obstet Gynecol 131:186, 1978.
2. Cunningham FG, MacDonald PC, Gant NF (eds): Williams Obstetrics, 18th ed. Norwalk, CT, Appleton & Lange, 1989.
3. Gabbe SG, Niebyl JR, Simpson JL (eds): Obstetrics: Normal & Problem Pregnancies. New York, Churchill Livingstone, 1986.
4. Minkoff H: Breech presentation. Postgrad Obstet Gynecol 3:1, 1983.
5. Myers SA, Gleicher N: Breech delivery: Why the dilemma? Am J Obstet Gynecol 155:6, 1986.
6. Newman RB, Peacock BS, VanDorsten JP, Hunt HH: Predicting success of external cephalic version. Am J Obstet Gynecol 169(2 Pt 1):245–249, 1993.
7. Savona-Ventura C: The role of external version in modern obstetrics. Obstet Gynecol Surv 41:393, 1986.

76. LABOR: INITIATION AND PROGRESSION

Louise Wilkins-Haug, M.D., Ph.D.

1. What factors in humans have been identified as crucial to the initiation of labor?

Although both the physiologic and biochemical changes associated with the onset of labor have been extensively documented, the link between the two, the actual trigger that initiates labor in humans, remains difficult to discern. In several species the fetal pituitary-adrenal system determines the onset of labor through alterations of estrogen and progesterone secretion. In humans, this pituitary-adrenal pathway may not be as instrumental; firm correlations between these hormonal levels and onset of human labor are not available. Prostaglandins, synthesized by the myometrium (PGI_2), the decidua ($PGF_{2\alpha}$), and the amnion and chorion (PGE_2) remain important mediators and possible initiators of uterine contractions.

2. How is chorioamnionitis believed to initiate labor?

Possibly through increased levels of platelet activating factor (PAF) and leukotrienes. Both are present in increased quantities when preterm labor is associated with chorioamnionitis. They are responsible for stimulating prostaglandin synthesis.

3. In which situations is induction of labor considered?

Awaiting the onset of normal labor may not be an option in certain circumstances. In preterm gestations indications for labor induction include preeclampsia, fetal growth retardation or other evidence of fetal compromise, and deteriorations of maternal disease so that continuation of pregnancy is believed to be detrimental. In the term or postterm pregnancy, induction of labor is often undertaken after rupture of membranes without labor (premature rupture of membranes) or post-datism (> 42 weeks' gestation). Unless maternal or fetal well-being is at risk, specific criteria should be met or fetal lung maturation established by amniocentesis.

One of the following parameters and fetal lung maturity assumed:
Positive fetoscope for 20 wks or Doppler tones for 30 wks
36 wks from positive test for beta human chorionic gonadotropin (urine or serum)
Early ultrasound (crown-rump length 6–11 wks) supports 39 wks
12–20 wk ultrasound confirms 39 wks from history or clinical exam

* American College of Obstetricians and Gynecologists 12/95.

4. What is Bishop's score? How is it used?

Based on the criteria in the table below, the cervical exam, as assessed by internal examination, is scored. In multiparous patients, scores are predictive of successful induction. No failures are expected with a score ≥ 9; 5% fail with scores 5–8; and 20% fail with a score < 4.

Bishop Scoring System

	SCORE			
FACTOR	0	1	2	3
Dilatation (cm)	Closed	1–2	3–4	≥ 5
Effacement (%)	0–30	40–50	60–70	≥ 80
Station	−3	−2	−1 or 0	+1, +2
Consistency	Firm	Medium	Soft	
Position of cervix	Posterior	Midposition	Anterior	

5. What other modalities have been proposed for predicting the potential success of induction?

The presence of fetal fibronectin in a cervical sample has been correlated with the onset of labor within a specific time frame. Some have proposed this method for ascertainment of a patient's suitability for induction, especially in term and postterm pregnancies.

6. What methods are available for preinduction cervical ripening?

Mechanical cervical ripening methods include placement of a Foley catheter with inflated balloon in the cervical canal and use of osmotic dilators (laminaria). Osmatic dilators, however, have been associated in some studies with higher rates of maternal and neonatal infection. Other options include nipple stimulation, amniotomy, low-dose oxytocin, and PGE_2. PGE_2 can be applied within the vagina in either gel or tablet form, and lower doses can be used intracervically. Studies both support and refute the efficacy of each of these modalities with regard to shortened duration of induction and percent of failed inductions. In particular, prostaglandin agents involve a low risk of maternal uterine hyperstimulation with possible resultant decreased perfusion and compromise to the infant. Nonetheless, some have advocated outpatient preinduction cervical ripening in low-risk patients.

7. Is preinduction ripening contraindicated in any particular group of patients?

For any of the agents described, including the newer prostaglandin gels, absolute contraindications apply only to patients for whom labor is contraindicated. Initial concerns about the use of prostaglandin agents in women with prior low transverse cesarean sections or rupture of membranes have not been confirmed in recent studies.

8. For the patient who is remote from term, how successful is induction of labor?

In women who require labor induction for preterm gestations, as often occurs in the setting of worsening maternal diseases such as preeclampsia, the success rate is less than in women who undergo induction at term. One study found that induction of labor led to vaginal delivery in only 15% of pregnancies < 30 weeks; the success rate for pregnancies from 30–34 weeks was 48%. Especially in patients with hemolysis, elevated liver enzymes, and low platelet count (HELLP) syndrome, decisions to proceed with cesarean section during induction often were influenced by nonreassurance of fetal well-being, and worsening maternal disease.

9. Does maternal intravenous magnesium sulfate for seizure prophylaxis lead to prolonged labor?

Probably not. Although magnesium sulfate is used as a tocolytic agent for suppression of contractions in women with preterm labor, once active labor is initiated, studies do not support prolonged labor in women receiving magnesium sulfate for seizure prophylaxis. Even in women undergoing induction of labor because of preeclampsia, concomitant use of maternal intravenous magnesium sulfate does not significantly prolong labor or result in increased cesarean delivery. Preeclamptic women randomized to seizure prophylaxis with magnesium sulfate or phenytoin demonstrated no differences in length of labor or number of cesarean deliveries.

10. What are the cardinal movements of labor?

1. Engagement
2. Descent
3. Flexion
4. Internal rotation
5. Extension
6. External rotation
7. Expulsion

11. What are Friedman curves?

In the late 1950s, Emmanual Friedman popularized the use of an objective measure of progress in labor. Often depicted graphically, Friedman curves plot cervical dilation against time passed, with varying expectations for nulliparous and multiparous patients. Used in conjunction with fetal descent, the curves provide clinical feedback about the normalcy of the parturient's progress in labor.

Labor Curve Abnormalities

	NULLIPAROUS	MULTIPAROUS
Prolonged latent phase	≥ 20 hr	≥ 14 hr
Protracted active phase	≤ 1.2 cm/hr	≤ 1.5 cm/hr
Active phase arrest	≥ 2 hr	≥ 2 hr
Protracted descent	≤ 1 cm/hr	≤ 2 cm/hr
Arrest of descent	≥ 1 hr	≥ 1 hr
Prolonged deceleration (8–10 cm)	≥ 3 hr	≥ 1 hr
2nd-stage arrest	≥ 2 hr	≥ 1 hr
(with CLE)	≥ 3 hr	≥ 2 hr

CLE = continuous lumbar epidural anesthesia.

12. What cervical changes generally take place during the latent phase?

Cervical ripening in the latent phase generally includes palpable softening, effacement, and anterior rotation of the cervix in the pelvic axis. Although only partially understood, these changes are most likely the result of prostaglandins with collagen degeneration.

13. When does conversion from latent to active phase occur?

The transition from latent to active phase is usually difficult to discern. It is generally characterized by increased regularity and intensity of contractions, accompanied by progressive and predictable cervical change. In nulliparous patients, the latent phase is generally longer, with active labor present at relatively minimal dilations (3 cm). In contrast, in multiparous patients the latent phase may be shorter, with the active phase not initiated until 6–7 cm; many multiparous patients have baseline cervical dilation of 3 cm at term even before the latent phase.

14. Is the degree of fetal descent before labor predictive of labor abnormalities?

The degree of fetal descent before labor is associated with both length of the latent phase and probability of vaginal delivery. The nulliparous patient with an unengaged fetal head entering labor may have as high as a 30% risk of cesarean section.

15. What is prolonged latent phase? Does it have any prognostic significance?

In nulliparous women, a prolonged latent phase is > 20 hours; in multiparous women, > 14 hours. It occurs in 5% of patients. Controversy exists as to whether a prolonged latent phase is predictive of labor curve abnormalities or increased rates of cesarean section. Although historically studies support no association, recent reviews that controlled for the influence of confounding variables such as macrosomia and parity found that prolonged latent phase alone is predictive of an increased rate of cesarean delivery.

16. What is the treatment of prolonged latent phase?

Two options are generally used—oxytocin stimulation of contractions or maternal sedation. Either has an approximate success rate of 85% in converting the patient into an active pattern. Choice of approach is generally governed by the clinical situation and the urgency with which delivery is to be accomplished.

17. What are abnormalities of the active phase? How are they treated?

Protracted active phase. Continued linear progression of dilatation, though at a subnormal rate, generally is not considered responsive to oxytocin stimulation. The majority of cases result from cephalopelvic disproportion. In addition, rupture of membranes has not been proved to be efficacious and may increase the rate of chorioamnionitis.

Arrest of dilation. Absence of further dilatation may follow protracted or normal active labor; generally such arrest is responsive to oxytocin stimulation.

18. What is considered full dilation?

Generally, 10 cm is considered full dilatation, because it is approximately the diameter of the fetal vertex at term. For preterm infants, however, full dilation may be < 10 cm, given the smaller presenting vertex and the fact that the cervix will not dilate past the maximal point of the presenting part.

19. What are abnormalities of the second stage of labor?

Protracted descent, arrest of descent and failure of descent. True descent can be difficult to discern if molding and caput obscure the true biparietal diameter. Suprapubic palpation may be helpful in these situations to assess the true degree of cephalic descent.

20. What is active management of labor?

Labor interventions, such as using strict diagnostic criteria for labor, early amniotomy, early use of oxytocin and continuous professional labor support, have been termed *active management of labor*. This approach originated at the National Maternity Hospital in Dublin. Early data suggested that such an approach could lower the rate of failure to progress in labor and resultant cesarean sections. More recently, reviews and randomized studies of this approach have failed to support a reduction in cesarean section delivery. The use of professional labor support appears to be perhaps the one component of the active management of labor that may decrease the cesarean section rate. A shortened duration of labor has been both supported and refuted in studies of active management of labor.

21. How is the pelvis assessed clinically?

The pelvic inlet (obstetric conjugate) is bounded by the sacral promontory and the pubic symphysis in the anterior-posterior dimension and laterally by the linea terminalis. An estimate of the inlet can be obtained by palpating the sacral promontory, which provides the measurement for the diagonal conjugate. The diagonal conjugate is approximately 1.5 cm greater than the obstetric conjugate. Assessment of the interspinous distance and outlet provides information about patients' overall pelvic dimensions and configuration. Most patients have an intermediate form of the four classically described pelvic types.

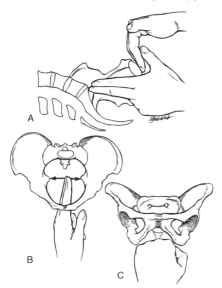

A, Sagittal view of the pelvis demonstrating clinical assessment of the diagonal conjugate. B, Superior view of the pelvis demonstrating clinical assessment of the mid-pelvic interspinous diameter. C, Frontal view of the pelvis demonstrating clinical assessment of the inter-tuberous diameter of the pelvic outlet. (From Repke JT (ed): Intrapartum Obstetrics. New York, Churchill Livingstone, 1996, with permission.)

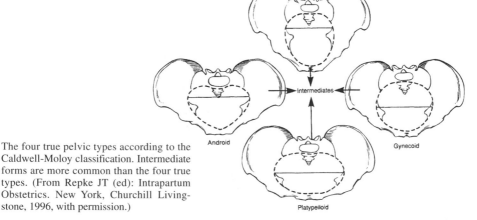

The four true pelvic types according to the Caldwell-Moloy classification. Intermediate forms are more common than the four true types. (From Repke JT (ed): Intrapartum Obstetrics. New York, Churchill Livingstone, 1996, with permission.)

BIBLIOGRAPHY

1. Adair CD, Sanchez-Ramos L, Gaudier FL, et al: Labor induction in patients with previous cesarean section. Am J Perinatol 12:450–454, 1995.
2. Atkinson MW, Guinn D, Owen J, Hauth JC: Does magnesium sulfate affect the length of labor induction in women with pregnancy-associated hypertension? Am J Obstet Gynecol 173:1219–1222, 1995.

3. Cammu H, Van Beckhout E: A randomized controlled trial of early versus delayed use of amniotomy and oxytocin infusion in nulliparous labor. Br J Obstet Gynecol 103:313–318, 1996.
4. Cohen W: Normal and abnormal labor. In Reece E, Hobbins J, Mahoney M, Petrie R (eds): Medicine of the Fetus and Mother. Philadelphia, J.B. Lippincott, 1992, pp 1370–1380.
5. Frigoletto FD, Lieberman E, Lang J, et al: A clinical trial of active management of labor. N Engl J Med 333:745–750, 1995.
6. Gonen R, Samberg I, Degani S: Intracervical prostaglandin E_2 for induction of labor in patients with premature rupture of membranes and an unripe cervix. Am J Perinatol 11:436–438, 1994.
7. Krammer J, Williams MC, Sawai SK, Brien WF: Pre-induction cervical ripening: A randomized comparison of two methods. Obstet Gynecol 85:614–618, 1995.
8. Magann EF, Roberts WE, Perry KG, et al: Factors relevant to mode of preterm delivery with syndrome of HELLP (hemolysis, elevated liver enzymes, and low platelets). Am J Obstet Gynecol 170:1828–1832, 1994.
9. Thorton JG, Lilford RJ: Active management of labour: Current knowledge and research issues. BMJ 309:366–369, 1994.
10. Uldbjerg N, Forman A, Peterson L, et al: Biomechanical and biochemical changes of the uterus and cervix during pregnancy. In Reece E, Hobbins J, Mahoney M, Petrie R (ed): Medicine of the Fetus and Mother. Philadelphia, J.B. Lippincott, 1992, pp 849–864.

77. INTRAPARTUM FETAL SURVEILLANCE

Robert S. McDuffie, Jr., M.D., and Albert D. Haverkamp, M.D.

1. How many years has fetal heart rate (FHR) monitoring during labor been practiced?

Auscultation of the fetal heart was begun by Marsac in 1650. By the turn of the 20th century, normal ranges had been established (100–160 bpm), and intermittent auscultation during labor was advocated. Continuous electronic fetal cardiac monitoring evolved during the 1950s and early 1960s. Clinical use began in the late 1960s.

2. How sensitive is continuous electronic fetal monitoring in detecting true hypoxia?

Relatively insensitive. Abnormal FHR patterns have a positive predictive value of only 15–25% for a compromised fetus. The strength of FHR monitoring lies in its ability to confirm well-being with reliability.

3. Which patients should have continuous FHR monitoring during labor?

Controversial. Typically most patients undergo continuous FHR monitoring during active labor. Many authorities, including the Food and Drug Administration, believe that this is unnecessary for low-risk patients. Most studies of continuous FHR monitoring vs. intermittent auscultation in low-risk and high-risk pregnancies have shown no significant difference in neonatal outcome measured by mortality, Apgar scores, or presence of seizures. The oft-quoted Dublin trial of randomized "selective" vs. "continuous" FHR monitoring of 13,000 patients showed a decrease in seizures in the second group. No other neonatal differences and no change in the incidence of cerebral palsy were noted. Shy's study of premature infants (< 1500 gm) showed a neurologic benefit of auscultation. Recently, Nelson reported an association of abnormal FHR tracings with cerebral palsy in neonates over 2500 gm. However, the false-positive rate of late decelerations and decreased beat-to-beat variability for prediction of cerebral palsy was over 90%. In an era of close scrutiny of fetal well-being during labor and careful, ongoing medicolegal documentation, a majority of obstetricians opt for continuous FHR monitoring of all patients.

4. What is the largest risk associated with continuous FHR monitoring?

Cesarean section. Continuous surveillance has increased the frequency of abnormal fetal heart rate patterns observed during labor. As described, the majority of abnormal patterns are false positives and do not reflect fetal hypoxia and acidosis. Unfortunately, further fetal evaluation by scalp pH determination is often not available or technically not possible (dilatation < 2 cm). In such cases, the inability to document fetal well-being may lead to emergent operative delivery.

5. What are the alternatives to continuous electronic FHR monitoring during labor?

Intermittent auscultation by either Doppler or stethoscope. For low-risk patients, no data determine optimal frequency of auscultation. Many obstetricians assess FHR every 30 minutes in the first stage and every 15 minutes in the second stage. For patients with risk factors, auscultation after contraction is recommended every 15 minutes during the first stage of labor and every 5 minutes during the second stage. Two important cautions are given relative to intermittent auscultation. First, it is critical to document fetal heart rates and times. If auscultation is not documented, it is presumed not to have occurred. Second, the difference between low-risk and high-risk patients is not well defined. In retrospect (e.g., medicolegal review) risk factors may be identified that mandate high-risk rather than low-risk guidelines for auscultation. If the reviewer finds that the presumed low-risk patient had risk factors, lawyers will argue that high-risk guidelines should be applied.

6. What problems, although rare, are encountered with continuous monitoring of all pregnancies with internal scalp electrodes and pressure catheters?

Uterine perforation and placental abruption with intrauterine tocometers. Problems with internal electrodes include scalp abscess, osteomyelitis, and transmission of herpes to the fetus.

7. What does the internal scalp electrode monitor? How does this differ from external fetal cardiac monitoring?

The internal monitors are applied with a small clip to the fetal scalp to register the fetal electrocardiogram. Intervals between the recorded R-R waves are calculated and the heart rate derived. The external FHR monitors use continuous Doppler detection of cardiac valve closure with a continuously changing rate recorded.

8. What are the benefits of internal cardiac monitoring? The disadvantages?

Advantages—truer representation of beat-to-beat variability; less chance of picking up maternal heart rate; technically easier to obtain monitoring uninterrupted by maternal or fetal movement.

Disadvantages—necessitates rupture of membranes for placement; small chance of fetal infection.

9. How does external monitoring of uterine activity differ from placement of a tocometer within the uterine cavity?

External tocodynamometers ("tocos") merely record movement of the anterior abdominal wall, with uterine contractions inferred. Clinical palpation is probably as good. Frequency and to some extent duration can be obtained but intensity of contractions can be assessed only with an intrauterine monitor. Uterine pressure is transmitted through a water-filled catheter to a monitor where the signal is converted to an appropriate readout.

10. Which parameters should be recorded when an FHR tracing is interpreted in labor?

Baseline—normal: 110–160 beats per minute (bpm)
Short-term variability—normal: 6–10 bpm
Long-term variability—normal: crude sine waves with a cycle of 3–6 per minute
Periodic changes—accelerations and decelerations

11. How are decelerations classically described?

Early—smooth, shallow decelerations appearing as a mirror image of the contraction. Nadir of the deceleration should match the peak of the contraction; heart rate returns to the baseline by the time the contraction has ceased. Typically ascribed to fetal head compression mediated through the sinoatrial node and the vagus nerve. These decelerations are not associated with fetal compromise or poor outcome.

Late—smooth, often shallow decreases of FHR with the nadir after the peak of the contraction. Classically the maximal deceleration of rate occurs > 18 seconds after the peak of the contraction. Ascribed to uteroplacental insufficiency, these decelerations may indicate poor fetal oxygenation and worsening acidosis.

Variable—mostly V-shaped decelerations with abrupt drop from baseline (> 30 bpm); usually occur with contractions (80–90%); variable in duration and degree of FHR depression and usually associated with acute cord compression. Although often relieved with position changes, persistent variable decelerations may signal worsening fetal compromise.

12. What factors should be considered when fetal tachycardia is present? Fetal bradycardia? Decreased or absent variability?

Tachycardia—chorioamnionitis, fetal anemia, maternal fever, illicit drug use, sympathomimetic drugs (terbutaline), fetal hypoxia and acidosis.

Bradycardia—rapid descent during labor, acute cord occlusion (prolapse), uterine hypercontractility (often iatrogenic with oxytocin stimulation), maternal hypotension, congenital heart block, tracing maternal pulse.

Decreased variability—hypoxia, narcotics, magnesium sulfate, central nervous system anomalies of fetus.

13. What is a sinusoidal pattern? When does it occur?

An undulating pattern of FHR with a frequency of 3–6 cycles per minute and variability within each peak of 5–30 bpm. Although short episodes (< 5 minutes) may be normal, a prolonged pattern suggests fetal anemia (Rh sensitization or fetomaternal hemorrhage). Some maternal narcotics also have been associated with this pattern. Absence of short-term variability may help to distinguish this pattern from normal long-term variability.

14. What are the three common causes of prolonged decelerations?

Cord compression with a tight nuchal or short umbilical cord
Hyperstimulation
Rapid descent of the fetal head during the second stage.
Less common causes include maternal hypotension secondary to epidural anesthesia, uterine dehiscence, and severe fetal hypoxia.

15. Does maternal oxygenation significantly increase fetal oxygenization?

Maternal oxygen administration at 8–10 L/min in a tight-fitting face mask increases fetal PO_2 by only a small amount. Some evidence suggests that prolonged oxygenization during the second stage of labor may result in neonates with more acidosis compared with untreated mothers.

16. When during labor should amnioinfusion by considered?

Presence of meconium or nonreassuring variable decelerations. In the setting of meconium, several randomized controlled trials have indicated that neonates born to mothers who had amnioinfusion in labor have lower rates of meconium below the vocal cords and of meconium aspiration syndrome. In addition, fewer cesarean deliveries were performed for the indication of suspected fetal stress. Other studies have indicated improved outcomes after amnioinfusion for preterm premature rupture of the membranes or oligohydramnios.

17. How is amnioinfusion performed?

Through a catheter placed into the intrauterine cavity. Both bolus and continuous infusions can be given. Normal saline or lactated Ringer's infusions of up to 800 ml can be given at 10–15 ml/min followed by additional 250-ml boluses at intervals thereafter. Alternatively, a continuous infusion can be initiated with 10 ml/min for 1 hour and a maintenance level of 3 ml/min. Warmed infusion has no benefit over room temperature infusion.

18. How are tocolytic agents used in the setting of suspected fetal stress?

As a treatment for nonreassuring FHR patterns, such as severe variable decelerations or bradycardia from uterine hyperstimulation, terbutaline, 0.25 mg subcutaneously or 0.125–0.25 mg intravenously, may be administered. A response to terbutaline allows time for continued observation, transport to another hospital, or preparation for cesarean delivery. Some evidence suggests that fetal acid-base status may be improved in neonates whose mothers receive terbutaline before emergent cesarean delivery. The use of terbutaline should not delay an otherwise appropriate intervention.

19. How is fetal scalp stimulation or vibroacoustic stimulation used in the assessment of fetal well-being in labor?

Accelerations of of 15 bpm lasting at least 15 seconds in response to either stimulus are associated with the absence of fetal acidosis. Failure to elicit accelerations with these maneuvers is associated with an increased chance of fetal acidosis. Fetal scalp sampling (FSS) may be considered in such settings. FSS is performed with the patient in lithotomy or Sims position. Under direct visualization, the fetal scalp is punctured and capillary blood obtained. Guidelines for interpretation: > 7.25, reassuring; 7.20–7.25, borderline (should be repeated in 15–30 minutes); < 7.20, acidosis; and < 7.00, critical or potentially damaging acidosis.

20. What options should be considered for FHR tracings associated with a high risk of fetal hypoxia and acidosis, such as persistent bradycardia below 90 bpm, repetitive severe variable decelerations, and repetitive late decelerations?

Improve the pattern with repositioning of the patient or with oxygen; validate fetal well-being with scalp stimulation or scalp sampling; or deliver the patient.

BIBLIOGRAPHY

1. American College of Obstetricians and Gynecologists: Guidelines for Perinatal Care, 3rd ed. Washington, DC, American College of Obstetricians and Gynecologists, 1991.
2. American College of Obstetricians and Gynecologists: Fetal heart rate patterns: Monitoring, interpretation, and management. ACOG Tech Bull 207, 1995.
3. American College of Obstetricians and Gynecologists: Utility of umbilical cord blood acid-base assessment. ACOG Committee Opinion. #138, 1994.
4. Burke MS, Porreco RP, Day D, et al: Intrauterine resuscitation with tocolysis: An alternate month trial. J Perinatol 9:296–300, 1989.
5. Dalton KJ, Dawes GS, Patrick JE: The autonomic nervous system and fetal heart rate variability. Am J Obstet Gynecol 246:456, 1983.
6. Haverkamp AD, Orleans M, Langendorf S, et al: A controlled trial of the differential effects of intrapartum fetal monitoring. Am J Obstet Gynecol 143:399, 1979.
7. Hon EH: An Atlas of Fetal Heart Patterns. New Haven, CT, Harty Press, 1968.
8. Katz M, Meizner I, Shani N, Insler V: Clinical significance of sinusoidal fetal heart rate pattern. Br J Obstet Gynecol 90:832, 1983.
9. Nelson KB, Dambrosia JM, Ting T, Grether JK: Uncertain value of electronic fetal monitoring in predicting cerebral palsy. N Engl J Med 334:613–618, 1996.
10. Shy KK, Luthy DA, Bennett FC, et al: Effects of electronic fetal heart rate monitoring, as compared with periodic auscultation, on the neurologic development of premature infants. N Engl J Med 322:588, 1990.
11. Thacker SB, Stroop DF, Peterson HB: Efficacy and safety of intrapartum electronic fetal monitoring: An update. Obstet Gynecol 86:613–620, 1995.

78. OBSTETRIC ANESTHESIA

Jonathan C. Berman, M.D., and Susan K. Palmer, M.D.

1. Why are anesthesiologists involved in labor and delivery?

Pain of varying intensity has always been a part of human parturition. Safe and effective pain relief for labor has been sought by birth attendants of all times and cultures. With the interest and expertise of anesthesiologists, modern anesthetic drugs and techniques can now be provided safely and effectively for most parturients. Choice of analgesia should be matched to the mother's needs and fetal condition. Anesthesiologists can provide invaluable consultation for the obstetrician and stress/pain relief for the mother. Appropriate pain relief can facilitate safe deliveries and can make some vaginal deliveries possible that would otherwise have been abdominal deliveries. The anesthesiologist also may act as a consultant for complex medical problems or as a perioperative internist for the critically ill parturient.

2. What important preoperative considerations regarding the parturient concern the anesthesiologist?

The physiologic changes of pregnancy are numerous and of importance to the anesthesiologist. Concurrent medical problems may be exaggerated during pregnancy (e.g., mitral valve disease, diabetes). The preanesthetic consultation for pregnant patients should consist of at least the following: (1) review of medical and anesthetic history, vital signs; (2) careful examination of maternal airway, heart, and lungs; (3) examination of maternal back; (4) assessment of fetal condition; (5) review of labor course and understanding of obstetric plans for delivery; and (6) presentation of anesthetic plan, procedures, risks, and choices to the patient. Particular attention must be paid to evaluating the maternal airway. Edema of the pharynx may alter the patient's voice or make intubation difficult to perform. Maternal cardiac workload peaks just after delivery, and in compromised patients this period can be hazardous and should probably be monitored by an anesthesiologist. Maternal changes in hemoglobin concentration, protein binding sites, drug distribution, and respiratory drive are all important in planning any exposure to anesthetics.

3. What important preanesthetic considerations regarding the fetus concern the anesthesiologist?

Fetal status should be evaluated before initiation of any anesthetic. Fetal heart rate tracings should be checked and abnormal conditions (growth retardation, postmaturity, breech presentation, heart failure) must be appreciated in order to plan maternal anesthesia that will not worsen the fetal condition.

4. What important considerations regarding labor status concern the anesthesiologist?

Epidural analgesia can be applied when labor is progressive and delivery expected in a reasonable time. It would be poor planning to give an epidural agent so early that maternal/fetal drug levels build dangerously, preventing proper use of the block for a comfortable delivery. Usually, epidural analgesia would be requested when the cervical exam shows at least 4 cm dilatation. In some cases of painful latent-phase labor, the epidural agent may be initiated earlier when the obstetric management is planned to ensure progress into active-phase labor.

5. What analgesic options are available for labor?

- None; education; focusing techniques; massage; hypnotism
- Intravenous opiates and sedatives
- Regional anesthesia—including epidural, caudal, and paracervical
- Intraspinal opiates

• Inhalational anesthetics—available in some regions and countries; usually self administered; thought to be hazardous and not generally popular in the United States

6. What are the goals of regional anesthesia?

The goal of regional anesthesia is to block the transmission of painful impulses that arise in
receptors of the uterine and perineal structures. Transmission of the pain of the first stage of labor
occurs in sympathetic nerve fibers that enter the neuraxis at the 10th, 11th, 12th thoracic and first
lumbar spinal levels. In the second stage of labor, pain impulses also enter the neuraxis at the
second to fifth sacral segments. The afferent sensory neural pathways can be effectively inacti-
vated with a block of pain and sympathetic afferents from T10–S5. See figure below.

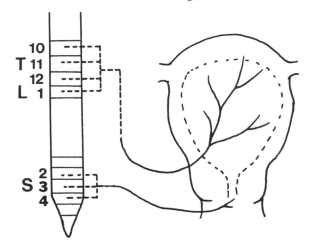

Pain pathways for the first and second
stages of labor. (From Datta S: The
Obstetric Anesthesia Handbook, 2nd
ed. St. Louis, Mosby, 1995, p 64, with
permission.)

7. What are the differences between the regional techniques?

Lumbar epidural block. The most popular for blocking the pain pathways associated with
labor and delivery. The technique allows blocking of the thoracic, lumbar, and sacral segments.
Advantages include safe reliable placement, choice of single shot or continuous catheter technique, slow onset of sympathetic blockade, and little maternal uptake of local anesthetic.

Caudal anesthesia. Placed in the sacral coccygeal hiatus, this anesthetic is useful for the
second stage of labor, but large doses are required to block up to T10 for the first stage of labor.
Toxic levels of local anesthetic are more common with this approach. Accidental puncture of the
fetal presenting part is possible through the sacral coccygeal membrane. There may be a theoretical increase of infection with this approach during labor.

Double catheter technique (lumbar epidural and caudal). This technique allows blocking of
T10–L1 with a lumbar epidural catheter for the first stage of labor and then use of caudal catheter
for blocking S2–S5 in the second stage of labor. This technique is not popular because of the
added hazard and discomfort of two needle and catheter insertions.

Spinal/saddle block. Highly effective but a single-shot technique. Analgesia may not last
until the time of delivery. Most effective when used in the second stage of labor immediately
before delivery. This technique is regaining popularity with subarachnoid opioids and with the
combined spinal/epidural technique.

Combined spinal/epidural or needle-through-needle technique. Now a popular technique
that allows placement of a subarachnoid opioid via a spinal needle that is placed through the
epidural needle, then removed; an epidural catheter is then placed. This technique allows (1) rapid
onset of pain relief, (2) opioid-only analgesia that may allow ambulating, and (3) flexibility in
later instituting an epidural block, if needed.

Continuous spinal. Microcatheters (26–32 gauge) were previously available for this technique; placement is still useful in selected cases with epidural catheters (18–20 gauge). This

technique offers continuous access to the subarachnoid space. Careful titration of sensory block is possible, thus decreasing the likelihood of cardiovascular instability. Segmented blockade of the sacral segments for the second stage of labor is possible. Rapid onset of surgical anesthesia is possible and reliable with this technique; it is also useful for the morbidly obese, delivery of twins, and management of the difficult-airway patient. Spinal headache and the potential for infection have been the main concerns with this technique.

Paracervical block. Blockade of uterine pain can be achieved by infiltration of the paracervical plexus. Rapid uptake of local anesthetics into maternal and fetal circulation occurs. The somatic sensory fibers from the perineum are not blocked and therefore this approach is ineffective for the second stage of labor. It became unpopular because of its association with fetal bradycardia and a few reported fetal deaths.

Pudendal block. This is a delivery room technique that is helpful just prior to delivery for perineal analgesia. Bilateral injection of pudendal nerves blocks S2–S4 only. Parts of the perineum are unblocked and uterine pain during delivery is unaffected.

8. What is a "walking epidural"?

Patients receive either opioid or opioid plus ultra-low-dose local anesthetic, usually in the epidural space. These combinations have minimal effects on lower extremity motor strength and allow the mother to ambulate. Some parturients still develop orthostatic hypotension, and ambulating should be allowed only after blood pressure has been checked and the ability to perform a deep knee bend demonstrated. There are many purported advantages, and patients enjoy being able to ambulate, if only to go to the bathroom. These low concentration drug combinations have varying success in providing adequate analgesia with progression to the second stage.

9. What are the complications of epidural analgesic techniques for labor and delivery?

In order of decreasing frequency, some complications are:

1. **Pain** at needle insertion site usually resembles tenderness from a small bruise. Many women have backaches unrelated to epidural analgesia after the strain of bearing down and positioning for vaginal delivery.

2. **Hypotension** caused by the sympathetic blockade can be expected if the patient is dehydrated. Most parturients should be hydrated with approximately 15–20 ml/kg of nondextrose-containing crystalloid prior to blockade.

3. **Spinal headache** may result from unintended dural puncture. Cerebrospinal fluid (CSF) is able to leak out, leading to a characteristic positional (upright) headache.

4. **Seizures** may occur if the local anesthetics are injected intravascularly owing to the placement of a catheter into a blood vessel in the epidural space.

5. **Total spinal** can occur from local anesthetics being deposited in the subarachnoid space instead of the epidural space. As for intramuscular injections, light aspiration of the catheter for blood or CSF should precede each injection.

6. **Allergic reaction** to local anesthetics has been reported in rare cases.

7. **Neurologic injury** is theoretically possible, exceedingly rare, and is seldom permanent. In reports of thousands of cases, no permanent neural injury could be attributed to epidural block.

10. Who is at risk for spinal headache? How are they treated?

The obstetric patient is at high risk for spinal headache. Incidence of spinal headache is inversely related to the size of the needle, and is affected by the direction of the needle bevel in relation to the dural fibers, the angle at which the needle punctures the dura, and whether or not second stage pushing is prolonged. The type of needle point is important. The pencil-point needle has a ten-fold less effect on headache rate compared with the standard Quincke needle. Treatment ranges from conservative to aggressive. Patients are treated with bed rest, fluids, and analgesics. Most headaches are self-limited and disappear within 1 week. Because the patient has a newborn infant to care for, spinal headache can be extremely aggravating. Recently, hydration and intravenous caffeine have been successful in treating spinal headache. Curative treatment can usually be obtained with an epidural blood patch. This technique involves aseptic placement of about 15 cc of autologous blood into the epidural space to help seal the dural hole.

11. Are there contraindications to epidural analgesia in obstetrics?

Untreated febrile illness and coagulation defects are relative contraindications. Many anesthesiologists decide on an individual basis if they use epidural blockade in patients with previous back surgery or a history of chronic low back pain. Patients who cannot understand the procedure or who cannot cooperate for the insertion may not be candidates.

12. Does epidural analgesia affect the course of labor?

In the few good studies in which patient selection bias has been eliminated or minimized, there appears to be no difference in the first stage of labor. However, second-stage labor appears to be prolonged an average of 20–25 minutes. Despite prolongation of the second stage, fetal/newborn condition is as good as or better than that of a non-epidural cohort. Most studies done retrospectively show a higher incidence of forceps use in patients given epidural analgesia. Whether this is causative or associative with regard to epidural analgesia remains an open question.

13. Does epidural analgesia affect the cesarean delivery rate?

No. Although epidural analgesia is associated with abdominal deliveries, a cause-and-effect relationship cannot be established from present studies. Epidural analgesia and anesthetic management are not generic procedures, and many variables may be important in determining whether there is a relationship between epidural analgesia and cesarean rates. Severe pain may be a predictor of a parturient's chance of operative delivery; such patients tend to receive epidurals. Obstetric practice and management, legal issues, pain, quality of labor, type and timing of epidural, and degree of motor blockade may affect the cesarean delivery rate. Resolving this issue will be difficult because a randomized controlled study would force a parturient to relinquish her choice of pain management plan for birth. This presents difficult personal and ethical dilemmas.

14. If a woman requires a cesarean delivery, what are her options for anesthesia?

Many factors can sway the patient or the anesthesiologist to choose one option over the other: patient's preference, fetal condition, surgical requirements, urgency of delivery, and the patient's physical, psychological, and medical condition.

General anesthesia is most often used for emergencies, such as in severe fetal distress, when time is of the essence. However, general anesthetics reach fetal blood and may depress neonatal respirations.

Major regional analgesia—spinal and epidural are the most popular forms of anesthesia for cesarean delivery. There is less fetal exposure to drugs. Recently spinal anesthesia has reemerged as the preferred choice for abdominal delivery when a parturient does not have an epidural block in place because of its quick onset, higher success rate, and dense sensory block.

15. Is fetal outcome any different between regional and general anesthesia?

Traditionally, neonates have been evaluated by: (1) Apgar score, (2) acid-base status (cord pH), and (3) neurobehavioral examination.

1. There appears to be a difference between general and regional anesthesia with regard to **Apgar scores**. Infants with general anesthesia from numerous studies have an increased incidence of slightly depressed scores at 1 minute and probably at 5 minutes. The factor that most likely causes this is transient sedation following induction of general anesthetic. The longer the exposure to nitrous oxide and general anesthetic before delivery, the more depressed the Apgar scores.

2. In elective cesarean sections, the differences in pH between regional and general anesthesia are not clinically significant. An important factor in **acid-base status** may be the time interval from uterine incision to delivery, and this has been shown to correlate inversely with fetal acidosis and hypoxia.

3. **Neurobehavioral scoring** shows some subtle early differences between general and regional anesthesia, with better scores in the regional group. There were essentially no differences at 24 hours. Well-performed anesthesia with surgically easy and rapid delivery of the infant will usually result in a vigorous infant.

16. What are the complications of general anesthesia?

Aspiration and failed intubation/ventilation are the most frequent life-threatening complications of general anesthesia in the obstetric population. Awareness and recall of the operation are more prevalent in this population than in the general population because of the desire to give the mother minimal anesthetics prior to delivery of the fetus. Rarely, anaphylaxis to anesthetic drugs or acute asthma may cause death or severe damage. Nausea, vomiting, sore throat, and lethargy are more common and less serious side effects.

17. Why are parturients at risk for aspiration?

Many of the physiologic changes of pregnancy contribute to this serious risk. Most important are the gastrointestinal changes that lead to delayed gastric emptying during pregnancy. These dangers are caused by increased levels of progesterone, decreased motilin, increased intragastric pressure, and displacement of the pylorus by the gravid uterus. Maternal response to fear, apprehension, and pain also may delay gastric emptying. These changes lead to increased gastric volumes > 25 ml with a pH of less than 2.5 in approximately 25–70% of parturients. Difficulty is often encountered in intubation and maintenance of the airway. The parturient may be obese, short-necked, or have mucosal congestion and edema. Cricoid pressure must be applied skillfully to avoid repeated attempts at intubation, which increase the risk of gastric aspiration.

18. What can be done to prevent aspiration?

The most important step in **safeguarding all pregnant patients is to have them refrain from eating once labor begins**. Of particular importance is the administration of nonparticulate antacids within 30 minutes of starting a general anesthetic. In elective situations H$_2$ blockers can be given the night before and morning of surgery to increase gastric pH. Metoclopramide may be administered to decrease gastric volume. Rapid sequence induction and intubation with cricoid pressure should be used in patients with normal airways. Patients with difficult airways should be identified and treated with alternative techniques such as awake intubation or regional anesthesia. Proper airway evaluation and management are the most effective ways of preventing airway problems during induction of general anesthesia.

19. Is an anesthesiologist needed for treatment of uterine inversion?

Uterine inversion is an obstetric problem that can cause life-threatening hemorrhage. If the uterus cannot be repositioned immediately, the anesthesiologist should be called to assist. The anesthesiologist can help to volume-resuscitate the mother, provide uterine relaxation if required, and treat the pain and circulatory reflex problems that occur with an inverted uterus. Traditionally general anesthesia with halothane has been given to achieve uterine relaxation. The halogenate anesthetic can produce rapid uterine relaxation when given in doses of two to three times the minimum alveolar concentration (MAC) needed to produce unconsciousness. At these high concentrations, the hemodynamic effects of these agents can cause vascular dilation and myocardial depression. The anesthesiologist may have to use vasopressor-like ephedrine or phenylephrine to maintain cardiovascular support. Of interest is the substitution of intravenous tocolytic agents such as terbutaline to provide uterine relaxation. This drug also has profound hemodynamic effects on a patient with hypotension and bradycardia. Recently intravenous and sublingual nitroglycerin has been used as a tocolytic. Its rapid onset and short half-life make it an attractive alternative when rapid relaxation of the uterus is required.

20. What is the anesthesiologist's role when uterine atony occurs after delivery?

Uterine atony can cause life-threatening hemorrhage. Anesthesiologists should be called as soon as atony is suspected. They can assist with resuscitation, monitoring, and treatment of side effects of drugs given to treat the atony. Anesthesiologists can also begin to prepare for laparotomy if that becomes necessary. Resuscitation of the mother hemodynamically is of highest priority. Administration of oxytocin, ergot derivatives, or prostaglandins may be necessary. A thorough understanding of their pharmacologic properties and how these drugs may affect parturients is critical. Oxytocin is administered intramuscularly or intravenously to improve uterine contractions; it may cause significant hypotension if given too rapidly in bolus form. Ergot derivatives are useful to promote sustained uterine contractions. These drugs should only be given intramuscularly. These drugs can cause severe hypertension and should be used cautiously in hypertensive patients. Headache and electrocardiographic changes often follow a dose of methergine 0.2 mg.

Prostaglandins can produce uterine contractions and have been successful in stopping postpartum uterine atony. Side effects include vomiting, dizziness, and elevated temperature. A recent report indicates that some prostaglandins may cause transient changes in arterial saturation due to intrapulmonary shunting. Patients should be monitored with oxygen saturation monitor and given supplemental oxygen while receiving this drug.

Uterine atony may become severe enough to require urgent laparotomy and ligation of the uterine blood supply or possible hysterectomy. These patients may require massive transfusions and are at risk for the sequelae of this therapy. Anesthesiologists must realize that if hysterectomy is contemplated, maternal mortality approaches 1%.

21. Is general anesthesia safer than regional?

In the United States there is no organized reporting of the total number and type of obstetric anesthetics; therefore an accurate rate of mortality cannot be computed at this time. We do know that among all maternal deaths, general anesthesia causes more than regional anesthesia. It is not possible to interpret this directly, because the most emergent cases are probably done with general anesthesia.

22. What is the anesthetic mortality in obstetric cases?

This is difficult to answer because of inconsistent reporting and handling of maternal mortality information in the U.S. The proportion of anesthesia-related deaths among all maternal deaths has increased. Airway problems, such as difficult intubation and aspiration, are the leading causes of anesthesia-related maternal deaths. When evaluated retrospectively, maternal deaths caused by airway problems are usually judged to be preventable. Anesthetic mortality for the general operating room has been reported to be as high as 1/3,000 cases or as low as 1/100,000 cases. Obstetric anesthetic deaths may be slightly more common.

23. What options are available for pain control after cesarean delivery?

This depends on the anesthetic technique used for surgery. If a general anesthetic was employed, the patient can be offered patient-controlled intravenous analgesia (PCA). A pump gives accurate amounts of narcotic at both a continuous and intermittent demand rate. This gives the patient control over analgesia and sedation.

If epidural analgesia was used for delivery, a narcotic may be placed in the epidural space to provide long-term analgesia. Recently, continuous infusions of narcotics into the epidural space postoperatively have been employed with great success. Patients may be given a controller device to augment a basal infusion rate, producing a patient-controlled epidural analgesic (PCEA).

If single-shot subarachnoid blockade was used, narcotics can be chosen and added to the subarachnoid space to provide good analgesia for up to 24 hours.

The use of intraspinal opiates has risen dramatically in obstetrics the past few years. They have proved to be safe and effective, but they are not without complications and controversy. Side effects from spinal opiates (both subarachnoid and epidural) include nausea, vomiting, itching, and urinary retention. Respiratory depression can occur from spinal opiates when narcotics migrate cephalad to affect respiratory centers in the brain stem. Because of this rare and severe possibility, monitoring of these patients must be appropriate and sustained.

BIBLIOGRAPHY

1. Check TG, Gutsche BB: Maternal physiologic affections during pregnancy. In Shnider SM, Levinson G (eds): Anesthesia for Obstetrics, 2nd ed. Baltimore, Williams & Wilkins, 1987.
2. Chestnut DC: The influence of continuous epidural bupivacaine analgesia in the second stage of labor and method of delivery in nulliparous women. Anesthesiology 66:774–780, 1987.
3. Endler GC: What obstetricians should know about anesthesia care standards. J Reprod Med 36:126–130, 1991.
4. Gibbs CP, Krischer J, Peckham BM, et al: Obstetric anesthesia: A national survey. Anesthesiology 65:298–306, 1986.
5. Gibbs CP, Modell JH: Aspiration pneumonitis. In Miller RD (ed): Anesthesia, 3rd ed. New York, Churchill Livingstone, 1990.
6. Giclen, Mathieu: Post dural puncture headache (PDPH): A review. Reg Anesth 14:101–106, 1990.
7. Marx GF, Luykx WM, Cohen S: Fetal neonatal status following cesarean section for fetal distress. Br J Anaesth 56:1009–1013, 1984.
8. Ong BY: Paresthesias and motor dysfunction after labor and delivery. Anesth Analg 66:18–22, 1987.
9. Palmer SK, Gibbs CP: Risk management in obstetrics. Int Anesthesiol Clin 27:188–199, 1989.
10. Shnider SM, Levinson G: Anesthesia for cesarean section. In Shnider SM, Levinson G (eds): Anesthesia for Obstetrics, 2nd ed. Baltimore, Williams & Wilkins, 1987.
11. Uitvlugt A: Managing complications of epidural analgesia. Int Anesthesiol Clin 28:11–16, 1990.

79. VAGINAL DELIVERY

Robert Goodlin, M.D.

1. What are the advantages of vaginal versus abdominal birth to the mother?
Less morbidity, fewer complications, shorter hospital stay, and less expense.

2. What are the advantages of vaginal versus abdominal birth to the fetus?
Less respiratory distress, better bonding, and fewer problems with iatrogenic prematurity.

3. In recording a vaginal exam, especially when preparing for a delivery, what observations should be included?
Fetal station (presenting part in relation to the maternal ischial spines), fetal position (orientation of fetal occiput), and cervical dilation and effacement.

4. What are the advantages of rotating an occiput posterior (OP) position to an occiput anterior (OA)?
Allows delivery of the fetal vertex by extension, with the vertex representing the smallest diameter.

5. Why does the OP position often fail to rotate to OA?
Because the vertex remains deflexed as it enters the pelvis. This can be clinically appreciated by determination that the fetal anterior fontanelle is relatively low in the pelvis (versus the flexed vertex with the anterior fontanelle appreciated more anteriorly).

6. What are the clinical signs of a persistent OP presentation in labor?
Protracted active phase, maternal "back labor," persistent anterior cervical lip, and fetal lie with back down as appreciated on abdominal exam or ultrasound.

7. Can a full-term infant with a face presentation safely deliver pelvically?
As many as one-third of mentum posterior face presentations rotate to mentum anterior. Mentum anterior presentations usually can be safely delivered pelvically.

8. What are the advantages of a routine episiotomy? The disadvantages?

Use of a routine episiotomy prevents excessive stretching of the maternal perineum with perhaps better perineal support in later life. However, an episiotomy produces a more painful postpartum course with potential subsequent sexual dysfunction as a result of pain at the introitus.

9. What are the advantages of the midline (median) versus the mediolateral episiotomy? The disadvantages?

Easier repair and less painful recovery but more frequent rectal extensions are characteristic of the midline episiotomy. The mediolateral episiotomy, which also begins at the introitus but extends at a 45° angle to the right or left, may be considered for large infants, a small perineal body, or in some cases of forceps delivery.

10. Which tissue layers are incised in a midline episiotomy? In a third-degree extension? In a fourth-degree extension?

A midline episiotomy extends posterior from the introitus through the vaginal wall and mucosa and is carried along the perineal raphe, separating the superficial transverse perineal muscles. Extensions of the incision through the rectal sphincter (third degree) or rectal mucosa (fourth degree) can occur. Such extensions at the perineal body are easily identified and repaired. However, both third- and fourth-degree extensions can occur higher in the vaginal vault as "buttonholes," which may not be appreciated; left unrepaired, they may predispose to formation of rectovaginal fistulas.

11. What is the Ritgen maneuver? What are its advantages? Disadvantages?

Extension of the fetal vertex prior to expulsion. This is achieved with operator extension of the fetal chin through rectal pressure. The maneuver serves to quicken delivery. The maneuver presents a greater fetal head diameter to the maternal vulva, leading to more frequent episiotomy or vaginal lacerations.

12. Why does shoulder dystocia occur? How can it be treated?

When either soft tissue or the fetal shoulder presents an excessive diameter to the maternal pelvic inlet, further descent of the fetus cannot occur. The easiest maneuver to correct this problem is marked flexion of the maternal thighs (McRobert maneuver).

The anterior shoulder can then be dislodged externally with suprapubic pressure (applied in an oblique fashion to rotate the shoulder under the pubic symphysis) or internally with the operator's hand on the fetal scapula of the impacted shoulder (Rubin maneuver). Other options include delivery of the posterior arm and the Woods maneuver, which converts the anterior shoulder to the posterior, followed by delivery of the posterior arm. If the anterior shoulder cannot then be delivered spontaneously, reverse rotation of the shoulder back to the posterior position usually accomplishes delivery. Extension of a midline episiotomy to a fourth degree often is needed for these maneuvers. Deliberate fracture of the clavicles is reserved as a last resort.

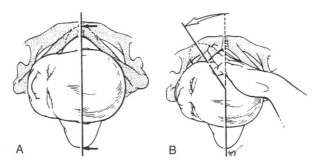

Rubin maneuver. *A*, Bisacromial diameter is shown as the distance between the arrows. *B*, Adduction of the most accessible shoulder, with rotation, tends to reduce the bisacromial diameter and facilitates delivery (From Cunningham F, Macdonald P, Gant N (eds): Conduct of normal labor and delivery. In Williams Obstetrics, 18th ed. Norwalk, CT, Appleton and Lange, 1989, with permission.)   A   B

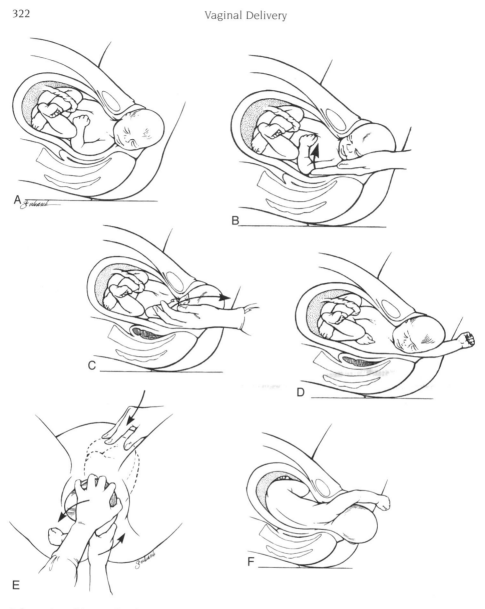

A, Impaction of the anterior shoulder against the symphysis pubis. *B*, Flexion of the fetal forearm brings the wrist within reach. *C*, The fetal forearm is swept across the chest and delivered. *D*, The posterior arm has been delivered and delivery of the trunk usually follows easily. *E*, More difficult impactions may require rotation of the vertex and of the posterior shoulder to the anterior position as an assistant pushes the fetal back over the midline to the other side of the maternal abdomen. *F*, Complete rotation results in disimpaction and delivery of the trunk. (From Nielsen PE, Gonick G: Shoulder dystocia. In Repke JT (ed): Intrapartum Obstetrics. New York, Churchill Livingstone, 1996, pp 196–197, with permission.)

13. How often does shoulder dystocia occur?

For infants of nondiabetic mothers, the risk is approximately 10% for infants weighing 4000–4499 gm and 23% for infants > 4500 gm. For infants of diabetic mothers the risk is 31% for infants > 4000 gm. Given the relative infrequency of both infants > 4500 gm and infants of diabetic mothers, shoulder dystocia occurs in only 2% of births, with 47% of infants < 4000 gm.

14. When should occurrence of shoulder dystocia be suspected?

When infants weigh more than 4,500 gm; excessive conduction anesthesia with maternal bearing-down ability impaired; with dysfunctional labor; and with operative vaginal delivery of the larger fetus; or with infants of diabetic mothers > 4,000 gm.

15. What is the Zavanelli maneuver?

Reported as having been successful in the delivery of shoulder dystocia in a small series, this maneuver involves flexion of the fetal head, replacement of the fetus within the uterine cavity, and emergent cesarean section delivery. Although advocated by some, this maneuver is reserved for rare situations that fail to respond to more conservative measures.

16. What are the fetal complications of shoulder dystocia?

Potential for prolonged hypoxia as the cord is compressed between the fetal body and the maternal pelvis until the shoulder can be dislodged. Fetal injuries include damage to the brachial plexus from excessive traction and fractures of the clavicles and humeri.

17. How is station generally defined when forceps applications are considered?

By current ACOG criteria, station is designated as the leading point of the bony vertex. The descent of the point in centimeters below the ischial spines (0 to +5 cm) is indicated. A previously used system divided the pelvis into thirds. Both systems are variable among examiners and for one examiner over time.

18. How does one evaluate the clinical situation for a low forceps delivery?

The fetal vertex must be engaged (with biparietal diameter through the inlet), with the fetal vertex filling the hollow of the maternal pelvis. Generally this occurs at +2 cm. A further modification, an outlet forceps delivery, is performed when the fetal vertex can be seen without separating the labia. Outlet forceps restrict rotation of the fetal head to < 45°.

19. What is the definition of a midforceps delivery? When is it indicated?

When the fetal vertex is engaged but not below a +2 station. A midforceps delivery may be undertaken as preparations for a cesarean section are under way and should be abandoned if undue traction is needed.

20. What are the advantages and disadvantages of elective forceps delivery?

Elective forceps delivery aids in a controlled vaginal delivery and a shortened second stage. The disadvantages include possible maternal and fetal trauma.

21. What are some of the indications for forceps deliveries?

After the above criteria for a forceps delivery have been met, indications include fetal distress, maternal exhaustion, or maternal disease such as cardiac, hypertensive, or neurologic dysfunction.

22. What are the requirements for a forceps delivery?

The position of the fetus must be established based on the pelvic exam. The station should be +2 or greater. The maternal pelvis is assessed as being adequate by clinical pelvimetry. The cervix should be dilated 10 cm. The bladder should be emptied with a catheter. The mother should have adequate pain relief.

23. What is asynclitism?

Asynclitism is failure of the vertex to descend with the sagittal suture in the midplane between the front and back of the pelvis. It is detected clinically on examination when either the anterior or posterior parietal bones precede the sagittal suture. When accompanied by molding, asynclitism can lead to erroneous assessments of the true fetal position with further implications for forceps applications.

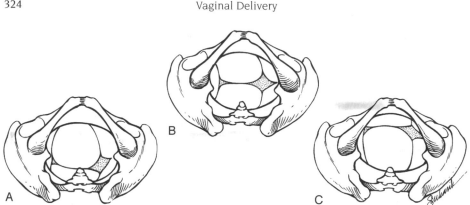

The fetal head can occupy varied positions in the maternal pelvis. A, Anterior asynclitism occurs when the anterior parietal bone is presenting. B, Normal synclitism occurs when the sagittal suture lies midway between the pubic symphysis and sacrum. C, Posterior asynclitism occurs with anterior displacement of the sagittal suture. (From Shipp T, Repke JT: Normal labor and delivery. In Repke JT: Intrapartum Obstetrics. New York, Churchill Livingstone, 1996, p 82, with permission.)

24. What are the characteristics of Simpson forceps? Elliot forceps? Tucker-McLane forceps?

Simpson—fenestrated blades with divergent handles; longer cephalic curve of blade is suited for the molded head and when traction is applied.

Elliot—fenestrated blades with convergent handles; short cephalic curve is suited for the un-molded head and when traction is desired.

Tucker-McLane—solid blade with convergent handles, short cephalic curve is suited for the unmolded head in situations requiring minimal traction (outlet forceps); the Luikart modification employs a pseudofenestrated blade and overlapping shanks.

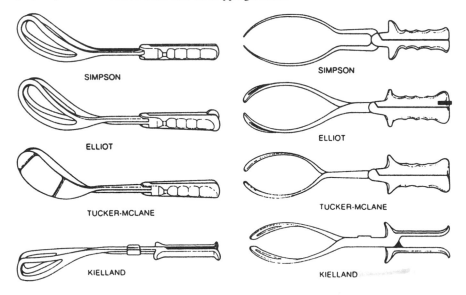

Lateral (left) and anteroposterior (right) views of various obstetric forceps. The pelvic curve, a prominent feature of the classic instruments, is lacking in the Kielland forceps. (From Gabbe SG, Niebyl JR, Simpson JL (eds): Obstetrics: Normal and Problem Pregnancies. New York, Churchill Livingstone, 1986, pp 364–365, with permission.)

25. What assessment should be made to ensure correct placement of forceps?

Sagittal sutures should be perpendicular to the plane of the shank and posterior fontannel, 1 cm above the shanks. For fenestrated blades, if the tip of the forefinger can be placed within the fenestration, blades are positioned too shallow on the fetal head and may pull off with traction.

26. When are Kielland forceps used?

Rotation of the vertex from OP or transverse to OA position can be accomplished with these forceps, given their minimal pelvic curve. Kielland forceps are less appropriate for traction for the same reason.

27. What is a Scanzoni maneuver?

Rotation from OP to OA with either Simpson or Kielland forceps, then reapplication of Simpson forceps for delivery from the OA position.

28. What are the indications, preparations, and prerequisites for vacuum cup (Silastic) application?

The indications for vacuum cup application are the same as for forceps applications. Cup placement ideally should occur over the sagittal suture about 3 cm in front of the posterior fontannel. Autorotation may occur to the occiput anterior position during descent. Operator-applied torque to accomplish such rotation is discouraged, because it may lead to injury of the fetal scalp.

29. What factors should be considered in vaginal delivery of the preterm infant?

Most authorities now believe that vaginal delivery of the vertex preterm infant is no more detrimental than cesarean section delivery. Consideration should be given to leaving the membranes intact to provide a cushion for the fetal vertex and use of an episiotomy to minimize perineal pressure against the head. Elective forceps for further protection of the fetal head has been advocated by some.

30. What is a nuchal cord? How does it complicate a vaginal delivery?

A cord wrapped around the fetal neck occurs in about 25% of vaginal deliveries. A loosely applied cord can often be slipped over the infant's head prior to cephalic extension or the infant may be delivered "through the cord" by passing the cord over the shoulders. Tight cords can significantly compromise the fetus and are best doubly clamped and cut before the body is delivered.

31. How are cord gases interpreted?

Arterial and venous cord blood can be obtained after delivery in order to provide an objective assessment of the fetal acid-base status. There is a correlation, although not particularly strong, with the infant's Apgar scores. Mean values are variable, but representative sea-level values are given below. Generally, when acidosis is present, a larger base excess (BE) suggests a more prolonged hypoxic episode than when acidosis occurs with only a minimally elevated base excess (deficit).

	Arterial	*Venous*
pH	7.26	7.34
pCO_2	45.98	35.66
pO_2	16.86	28.49
BE	−6.0	−5.03

BIBLIOGRAPHY

1. Acker DB, Sachs BP, Friedman EA: Risk factors for shoulder dystocia. Obstet Gynecol 66:762, 1985.
2. American College of Obstetricians and Gynecologists: Operative Vaginal Delivery. ACOG Tech Bull 196, 1994.
3. Bowes WA: Clinical aspects of normal and abnormal labor. In Creasy RK, Resnik R (eds): Maternal-Fetal Medicine, 3rd ed. Philadelphia, W.B. Saunders, 1994.
4. Seeds JC: Malpresentations. In Gabbe SG, Niebyl JR, Simpson JL (eds): Obstetrics: Normal and Problem Pregnancies, 2nd ed. New York, Churchill Livingstone, 1996.

80. ABDOMINAL DELIVERY

Jean E. Dwinnell, M.D., and Marshall R. Gottesfeld, M.D.

1. What is a cesarean section?

The delivery of a fetus by abdominal surgery (laparotomy) requiring an incision through the uterine wall (hysterotomy).

2. What is the origin of the term *cesarean*?

Some believe that the term *cesarean* best describes a postmortem delivery and that the term should therefore be replaced. However, three principal explanations have been suggested: (1) According to legend, Julius Caesar was born in this manner. However, in 100 B.C., this operation would have been fatal, and the mother of Julius Caesar lived many years after his birth. (2) The term was derived from Roman law, when Rome was ruled by Numa Pompilius (8th century B.C.). The law decreed that the operation be performed upon women dying in childbirth; hence the term *lex caesarea*. (3) Another explanation is based on the Latin verb *caedere*, to cut; an abdominal birth is termed *partus caesareus*.

3. What are the indications for cesarean section?

There are few absolute indications for cesarean section; most are relative, depending on the skill and judgment of the obstetrician.

Fetal	Nonvertex presentations that persist after attempt at external cephalic version, such as transverse lie, breech presentation
	Face presentation—mentum posterior
	Multiple gestations—triplets or greater, twins in which the presenting twin is nonvertex
	Macrosomia—fetus weighing > 4500 gm
	Fetal abnormality—spina bifida, hydrocephaly
	Fetal distress (a term that is falling out of favor), which may refer to prolonged fetal bradycardia, decreased fetal heart rate variability, repetitive late decelerations, severe variables, fetal scalp blood pH < 7.20
Placental	Previa, vasa previa, abruption leading to fetal distress
Uterine	Previous classic cesarean section, previous uterine surgery (e.g., myomectomy) in which endometrial cavity was entered
Vaginal	Complications of a previous fourth-degree laceration, vaginal reconstructive surgery, obstructive condylomata
Pelvic	Obstructive pelvic tumors (uterine myoma, pelvic kidney, neurofibroma), constricted bony structure
Maternal	Worsening preeclampsia in which delayed delivery may be harmful to the mother, symptomatic genital herpes simplex virus, cervical cancer
Abnormal labor	Arrest of dilatation in the active phase of labor, arrest of descent in the second stage of labor

4. What is the most common abdominal incision performed for cesarean section in the United States?

The Pfannenstiel incision.

5. How is a cesarean section performed?

1. A horizontal incision is made in the skin and subcutaneous tissue down to the layer of the fascia, approximately 3–5 cm above the pubic symphysis.

2. The fascia is composed of the aponeurosis of the external and internal oblique muscles and the aponeurosis of the transverse abdominal muscle. These layers are incised transversely, exposing the rectus muscles.

3. The rectus muscles are dissected off the fascia superiorly and inferiorly and divided in the midline.

4. The peritoneum is entered, exposing the uterus.

5. The vesicouterine serosa overlying the uterus is incised, and the bladder is bluntly dissected off the lower uterine segment.

6. The uterus is entered with a transverse incision, and the infant is delivered.

6. What types of abdominal incisions can be used in grossly obese patients?

A transverse skin incision can be performed above the panniculus, or a supraumbilical vertical skin incision can be used.

7. What types of uterine incisions are used in cesarean section? Why?

1. The most common incision is a transverse incision in the lower uterine segment (Kerr). This type of incision is least likely to rupture in subsequent pregnancies.

2. The classic incision is a vertical incision into the contractile portion of the uterus. It is used for back-down transverse lie or for the extremely premature fetus. It has a greater risk for uterine dehiscence with subsequent pregnancies and usually warrants elective repeat cesarean section.

3. A low vertical incision on the uterus can be performed; it is the same as above but made in the lower uterine segment. Subsequent pregnancies can be offered a trial of labor.

8. What is the current rate of abdominal delivery in the United States?

22.6% (1992).

9. What is the most common complication of cesarean section?

Endometritis. The incidence varies from 5–85% (mean incidence of 35%). Endometritis is more likely in patients with prolonged labor, numerous vaginal exams, and prolonged rupture of membranes.

10. What is the American College of Obstetrics and Gynecology guideline for the time in which an emergent cesarean section should be performed?

30 minutes.

11. What complications should be covered in the consent of a woman undergoing a cesarean section?

Bleeding

Infection

Injury to internal organs, including uterus, ovaries, fallopian tubes, bowel, ureters, and blood vessels

Injury to infant

Possible need for blood transfusion

12. What risks are faced by women undergoing cesarean section for placenta previa? How does this change with an additional history of prior abdominal delivery (or deliveries)?

Bleeding is a risk for a woman with placenta previa because of the higher incidence of abnormal placental implantation, including placenta accreta. With a previous history of multiple cesarean section, there is up to a 67% risk of placenta accreta in a patient with a placenta previa.

13. Should fibroids be removed at the time of cesarean section?

Elective myomectomy should not be performed during a cesarean section. If, however, a myoma is incised in entering the uterine cavity, it may be advantageous to remove the myoma to close the uterine incision.

14. How should an unsuspected adnexal mass be addressed at the time of cesarean section?
Any suspicious adnexal mass > 2 cm should be removed.

15. A woman is undergoing her fourth cesarean section and desires permanent steriliza-tion. She has a history and clinical evidence of uterine fibroids. She requests a hysterec-tomy at the time of the cesarean section. What is your response?
Bey and colleagues performed a prospective study of 82 elective cesarean hysterectomies and 102 matched cesarean tubal ligations. They found significantly greater blood loss and operat-ing time in the hysterectomy patients but significantly greater febrile morbidity in the tubal liga-tion patients. Blood transfusions, mean hospital stay, and perioperative complications were not significantly different between the two groups. However, the risk of long-term complications such as vaginal fistula were not assessed.

16. What types of anesthesia may be used for cesarean section?
Anesthesia may be general or regional (e.g., spinal or epidural). In an emergent cesarean sec-tion, a general anesthetic needs to be used because of the time needed to place an effective epidural. The risks relate mainly to aspiration of gastric contents because the patient may not be fasting. Pregnant women have loss of tone of the cardiac sphincter of the stomach, increasing the chance of gastric reflux.

17. What are the chances of having a successful vaginal birth after cesarean section (VBAC) after a previous low transverse cesarean section?
Approximately 60–80%, depending on the previous indication for cesarean section.

18. What is the average blood loss at the time of cesarean section?
1000 ml.

19. What is the maternal mortality rate with cesarean section?
Maternal mortality after cesarean section has been quoted as 4 times greater than after vagi-nal delivery (approximately 40/100,000 births vs. 9/100,000 births). If only elective repeat sec-tions are considered, the rates are 2 times that of vaginal delivery.

20. If emergent hysterectomy is needed at the time of cesarean section (puerperal hysterec-tomy), what are the associated morbidity and mortality rates?
Maternal mortality is 0.7%, with 3% experiencing a bladder injury and 1% requiring re-exploration for bleeding.

BIBLIOGRAPHY

1. Flamm BL, Quilligan EJ: Cesarean Section: Guidelines for Appropriate Utilization. New York, Springer-Verlag, 1995.
2. Hankins GD, Clark SL, Cunningham FG, et al (eds): Operative Obstetrics. Norwalk, CT, Appleton & Lange, 1995.
3. Katz VL, Wells SR, Kuller JA, et al: Cesarean delivery: A reconsideration of terminology. Obstet Gynecol 86(1):152–153, 1995.
4. Litta P, et al: Risk factors for complicating infection after cesarean section. Clin Exp Obstet Gynecol 22:71–75, 1995.
5. Naef RW, Ray MA, Chauhan SP, et al: Trial of labor after cesarean delivery with a lower-segment, vertical uterine incision: Is it safe? Am J Obstet Gynecol 172:1666–1673, 1995.
6. Paul RH, Miller DA: Cesarean birth: How to reduce the rate. Am J Obstet Gynecol 172:1903–1907, 1995.
7. Plauche WC: Cesarean section. Obstet Gynecol Clin North Am 15(4):591–795, 1988.
8. Seidman DS, Paz I, Nadu A, et al: Are multiple cesarean sections safe? Eur J Obstet Gynecol Reprod Biol 57(1):7–12, 1994.

81. THIRD STAGE OF LABOR AND POSTPARTUM HEMORRHAGE

Sue Anne Murahata, M.D.

1. What is the third stage of labor?

The third stage of labor begins at the completion of the delivery of the infant and ends with the delivery of the placenta. A prolonged third stage lasts > 30 minutes.

2. What is the appropriate management once the infant has delivered?

Patience. Undue traction on the umbilical cord and/or fundal pressure may contribute to a uterine inversion. Watch for an increase in vaginal bleeding and lengthening of the umbilical cord as signs of placental separation. Gentle traction on the umbilical cord at this time (along with gentle counterpressure upward on the uterine fundus to prevent uterine inversion) will result in delivery of the placenta and membranes.

3. What if the placenta does not separate spontaneously?

After waiting 30 minutes (most placentas deliver within 10–15 min), manual removal of the placenta may be indicated. Using antiseptic solution on the glove (e.g., Betadine), the hand is placed within the uterine cavity and the natural cleavage plane developed. The placenta and membranes need to be carefully inspected to ensure that they have been removed completely. If there is any question, curettage may be needed. Consideration should be given to placing such patients on prophylactic antibiotics, as they are at risk for endometritis. Appropriate analgesia and/or anesthesia is also indicated.

4. The placenta has delivered. On inspection, it is found to be complete and intact. What should be done next?

Routinely, an oxytocic agent (e.g., Pitocin) is administered to minimize bleeding. The cervix, vagina, and perineum are inspected for lacerations. The episiotomy and lacerations, if present, are repaired with absorbable suture.

5. What is postpartum hemorrhage?

It is generally described as an estimated blood loss > 500 cc at the time of delivery. It accounts for roughly 10% of nonabortive maternal deaths and occurs in approximately 8% (range of 0.4–10%) of deliveries.

6. Why does postpartum hemorrhage occur?

The normal mechanism for hemostasis after delivery of the placenta is contraction of the uterine muscle to occlude the open sinuses that previously fed blood into the placenta. Any event that interferes with contraction of the uterus will contribute to postpartum blood loss. The most common interferences are uterine atony, lacerations of the genital tract (including rupture of the uterus), and retained products of conception. Less common causes may be related to an abnormal placenta implantation site or a coagulation disorder.

Keep in mind that while trying to diagnose and treat the cause of postpartum hemorrhage, the appropriate measures for the management of a patient in shock must also be taken (e.g., central venous lines, fluid and blood replacement).

7. How can the cause be diagnosed?

Palpate the uterus. If it is boggy, the cause is probably uterine atony. This problem is more common after a rapid or prolonged labor, uterine overdistention (multiple gestations, polyhydramnios, large infant), use of oxytocin for induction or augmentation of labor, use of magnesium sulfate, or chorioamnionitis.

8. How is uterine atony treated?

Initiate uterine massage. If no intravenous access is present, it should be placed and intravenous oxytocin administered. The bladder should be emptied, as a full bladder may interfere with uterine contraction. Emptying can be accomplished either with single, straight catheterization or placement of a Foley catheter. If this is not effective, methylergonovine, 0.2 mg, may be administered intramuscularly. Onset is within 7 minutes and lasts for several hours. Methylergonovine must be used with caution in patients with an elevated or labile blood pressure. If bleeding is still excessive, 15 methyl $F_{2\alpha}$ prostaglandin should be given intramuscularly or as a direct intrauterine injection. Although not available in the United States, prostaglandin-containing pessaries have been used in cases of uterine atony.

9. What if the uterus is firm but the patient is still bleeding?

Other causes must be investigated. The vagina, cervix, and perineum must be carefully reinspected. If no abnormalities are found, the uterus should be explored. Gentle curettage should ensure that no products of conception are retained and that the uterus is intact (not ruptured). Coagulation studies should be checked and abnormalities corrected. If a defect in the uterine wall is detected, an exploratory laparotomy must be performed for repair.

10. What leads to retained products of conception?

If the placenta has had a disruption in the development of the fibrinoid layer (Nitabuch's layer), the natural cleavage plane for placental separation may not exist. This is known as placenta accreta, percreta, or increta. The differentiation is based on the increasing extent of invasion of trophoblastic tissue through the myometrium.

11. What should be done if one of the placental abnormalities is suspected?

Curettage should be done to remove as much of the tissue as possible. Oxytocin should be used. Because of the tissue remaining in the uterine cavity, such patients are at high risk for developing endometritis and should be given antibiotics.

12. And what if the patient is still bleeding?

Surgical correction must be considered. An exploratory laparotomy is performed, and the uterine artery is ligated bilaterally. Some physicians believe that the hypogastric arteries should be ligated first. Ligation of both hypogastric arteries results in approximately 77% reduction in the pulse pressure in the vessels distal to the ligation, allowing other clotting mechanisms to occur. In extreme cases, a hysterectomy must be done to preserve the patient's life.

13. Are there any alternatives?

There has been some measure of success with infusion of vasopressin into the uterine artery as well as hypogastric artery embolization, although this approach is not routinely done. Uterine packing has been done in the past and at some institutions continues to be used, though less commonly. The uterine cavity is packed tightly with gauze. Many physicians believe that the packing in the uterine cavity will mask continued blood loss; the original concept was that it provided direct pressure on the open sinuses.

14. What type of coagulation defects should be suspected?

Disseminated intravascular coagulation (DIC) should always be suspected in a patient who bleeds excessively. Keep in mind that patients with preeclampsia often have abnormal platelet counts, that placental abruption can predispose a patient to a coagulopathy and that an amniotic fluid embolus can lead to DIC. The usual studies, including prothrombin time, partial thromboplastin time, platelet count, and fibrin split products, should be done. In addition, any patient receiving large quantities of crystalloid or packed red blood cells (> 5 units) in such situations is at risk for dilutional coagulopathy and requires adequate coagulation replacement.

15. Significant postpartum hemorrhage may require blood product replacement. What are general guidelines for replacement?

Provided that the source of hemorrhage is controlled, a healthy woman can tolerate a hematocrit (Hct) as low as 21%; if perfusion and volume are adequate, this Hct allows adequate oxygen perfusion to continue. Higher Hcts are needed if massive transfusions have been performed, because the oxygen-carrying capacity of transfused blood is lower. Additionally, some women, such as those with unrecognized coronary artery disease or cardiac valve abnormalities, may not tolerate the same lowering in Hct without becoming symptomatic.

Packed red blood cells—in general, 1 unit should raise the Hct by 3%. Other guidelines include transfusion of 1 unit fresh frozen plasma for every 4 units of packed red blood cells.

Platelet transfusions—should be initiated if platelet count is < 20,000 and for patients with counts < 50,000 who are undergoing surgery. A "six-pack" of platelets increases the count by approximately 60,000. Further transfusion should be based on count.

Fresh frozen plasma (FFP)—for prothrombin or partial thromboplastin times > 1.5 times normal, 2–4 bags of FFP is usually adequate.

Cryoprecipitate—concentrated source of fibrinogen, factor VIII, von Willebrand factor, factor XIII, and fibronectin; one bag per 5 kg increases fibrinogen by 100.

16. What risks does the patient face from blood product replacement?

Risks of leukocyte reactions and cytomegalovirus infection can be decreased by using a leukocyte filter in the blood product IV line. Approximate risks for hepatitis B are 1:50,000; for hepatitis C, 1:3,300; for HIV-I,II, 1:150,000–1,000,000; and for HTLV-I,II, 1:50,000. An acute hemolytic reaction occurs in 1:6000 units with a 1:17 mortality rate. Alternatives, especially when blood loss is anticipated, include autologous or directed donation, intraoperative blood salvage and acute normovolemic hemodilution. Intraoperative salvage requires specialized equipment and training often not available in obstetric emergencies. A newer procedure, acute normovolemic hemodilution, involves intervention just before the anticipated time of acute blood loss. A portion of the woman's blood volume is removed and volume is maintained with crystalloid volume expanders. This provides a source of RBCs for autotransfusion if needed.

17. What is uterine inversion?

The uterine fundus turns "inside out." Inversion occurs in 1 of 2,000 deliveries and is associated with uterine hypotonia and fundal implantation of the placenta.

18. What is to be done?

Treatment for uterine inversion depends on prompt recognition of the problem. By the time the extent of the problem is appreciated, the cervix has often begun to close down, effectively trapping the uterine fundus in the vagina or at the introitus. To facilitate replacement of the fundus, tocolytic drugs (ritodrine, terbutaline) as well as anesthetics with uterine-relaxing qualities (halothane) can be given. Pressure is applied around the edges of the inversion to gently replace the fundus to its normal anatomic position. Once it has been replaced, pressure within the fundus should be maintained until uterine tone returns. Administration of oxytocic agents at this point is helpful. On rare occasions, laparotomy is required to accomplish reinversion. The fundus is grasped abdominally with simultaneous pressure from below. If the placenta is still attached to the fundus at the time of inversion, it should be removed before attempting replacement of the fundus.

19. What is Sheehan syndrome?

Postpartum hemorrhage may be associated with hypotension and can lead to ischemic necrosis of the pituitary. Present in varying degrees, it can result in panhypopituitarism with onset of symptoms during the postpartum period. Subtle changes such as nausea, weakness, and fatigue are often attributed to the postpartum state. The lack of lactation because of decreased secretion of prolactin is usually the first recognized pituitary deficiency. Symptoms of hypothyroidism, hypoandrenalism, and hypogonadotropism may follow.

BIBLIOGRAPHY

1. American College of Obstetrics and Gynecology: Blood component therapy. ACOG Tech Bull No. 199, 1994.
2. Andersen HF, Hopkins M: Postpartum hemorrhage. In Sciarra JJ (ed): Gynecology and Obstetrics, vol 2. Philadelphia, J.B. Lippincott, 1993, pp 1–10.
3. Buttino L Jr, Garite TJ: The use of 15 methyl F_2 alpha prostaglandin (Prostin 15M) for the control of postpartum hemorrhage. Am J Perinatol 3:241–243, 1986.
4. Barrington JW, Roberts A: The use of gemeprost pessaries to arrest postpartum haemorrhage. Br J Obstet Gynaecol 100:691–692, 1993.
5. Ferland RJ, Adler LM: Management of postpartum uterine atony. Rhode Island Med J 73:626–627, 1990.
6. Katesmark M, Brown R, Raju KS: Successful use of a Sengstaken-Blakemore tube to control massive postpartum haemorrhage. Br J Obstet Gynaecol 101:259–260, 1994.
7. Maier RC: Control of postpartum hemorrhage with uterine packing. Am J Obstet Gynecol 169:317–323, 1993.
8. Mitty HA, Sterling KM, Alvarez M, Gendler R: Obstetric hemorrhage: Prophylactic and emergency arterial catheterization and embolotherapy. Radiology 188:183–187, 1993.
9. VanDongen PWJ, Van Roosmalen J, DeBoer CN, Van Rooij J: Oxytocics for the prevention of postpartum haemorrhages. Pharmaceutisch Weekblad 13:238–243, 1991.
10. Varner M: Postpartum hemorrhage. Crit Care Clin 7:883–897, 1991.
11. Zahn CM, Yeomans ER: Postpartum hemorrhage: Placenta accreta, uterine inversion and puerperal hematomas. Clin Obstet Gynecol 33:422–431, 1990.
12. The management of postpartum haemorrhage. Drug Ther Bull 30:89–92, 1992.

82. VAGINAL DELIVERY AFTER CESAREAN SECTION

Robert M. Silver, M.D.

1. What was the initial impetus for elective repeat cesarean section?

Reports of uterine rupture during labor with a scarred uterus led to the dictum, "Once a cesarean, always a cesarean." This has influenced American obstetrics for much of the last century. However, recent medical advances have markedly decreased the fetal and maternal risks of vaginal birth after cesarean section (VBAC).

2. What is uterine rupture?

To assess the risk of VBAC accurately, it is necessary to differentiate between complete or true uterine rupture and incomplete rupture, often termed occult rupture, uterine dehiscence, or uterine window. Complete uterine rupture is a separation of the previous scar and overlying peritoneum with extrusion of intrauterine contents into the peritoneal cavity. If is often sudden and associated with pain, blood loss, and fetal morbidity. Complete rupture is most commonly seen in spontaneous or traumatic rupture of the unscarred uterus. It also has been associated with classic uterine scars, often before onset of labor.

Conversely, uterine dehiscence refers to a partial separation of the uterine wall with intact overlying serosa and no expulsion of the fetus or placenta. It is usually asymptomatic and rarely contributes to fetal or maternal morbidity. This type of separation is seen in lower segment scars and usually occurs during labor. Often asymptomatic uterine windows are incidentally noted at the time of repeat cesarean delivery.

3. What are the risks of uterine dehiscence and rupture with VBAC? Are there differences in these risks in women with classic vs. lower segment uterine scars?

There is little difference in the rate of uterine dehiscence between the scar types, approximately 1–2% for both. However, the data are difficult to interpret. Many studies fail to distinguish between rupture and dehiscence. Furthermore, investigations wherein the uterus was routinely examined after delivery (either postpartum or at the time of cesarean section) noted higher dehiscence rates than studies including only symptomatic cases. Overall, the incidence of dehiscence ranged from 0.4–9%.

However, there is a large difference in the rates of uterine rupture associated with different scars. Uterine rupture has been reported in 0.2–2.3% of VBACs in women with lower segment uterine scars compared with 4.3–8.8% in women with prior classic incisions. The most accurate estimation of risk is derived from two recent publications of large experiences with VBAC. Uterine rupture was reported in 10 of 5733 (0.17%) and 95 of 12,707 (0.7%) of VBACs with prior lower uterine segment and unknown scar incisions, respectively.

4. What is the morbidity associated with uterine rupture?

In reviews before 1987, encompassing almost 10,000 VBACs, there were no maternal deaths from rupture of either scar type. Of 20 fetal deaths, 17 were associated with classic scars. Of the three from lower segment rupture, all occurred over 25 years previously in unmonitored patients. These data led obstetricians to conclude that rupture of a lower transverse uterine scar rarely carries significant fetal morbidity. As such, VBAC was strongly recommended for all patients with a previous lower segment incision.

Over the past few years, however, it has become clear that uterine rupture in women with prior lower segment incisions can be catastrophic and is associated with perinatal death, neonatal asphyxia, hysterectomy, bladder laceration, and blood transfusion. In addition, maternal deaths have now been reported after uterine rupture. The rupture-related perinatal and maternal mortality rates associated with VBAC in women with prior lower segment scars is estimated at 0.24 per 1,000 and 7.9 per 100,000, respectively. Because these events are rare, they have been recognized only in the face of increasing experience with VBAC.

5. What risks are associated with a previous low vertical incision? A "T" incision? What about unknown uterine scars?

The risk of uterine rupture in women with low vertical incisions is reported as 0.5–6.5%. If the scar is truly in the lower segment, the risk approaches that of a low transverse incision. If it involves the muscular portion of the uterus, the risk of rupture is similar to that for classic incisions. This issue should be addressed in detail in operative reports of low vertical incisions. The risk in women with "T" incisions is unknown but estimated as 4.3–8.8% (the same as classic scars).

6. What are the symptoms and signs most commonly associated with uterine rupture?

Unfortunately, no single symptom or sign can reliably predict uterine rupture. The most consistent presenting sign of uterine rupture is an abnormal fetal heart rate tracing, occurring in 50–70% of ruptures. A common scenario is the presence of variable decelerations that progress to repetitive late decelerations or bradycardia. Other findings may include vaginal bleeding, uterine pain, and less commonly, loss of fetal station, hematuria, shock, or cessation of uterine contractions. Because these findings are unreliable, clinicians must have a high index of suspicion for uterine rupture and a low threshold for exploratory laparotomy.

7. Aside from uterine rupture, are there other significant risks of VBAC?

No. Several studies have shown no increase in perinatal or maternal morbidity in women undergoing VBAC compared with repeat cesarean section.

8. What are the benefits of VBAC?

Several investigators have reported a marked decrease in maternal morbidity such as postpartum transfusions, febrile morbidity, and length of hospital stay in women undergoing VBAC.

Available evidence clearly indicates that the benefits of a trial of labor outweigh the risks. VBAC is also substantially cheaper than repeat cesarean section. In most facilities, cesarean section is approximately twice as costly as vaginal birth.

9. What are the success rates of VBAC?

The success rate or proportion of vaginal births after a trial of labor in women attempting VBAC ranges from 60–80%. These rates are influenced by the cesarean rates of clinicians as well as selection bias. For example, women choosing VBAC are likely to be more motivated to achieve a vaginal birth than those electing repeat cesarean section.

10. Is the VBAC success rate different for patients with prior cesarean because of labor disorders or cephalopelvic disproportion? Should such patients be allowed a trial of labor (TOL)?

There are significant differences in success rates. For patients with nonrecurring causes for cesarean section (e.g., breech, fetal distress, placental abruptions), the success rate of VBAC is 70–89%. The incidence of vaginal birth is essentially the same as the overall incidence of laboring patients without uterine scars. For recurring causes (cephalopelvic disproportion, first-stage arrest, second-stage arrest), the success rate is only 65–70%. However, even a success rate of 65% does not justify repeat cesarean section. Such patients should be allowed TOL. In fact, even patients with larger infants during a subsequent pregnancy have over a 50% chance of successful VBAC.

11. What are some of the predictors of vaginal delivery in patients undergoing VBAC?

Several investigators have attempted to predict vaginal delivery in women attempting VBAC. No single characteristic or group of variables definitively predicts successful VBAC. Nonetheless, several characteristics strongly correlate with vaginal birth. Variables positively correlated with successful VBAC include previous vaginal delivery, previous successful VBAC, spontaneous labor, nonrepetitive cause for previous cesarean, normal fetal heart rate tracing, favorable cervical examination upon admission, lack of oxytocin, lower estimated fetal weight, and earlier gestation. Models have been based on these parameters to counsel women about their precise chance of vaginal delivery. One group used ultrasound and x-ray pelvimetry to determine a fetal-pelvic index to predict successful VBAC. Although promising, this method requires further study before widespread use is recommended.

12. Is it appropriate to use oxytocin in patients having a VBAC?

Yes. Most authors have found no increase in maternal or fetal morbidity with oxytocin. Meta-analysis failed to show an association between oxytocin use and uterine dehiscence or rupture. However, oxytocin use has been associated with a large number of uterine ruptures, and one case-control study correlated high-dose oxytocin with uterine rupture. Although the requirement for oxytocin decreases the likelihood of successful VBAC, 60–80% of such women have vaginal births. Overall, the indications, protocols, and precautions for the use of oxytocin should be the same in these patients as for patients without uterine scars. It is prudent to optimize uterine contractions with the use of an intrauterine pressure catheter and to avoid hyperstimulation. Most importantly, clinicians should be alert for evidence of uterine rupture when using oxytocin during attempted VBAC.

13. Can labor be induced in patients with prior cesarean section?

Yes. Numerous studies have shown no increase in morbidity in women attempting VBAC and undergoing labor induction with either oxytocin or prostaglandin E_2. Cesarean rates have been higher in some cohorts of women undergoing induction and VBAC (compared with spontaneous labor). However, these rates are similar to those for women with unscarred uteruses undergoing induction of labor.

14. Can regional anesthesia be used in patients having VBAC?

Yes. Theoretical concern for potentially masking the symptoms of uterine rupture has not been supported by available data. Several case reports of uterine rupture in patients with epidural anesthesia noted that patients were well aware of uterine pain despite anesthesia. Furthermore, in large reviews of intrapartum uterine rupture, most patients (over 75%) did not experience pain. There has been no documented increase in morbidity among the thousands of patients who received epidural anesthesia while undergoing VBAC.

15. Is it possible to allow TOL in a patient with multiple cesarean sections?

Yes. Thousands of women with two or more previous cesarean sections have had successful VBAC. Several studies have demonstrated that VBAC is less successful in women with more than one previous cesarean than in those with one prior operation. Success rates for VBAC in women with more than one previous cesarean have ranged from 64–75%. There also appears to be an increased risk of uterine rupture associated with TOL in women with two or more previous cesareans. Because uterine rupture is rare, most studies have not shown a statistically significant increase in uterine rupture in women with more than one prior cesarean. Nonetheless, several reports have noted a 2–3-fold increase in risk of uterine rupture during attempted VBAC in women with more than one (vs. one) prior abdominal delivery. Uterine rupture is still rare in women with multiple previous cesareans, ranging from 1–2%. There have been reports of successful VBAC after three or more prior cesareans in a small number of patients. Data support a trial of labor for selected women with more than one previous cesarean. However, such women should be motivated to achieve vaginal birth and counseled about the slightly increased risk of uterine rupture and decreased chance of success.

16. Are VBACs safe in twin gestations? Breech presentations?

Data are inadequate to support or refute the safety of such procedures, although successful VBACs have been reported in women with twins and breech presentations. The question of whether to allow a TOL must be assessed on an individual basis. Limited data support the safety of external cephalic version for breech presentation, as well as breech extraction, in twin gestations in women with previous lower segment uterine incisions.

17. Who are candidates for VBAC? When is VBAC contraindicated?

VBAC should be offered and perhaps actively promoted for most women with one previous low transverse uterine incision. In addition, VBAC is a reasonable option for motivated patients with two or more previous lower segment incisions as well as those with prior low vertical incisions that did not enter the muscular portion of the uterus.

Contraindications to VBAC include prior classic or "T" uterine incisions, prior uterine ruptures or dehiscences, or medical or obstetric contraindications to labor. Classic scars frequently separate before delivery, whereas lower segment scars tend to separate during delivery. Patients with vertical uterine incisions should be aggressively delivered by cesarean section, before the onset of active labor, and after documentation of fetal pulmonary maturity. Multiple gestation, breech presentation, macrosomia, epidural anesthesia and need for induction are not absolute contraindications for TOL.

18. What are the guidelines of the American College of Obstetricians and Gynecologists (ACOG) for VBAC?

Guidelines include the availability of a physician capable of evaluating labor, performing a cesarean, and managing the complication of uterine rupture, the capability of carrying out a cesarean section within 30 minutes, and fetal monitoring.

19. What special management is required for VBAC?

Some authorities believe that the ACOG guidelines are insufficient and that management of attempted VBAC is safest when anesthesia, obstetric, and blood bank personnel are immediately available. Although rare and unpredictable, there have been numerous cases of uterine rupture wherein delaying laparotomy for 30 minutes would have compromised both mother and fetus. Indeed, the majority of perinatal mortality associated with uterine rupture occurred in patients laboring outside of a traditional hospital labor and delivery setting. Other reasonable measures include intravenous access, no oral intake, continuous electronic fetal monitoring, intrauterine pressure catheter, and blood type and screen. Again clinicians must have a high index of suspicion for uterine rupture. These conditions are met easily at most community hospitals, and VBAC should not be limited to large tertiary care centers. Management by certified nurse midwives and delivery in birthing rooms are appropriate and safe in the setting of the above requirements.

20. How should dehiscence or rupture be managed?

There are insufficient data to allow definitive recommendations for the management of uterine dehiscence or rupture. Scar dehiscence is usually asymptomatic, and most heal adequately without repair. Although the necessity for routine palpation of the uterine scar is controversial, no evidence suggests that surgical repair improves outcome in subsequent pregnancies. We do not routinely assess the integrity of the uterus in asymptomatic women after successful VBAC.

It is unclear whether hemostatically stable dehiscences that are confined to the lower uterine segment should be repaired in asymptomatic patients at the time of repeat cesarean section. Although the benefits of such repair are unproved, it is easy to accomplish and carries little morbidity in the setting of laparotomy. Most cases of symptomatic ruptured uterine scars are amenable to surgical repair. Occasionally this is not feasible because of uterine damage or extension into the broad ligament, and hysterectomy is required.

If the ruptured or separated scar is confined to the lower uterine segment, the recurrence risk of rupture of dehiscence is reported as 6.4%. If the scar or rupture involves the upper part of the uterus, the recurrence risk is 32.1%. Permanent sterilization by hysterectomy or tubal ligation should be considered in cases of upper segment rupture because of the high rate of recurrence. This issue is best addressed with the patient before laparotomy.

BIBLIOGRAPHY

1. Asakura H, Myers SA: More than one previous cesarean delivery: A 5-year experience with 435 patients. Obstet Gynecol 85:925–929, 1995.
2. Flamm BL, Newman LA, Thomas SJ, et al: Vaginal birth after cesarean delivery: Results of a 5-year multicenter collaborative study. Obstet Gynecol 76:750–754, 1990.
3. Jones RO, Nagashima AW, Hartnett-Goodman MM, Goodlin RC: Rupture of low transverse cesarean scars during trial of labor. Obstet Gynecol 77:815–817, 1991.
4. Leung AS, Farmer RM, Leung EK, et al: Risk factors associated with uterine rupture during trial of labor after cesarean delivery: A case control study. Am J Obstet Gynecol 168:1358–1363, 1993.
5. Miller DA, Diaz FG, Paul RH: Vaginal birth after cesarean: A 10-year experience. Obstet Gynecol 84:255–258, 1994.
6. Pickhardt MG, Martin JN, Meydrech EF, et al: Vaginal birth after cesarean delivery: Are there useful and valid predictors of success or failure? Am J Obstet Gynecol 166:1811–1819, 1992.
7. Pruett KM, Kirshon B, Cotton DB: Unknown uterine scar and trial of labor. Am J Obstet Gynecol 159:807–810, 1988.
8. Rosen MG, Dickinson JC: Vaginal birth after cesarean: A meta-analysis of indicators for success. Obstet Gynecol 76:865–869, 1990.
9. Scott JR: Mandatory trial of labor after cesarean delivery: An alternative viewpoint. Obstet Gynecol 77:811–814, 1991.
10. Troyer LR, Parisi VM: Obstetric parameters affecting success in a trial of labor: Designation of a scoring system. Obstet Gynecol 167:1099–1104, 1992.

83. NEWBORN RESUSCITATION

Sharon Langendoerfer, M.D.

1. Have newborn resuscitation procedures been standardized?

Yes. The information in this chapter agrees with but is not a substitute for the Neonatal Resuscitation Program (NPR) developed by the American Heart Association and the American Academy of Pediatrics.

2. What are the requirements of successful newborn resuscitation?

Anticipation of the problem, careful planning, standard resuscitation equipment, and trained personnel. Both prenatal and intrapartum histories can suggest the possible need for resuscitation of the infant. Equipment and personnel should be prepared for many more resuscitations than are actually required. Equipment that should be available for every delivery includes a heated infant warmer and dry blankets, 100% oxygen, wall suction (−80 to −120 mmHg) with a DeLee trap or sideport suction catheter, stethoscope, self-inflating infant size bag with attached oxygen reservoir, premature and term-size masks, endotracheal tubes sizes 2.5, 3.0 and 3.5 cm with wire stylets, and laryngoscope with size 0 blade and bright light.

An 8-Fr feeding tube is taped under the lamp on the laryngoscope blade to deliver oxygen during laryngoscopy and intubation. This allows the infant to tolerate the procedure for several seconds longer before becoming more hypoxic and bradycardic. Medications for resuscitation also should be immediately available: epinephrine, 1:10,000; 5% albumin-saline solution; normal saline; naloxone, 0.4 mg/ml or 1.0 mg/ml; and sodium bicarbonate, 0.5 mEq/ml. Two trained staff are required for newborn resuscitation. Both must be able to suction, stimulate, and assess the infant; to deliver effective bag and mask ventilation; and to perform chest compressions. One of the two also must be able to intubate and order correct medication doses. Roles should be decided before delivery. (For an anticipated resuscitation, the two people should have no other responsibilities except care of the infant.)

3. How can I determine how much resuscitation is needed and when?

The infant must be evaluated repeatedly during resuscitation, starting at the moment of birth. Stepwise assessment and treatment ensure the needed resuscitation and prevent overtreatment. **Note:** Do not interrupt resuscitation for more than 6-second intervals unless the infant is vigorous. To assess need for resuscitation, use three Apgar criteria:

1. Are respirations adequate to maintain heart rate?
2. Is heart rate > 100 bpm (≥ 10 in 6 seconds)?
3. Does infant have central cyanosis (cyanosis of body and mucous membranes)?

To assess effectiveness of resuscitation, use the Apgar score at 1 minute and 5 minutes. If 5-minute score is < 7, continue to assign a score every 5 minutes until two successive scores are ≥ 8. Use the mnemonic **APGAR** to remember the five criteria:

Apgar Criteria

COMPONENT	SCORE		
	0	1	2
Activity = tone	Limp	Some flexion	Active
Pulse = heart rate	Absent × 6 sec	< 100 bpm	> 100 bpm
Grimace = reflex irritability (with suctioning)	No response	Grimace	Cough or sneeze
Appearance = color	Blue or pale	Body pink, extremities blue	All pink
Respirations	Absent	Weak cry, hypoventilation	Strong cry

Note: Apgar scores are affected by a number of factors besides hypoxia/ischemia, including gestational age, maternal medications, and congenital disorders. Therefore, Apgar scores alone are not evidence of sufficient hypoxia to result in neurologic damage.

4. What are the steps of resuscitation?

Resuscitation of the newborn infant follows the basic pattern used for persons of all ages with one notable exception: **preventing heat loss** is a much more critical issue for the neonates and requires attention from the moment of birth. Prevent heat loss in two ways:
1. Place the infant immediately under a heated infant warmer.
2. Wipe body and scalp dry with absorbent towels and discard wet ones.

These quick steps prevent the serious metabolic problems resulting from cold stress and provide stimulation to breathe. Now proceed with the ABCs of resuscitation as needed.

5. How is airway management different for a newborn infant?

The newborn airway is opened by:
1. Proper positioning—supine on the warming table, tilted head down, with neck only slightly extended (less extended than for an older child).
2. Suctioning—first the mouth and then the nose, with a bulb aspirator or catheter attached to wall suction.

Note: If a large amount of mucus is present, turn the head to the side so that the secretions pool in the cheek rather than in the posterior pharynx. Also avoid producing gag and vagal bradycardia, if possible.

6. How should airway management differ when meconium is present?

Regardless of the severity of meconium staining of the amniotic fluid, it is important to suction the nasopharynx and mouth before delivery of the thorax and the first breath. Use a 10-Fr DeLee trap (requires only one hand) or a whistle-tip suction catheter (requires a second hand to occlude the sideport) attached to wall suction (–80 to –120 mmHg). While the head is on the perineum, suction the nasopharynx first, because the volume of secretions is greater than in the closed mouth. Insert the catheter tip into the nostril, lift gently, then push the catheter straight back along the floor of the nose. Suction the second nostril, then the oropharynx.

After delivery is accomplished, laryngoscopy, intubation, and tracheal suction are indicated. Tracheal suction is not recommended for vigorous infants who are making good respiratory effort immediately after birth because the procedure is more hazardous in infants who resist, and the potential for preventing subsequent respiratory disease is limited. Laryngoscopy is indicated only for intubation and suctioning, not for examining the cords for meconium staining, because clear cords do not ensure that there is no meconium in the trachea.

Intubate the trachea (see question 16 for technique); apply suction directly to the endotracheal (ET) tube connector, either by an adaptor that fits over the connector or by the wall suction tubing pressed against the connector. (A suction catheter inserted through the ET tube is too small to aspirate particulate meconium.)

Stop the negative pressure before withdrawing the ET tube from the trachea to avoid a false-positive impression of meconium in the trachea when in fact it was aspirated from the posterior pharynx as the tube was withdrawn. If a large amount of thick meconium is found in the trachea, consider a second intubation and suctioning before proceeding with further resuscitation.

7. Should I take the time to intubate and suction a severely depressed infant with moderate-to-severe meconium-stained fluid?

Yes. Intubate and suction at least once, because the risk of in utero aspiration of meconium is high in such infants. Intubation is usually easier, and therefore faster, in hypotonic infants.

8. If meconium is not present, what is the next step of the resuscitation?

With the airway open, the infant should begin breathing. If the stimulation of rubbing to dry and of suctioning the pharynx has not initiated respirations, make two quick attempts to stimulate baby by either slapping the soles of the feet (may bruise a premature infant) or rubbing the back. (Move the skin over the ribs; do not rub off the skin.) Deliver free-flow oxygen near the nose and mouth at this time. If breathing begins, continue to deliver oxygen and check heart rate to assess adequacy of respiratory effort. If heart rate does not quickly increase to 100 bpm, then begin bag and mask ventilation. If infant remains apneic after brief stimulation, begin bag and mask ventilation with 100% oxygen (bag with reservoir attached) at once: (1) check again for patency of airway; (2) apply the proper size mask to the infant's face over the chin first and then over the nose; and (3) deliver breaths adequate to move the chest gently (15–30 cm H_2O) at a rate of 40 breaths/min (squeeze–two–three). Heart rate should increase after only 15–30 seconds of adequate ventilation. Color should begin to improve, and the infant may attempt spontaneous respirations. After 30 seconds of ventilation, count the heart rate for 6 seconds (8–10 = 80–100 bpm).

9. What if I am unable to ventilate the baby?

First check the airway again for patency (position and suction); then reapply the mask to the face and check for seal (listen for air leaks around the mask). If the chest still does not move, apply more pressure to the bag with each breath. Expect to use significantly more pressure (30–40 cm H_2O) if the infant has not taken a first spontaneous breath or if lung disease is present.

If these steps are not successful, recheck the heart rate to see if chest compressions are now needed and make a third attempt to ventilate with bag and mask before trying to intubate. When more than 2 minutes of bag and mask ventilation is required, an orogastric tube should be placed in the stomach (length from bridge of nose to ear lobe to xiphoid). Remove air and mucus with a 10-ml syringe; then leave tube in place open to the air.

10. When bag and mask ventilation is adequate, what next?

When the heart rate is > 100 bpm, the color is beginning to improve, and the infant is attempting to breathe spontaneously, discontinue bag and mask ventilation and offer the infant oxygen and gentle stimulation. If spontaneous breaths fail to maintain heart rate > 100 bpm, resume bag and mask ventilation.

11. When are chest compressions indicated?

After the initial 30 seconds of adequate bag and mask ventilation (i.e., good chest movement and 100% oxygen), if the heart rate remains < 60 bpm (< 6 in 6 sec) or between 60–80 bpm and is not increasing, chest compressions should be begun.

12. How should chest compressions and ventilation be given?

Ventilation must always be given with chest compressions. Some data suggest that chest compression can interfere with full respiration if delivered simultaneously. Therefore, the current recommendation is that chest compressions should be delivered at a rate of 90/minute, interposed with 30 breaths/minute; i.e., give 3 compressions followed by 1 breath in each 2-second interval. Count "ONE and TWO and THREE and BAG and ONE and TWO and . . . ."

Place the fingers of one hand under the infant's spine for support and, using second and third or third and fourth fingertips over the lower one-third of the sternum (just below an imaginary line between the nipples), depress the sternum by one-half to three-quarter inch, then release the pressure (without completely removing the fingertips from the chest wall) to allow the heart to refill.

A second technique involves holding the infant's chest in both hands with fingers along the spine and both thumbs over the lower sternum. Take care not to squeeze the ribs and lungs while compressing the heart with this method.

If possible, have a third person palpate the femoral pulse to check the effectiveness of the compressions. Discontinue compressions when the infant's heart rate is > 80 bpm.

13. Are chest compressions dangerous?

Dangerous enough that the technique should be practiced only on an infant manikin and never on a real baby. Broken ribs may cause pneumothorax or hemothorax, and the liver can be lacerated by pressure on the xiphoid.

14. What are the indications for endotracheal intubation?

1. If tracheal suctioning is required (see questions 6 and 7 about meconium).
2. If bag and mask ventilation is ineffective.
3. If diaphragmatic hernia is suspected (intubate immediately to avoid distention of the gut in the chest).
4. If prolonged ventilation is required. (When bag and mask ventilation is effective, intubation becomes semielective and can be delayed until conditions are optimized.)

15. What final preparations are necessary?

Choose the proper size ET tube for the infant: 2.5 cm for < 1000 gm/< 28 wks; 3.00 for 1000–2000 gm/28–34 wks; and 3.5 for > 2000 gm/> 35 wks. Make sure that suction is immediately available.

16. How to proceed?

Position the infant the same as for bagging, with neck only slightly extended. Hold the laryngoscope in the left hand and insert the blade gently over the tongue; then press the tongue into the floor of the mouth with the entire blade (in the direction of the handle) to visualize the glottic area. Do not pry open the throat by tilting the blade against the upper alveolar ridge. Place the tip of the blade in the valecula to lift the epiglottis and reveal the cords. (For small infants it may be necessary to lift the epiglottis itself gently with the tip of the blade.) Gentle pressure on the neck over the trachea may improve visualization of the glottic area.

The assistant should remind the operator to interrupt the attempt after 20 seconds or sooner if the infant becomes bradycardic. The infant should be stabilized with oxygen or bag and mask ventilation as needed before the next attempt. When the vocal cords are clearly in view, place the ET tube into the right side of the mouth so that the cords remain in view until the tube has been passed between them to the level of the vocal cord marker.

17. What are reliable signs that the tube is in proper position?

- Infant's oxygenation is as good as or better than that provided by bag and mask ventilation.
- Chest movement is symmetrical.
- Breath sounds are equal in both axillae.
- Breath sounds are faint over the stomach, without obvious gastric distention.
- Cm marker at the lip is 7 cm for < 1000 gm infants, 8 cm for 1000–2000 gm, 9 cm for 2000–3000 gm, and 10 cm for > 3000 gm infants.

If the condition is deteriorating, remove the tube and resume bag and mask ventilation! If the infant is stable or improving, secure the tube to the face with tape and recheck tube position.

18. What are the possible complications of endotracheal intubation?

Possible complications include hypoxia from the duration of the attempt or incorrect tube placement; bradycardia or apnea from hypoxia or vagal stimulation; pneumothorax from over-ventilating one lung with the tube in a mainstem bronchus; injury to oropharyngeal structures, esophagus or trachea, including perforation by the protruding stylet; and infection.

19. Is the laryngeal mask airway (LMA) a better choice than endotracheal intubation?

Limited data about its use in newborns suggest that the LMA is effective for delivering positive pressure ventilation to almost all newborns and that the technique for correct placement is easier to learn than endotracheal intubation. Thus it has been suggested that the LMA should be further assessed as an alternative to endotracheal intubation.

20. How should medications be used in newborn resuscitation?

Medications and volume expanders are required for few resuscitations because most newborns' problems can be corrected by oxygenation and ventilation.

21. Which medications are indicated? When?

Epinephrine should be given when the heart rate remains < 80 bpm after 30 seconds of adequate bag and mask ventilation with chest compressions or when there is no heart beat at birth (for 6 seconds). Obviously, there will be no available route of administration at the time recommended! Therefore, endotracheal intubation and/or placement of an umbilical vein catheter should be accomplished as soon as the likely need for medication is established. Epinephrine, 1:10,000, 0.1–0.3 ml/kg, should be given rapidly via trachea or intravenous line. Dose may be repeated every 3–5 minutes if heart rate remains < 100 bpm. If response is inadequate to intratracheal dose, try 1.0 ml/kg via the trachea.

A volume expander (5% albumin-saline solution, normal saline, or Ringer's lactate) is indicated for evidence of acute bleeding with signs of hypovolemia: pallor despite good oxygenation; weak pulses with good heart rate; and poor response to resuscitation. The presence of placenta previa, abruption or fetal monitor evidence of cord compression, or a sine wave suggests fetal blood loss. Give 10 ml/kg intravenously over 5–10 minutes.

Naloxone (Narcan) (0.4 mg/ml or 1.0 mg/ml solution, 0.1 mg/kg intramuscularly or intravenously) is indicated only if there is a history of narcotic administration to the mother within the previous 4 hours and severe respiratory depression. The latter should be treated immediately with bag and mask ventilation until the drug becomes effective. **Caution:** This narcotic antagonist can precipitate withdrawal symptoms, including seizures, in addicted infants.

Sodium bicarbonate (4.2% solution = 0.5 mEq/ml) should be given only for documented metabolic acidosis during prolonged resuscitation. It should not be given without telephone consultation with a neonatologist except when this is not possible. The dose is 2 mEq/kg, administered intravenously and slowly over at least 2 minutes.

BIBLIOGRAPHY

1. American Academy of Pediatrics, Committee on the Fetus and Newborn: Use and abuse of the Apgar score. Pediatrics 78:1148, 1986.
2. Bloom RS, Cropley C: AHA/AAP Neonatal Resuscitation Program Steering Committee: Textbook of Neonatal Resuscitation. American Heart Association and American Academy of Pediatrics, 1994.
3. Brimacombe J: The laryngeal mask airway for neonatal resuscitation [letter]. Pediatrics 93:874, 1994.
4. Burchfield D, Erenberg A, Mullett MD, et al: Why change the compression and ventilation rates during CPR in neonates? Pediatrics 93:1026, 1994.
5. Catlin EA, Carpenter MW, Brann BS, et al: The Apgar score revisited: Influence of gestational age. J Pediatr 109:865, 1986.
6. Paterson SJ, Byrne PJ, et al: Neonatal resuscitation using the laryngeal mask airway. Anesthesiology 80:1248, 1994.
7. Yoder BA: Meconium-stained amniotic fluid and respiratory complications: Impact of selective tracheal suction. Obstet Gynecol 83:77, 1994.

84. POSTPARTUM ISSUES

Susan A. Arnold-Aldea, M.D., and Deborah Cohen, R.N.

1. What is the puerperium?

The word *puerperium* originates from the Latin words *puer* (child) and *parere* (to bear). Although puerperium refers only to the period around delivery, it has come to include the period during which the reproductive tract returns to its nonpregnant state, commonly considered to be the first 6 postpartum weeks. This definition may be misleading, because some organ systems resume their nonpregnant functions more rapidly than others, which are still altered 6 weeks after delivery, especially in the lactating mother.

2. After a term delivery, when does the serum level of beta human chorionic gonadotropin (βhCG) become negative?

On average the βhCG becomes negative 2 weeks after delivery. During the first trimester serum βhCG is much higher than at term. After a first trimester loss, it takes an average of 5 weeks for the βhCG to become negative.

3. How rapidly does the pregnant uterus return to its nonpregnant size?

The largest reduction in uterine size occurs immediately after expulsion of the placenta. At that time the uterus shrinks to midway between the umbilicus and the symphysis pubis. This initial reduction in uterine size is due almost exclusively to contraction of the myometrium. The myometrial wall is greatly thickened and on exam feels very firm. The middle layer of the myometrium is arranged as a dense network of many myometrial cells that are curved around perforating vessels. This unique and characteristic anatomic arrangement of myometrial muscle fibers facilitates the postpartum strangulation of the perforating vessels, allowing the contracting uterus to shut off the large blood flow to the placenta.

4. When is postpartum hemorrhage most likely to occur?

Postpartum hemorrhage is most likely to occur in the delivery room or within 1 or 2 hours of delivery. It is the result of suboptimal contractions of the uterus or an abnormal implantation site at which bleeding cannot be controlled by uterine contraction. Occasionally severe uterine bleeding occurs several days after delivery. This type of bleeding is due to transient myometrial relaxation and may be associated with endomyometritis or retained products of conception. It is often associated with large intrauterine clots that need to be expelled before adequate uterine contraction can be achieved. Active uterine massage through the abdominal wall and administration of oxytocin, methergine, or prostaglandins are usually sufficient to promote uterine contraction. Rarely curettage is necessary.

5. Do some types of episiotomy cause more pain than other?

Mediolateral episiotomies cause a great deal more pain after delivery than median episiotomies. Most of the pain from median episiotomies is due to superficial skin abrasions or tears of the perineum. The pain is burning in nature, is made much worse by urination, and improves within 2–3 days of delivery. Avoiding direct contact of acidic urine with skin tears is an important way to reduce pain. This goal is accomplished by urinating in water (e.g., Sitz bath, bidet, or bath tub) or squirting the perineum with water immediately after urinating. Local anesthetic sprays are often necessary. A great deal of vaginal or perineal pain not relieved by local measures is a concerning symptom. A careful exam is essential to exclude large vulvar, paravaginal, or ischiorectal hematomas or abscesses.

6. Is urinary retention common after delivery?

Yes. During labor, the bladder wall becomes edematous and hyperemic. This causes an increase in bladder capacity and a decrease in sensitivity to intravesicle volumes. Impairment in bladder function can be compounded by the occasional paralyzing effect of epidural anesthesia. The bladder can thus become overdistended or empty incompletely. Excessive postvoid residual urine can further compromise the ability of the bladder to contract and predisposes to the development of urinary tract infections. Postpartum bladder function needs to be monitored carefully to prevent overdistention. If the patient does not void at all in a 6–8-hour period or if she has frequent small voids, she needs to be catheterized. Often one catheterization is sufficient to restore normal bladder function; occasionally, however, the placement of a Foley catheter may be necessary to provide complete bladder drainage for 24–48 hours.

7. What are the common sources of fever in the postpartum patient?

Severe breast engorgement, urinary tract infections, and endomyometritis are common sources of fever within the first few postpartum days. Endomyometritis, infection of the decidual lining of the uterus and the adjacent myometrium, is diagnosed when postpartum fever is accompanied by uterine tenderness. These symptoms develop most commonly 2–5 days after delivery. Endomyometritis is more common after cesarean section than after vaginal delivery. In most cases, it is a polymicrobial infection of organisms that have ascended from the lower genital tract. Anaerobic organisms are present in as many as 80% of cases. With antibiotic therapy most patients improve within 2–3 days. In a patient with persistent fever despite appropriate antibiotic therapy, wound infection, intraabdominal or retroperitoneal masses, and pelvic thrombophlebitis need to be excluded.

8. What is pelvic thrombophlebitis?

Septic pelvic thrombophlebitis was first recognized in 1919 from autopsies of patients dying of puerperal infections. About 50% of cases had thrombosis and inflammation of pelvic veins, the most common of which were the right ovarian veins. Patients characteristically remain febrile after a protracted course of antibiotics, appear nontoxic, and have poorly localized discomfort. Occasionally, patients present with severe lower abdominal or flank pain. Although in most cases the diagnosis is presumptive, occasionally magnetic resonance imaging or computed tomography of the pelvis may show obstructed ovarian veins. Characteristically, patients defervesce after 2–3 days of intravenous heparin therapy.

9. How does mastitis present?

Mastitis presents with localized tenderness and redness, fever, and malaise. Mastitis occurs most often in the second or third week after delivery. High fevers and localized tenderness and redness allow mastitis to be distinguished from the bilateral redness and generalized tenderness of breast engorgement or the localized redness of a blocked milk duct. The treatment of mastitis relies on emptying the breast either by continued breastfeeding or, if too painful, by using a hospital-type electric pump. Local moist heat applications, analgesics and antibiotics are also used in the treatment of mastitis. Only rarely does mastitis progress to abscess formation that requires surgical drainage.

10. Which hormones control lactation?

For lactation to occur, first the mammary glands need to grow; then the alveoli need to synthesize milk; and finally the milk needs to be ejected from the alveoli into the ductules. Early in pregnancy, chorionic somatotropin, prolactin, and chorionic gonadotropin cause a marked increase in ductular sprouting and branching. Estradiol and progesterone cause the mammary gland to become richly arborized. Serum growth factor and insulin cause cell proliferation at the end of the ducts, which, under the influence of prolactin and corticosteroids, differentiate to form alveoli. Placental lactogen and prolactin stimulate the secretion of colostrum. The withdrawal of estrogen, with delivery of the placenta, allows lactation to begin. Lactation is in large part sustained by the stimulus of nursing that causes a transient increase in prolactin and oxytocin. Prolactin is necessary for the synthesis of milk, and oxytocin is important for its release. A delay in initiation of nipple stimulation or lack of regular stimulation (every 3–4 hrs) by either infant or breast pump may adversely effect the long-term outcome of breastfeeding.

11. Is the composition of human milk always the same?

The composition of milk varies with the gestational age at delivery, stage of lactation, sampling time during feeding, and time of day. Preterm milk has a higher content of protein, fat, and possibly sodium and chloride. Preterm milk is easier for the immature intestine to absorb.

The first milk produced after delivery is colostrum. It is produced in small quantities and has a thicker and yellower appearance than mature milk. It provides fewer calories and has more beta-carotene, sodium, potassium, and chloride and a higher percentage of protein, fat-soluble vitamins, and minerals. Colostrum is rich in antibodies and facilitates the colonization of the sterile newborn gut by normal intestinal flora, protecting it from pathologic bacterial invasion.

Three to five days after delivery, milk changes from colostrum to transitional milk. This change is accompanied by a sudden increase in milk volume and often painful filling of the breasts. Mature milk is not produced until 1–2 weeks after delivery. During the transitional phase milk gradually loses some of its proteins, specifically immunoglobulins, and increases its lactose, fat, and total caloric content.

The milk ejected at the beginning of a feed, foremilk, is less concentrated. Hindmilk, milk ejected towards the end of the feed, has a higher fat and caloric content. Both the volume of milk produced and its fat content are highest at midday. Although maternal malnutrition changes breast milk by decreasing water-soluble vitamins, ascorbic acid, thiamin, and B12 and by decreasing its total production, it has little effect on protein, fat, or carbohydrate composition.

12. Does breastfeeding increase the infant's resistance to infections?

Many components of breast milk are thought to protect the infant from infections. Breast milk IgA has antitoxin activity against the enterotoxins of *Escherichia coli* and *Vibrio cholerae*. Maternal antibodies against most of the infant's strains of intestinal bacteria are also found in the milk as well as many antiviral antibodies. Furthermore, some evidence suggests that cell-mediated immunity can also be transmitted from mother to infant across breast milk. Despite such encouraging data, the only infection that has been proved to be less prevalent in breastfed infants is otitis media.

13. Do infants with strong family histories of allergic diseases benefit from breast milk?

Bovine milk is the single most common allergen. Proteins in bovine milk that act as allergens include lactoglobulin, casein, bovine serum albumin, and lactalbumin. Modern processing of cow's milk to make formula has reduced but not eliminated the allergenic potential of these proteins. Although studies on the benefits of breastfeeding in allergenic diseases are conflicting, the majority show a protective effect. Mothers with a family history of severe atopic eczema or other allergic disorders can be advised to breastfeed their infants and delay solid food supplement for at least 6 months. Cow's milk antigens can be found in breast milk from maternal ingestion. Limiting maternal ingestion of cow milk, peanuts, and other allergenic foods during the third trimester and during lactation is also recommended in families with a strong history of atopic diseases as an unproved method to prevent the development of atopic diseases in the infant.

14. Is breastfeeding painful?

When transitional milk begins, it is common for the initial suck of the infant to cause a few seconds of nipple pain. After a few days, when lactation is well established, the pain subsides. Persistent pain with breastfeeding should be investigated; it may be due to cracked nipples that require better care as well as better positioning of the infant during feeding. Healing of a cracked nipple can be promoted by expressing milk, applying it to the nipple, and allowing it to air-dry. Severe nipple soreness associated with red nipples can be a sign of candidal infection, which can be transmitted between the mother and the infant. Both the mother's nipples and the infant's mouth need to be treated with antifungal preparations.

15. Are drugs ingested by the mother present in breast milk?

Usually drug dose in maternal milk is 1–2% of total maternal dose. Drugs with increased lipid solubility and low plasma protein-binding may concentrate in milk. Drugs that are rapidly metabolized are unlikely to achieve a significant concentration in the infant's circulation.

16. Which maternally ingested drugs contraindicate breastfeeding?

A number of pharmacologic agents are incompatible with breastfeeding because of the recognized risks to the infant. Examples include amphetamines, lithium, cyclophosphamide, methotrexate, cyclosporine, doxorubicin, phencyclidine, and phenindione. Other drugs that are relatively contraindicated include chloramphenicol, erythromycin, or metronidazole in preterm or young infants. Sulfa drugs can increase the incidence and severity of neonatal jaundice during the first month of life. Ciprofloxacin has been associated with arthropathies in children and is excreted at high levels in human milk. Propylthiouracil and methimazole may cause goiter and inhibit synthesis of infant's thyroid hormones. Infant thyroid functions should be periodically monitored. When radioactive compounds (e.g., I125, Ba67) are administered to the mother, nursing should be discontinued for 48 hours. For the most current listing refer to the American Association of Pediatrics *Guidelines for Drugs and Breastfeeding.*

17. Which viral infections or vaccines are contraindications for breastfeeding?

Small pox vaccine is a live virus that, although not excreted in breast milk, is contraindicated when the mother has an infant under 1 year of age. In contrast, rubella vaccination causes attenuated virus to be excreted in breast milk but causes no harm to the infant. The human immunodeficiency virus (HIV) has been detected in breast milk; therefore, HIV-positive mothers should be advised not to breastfeed. Pasteurization at 56°C for 30 minutes is reported to inactivate the virus. Breast feeding does not increase the rate of infection among infants born to hepatitis antigen-positive mothers.

18. Is hormonal contraception contraindicated in nursing mothers?

Oral contraceptives may diminish milk supply and decrease the milk's content of vitamins, proteins, and fat. Although some case reports suggest that oral contraceptives in breast milk can cause feminization of the male infant, oral contraceptives may be the contraceptive method of choice for many breastfeeding women. Most of the side effects ascribed to oral contraceptives in regard to breastfeeding depend on the presence of estrogen and can be potentially lessened with the use of progestational contraceptives. Provera, administered intramuscularly, is not excreted in breast milk.

19. Which maternal conditions may worsen or present for the first time after delivery?

Many maternal conditions worsen after delivery. The large increases in intravascular volume that occur during the first 48 hours after delivery make this a particularly critical period in the care of any patient with severe cardiovascular disease. Neuromuscular diseases such as multiple sclerosis or myasthenia gravis frequently worsen during the puerperium. The reason is largely unknown.

Venous thrombosis is most likely to occur after delivery. Although the most common sites are pelvic veins and veins of the lower extremities, intracranial venous thrombosis has also been observed. Sagittal sinus or cortical vein thrombosis classically presents with headaches followed by seizures and may result in hemiplegia, aphasia, or coma.

Sudden idiopathic cardiomyopathy may present within the first few months after delivery. Typically women present with cough or abdominal pains of unclear etiology and eventually shortness of breath. Peripartum cardiomyopathy is most commonly misdiagnosed as bronchitis. Prompt intervention with critical care support can be life-saving.

Acute irreversible renal failure occurring within the first 6 weeks after delivery has been referred to as postpartum hemolytic uremic syndrome. Although the mortality rate with this condition is as high as 80%, favorable outcomes have been reported with repeated plasma exchange transfusions and hemodialysis.

BIBLIOGRAPHY

1. Creasy RK, Resnik R (eds): Maternal Fetal Medicine: Principles and Practice, 3rd ed. Philadelphia, W.B. Saunders, 1994.
2. Cunningham FG, MacDonald PC, Gant NF (eds): Williams' Obstetrics, 19th ed. Norwalk, CT, Appleton & Lange, 1993.
3. Lawrence RA: Breastfeeding: A Guide for the Medical Profession, 4th ed. St. Louis, Mosby, 1994.
4. Riordan J, Auerbach KG (ed): Breastfeeding and Human Lactation. Boston, Jones & Bartlett, 1993.

INDEX

Page numbers in **boldface type** indicate complete chapters.